Infections of the Foot

Diagnosis and Management

Infections of the Foot

Diagnosis and Management

David Edward Marcinko, D.P.M., M.B.A.

Founder and Chairman,
Foot and Ankle Research Consortium, Inc.,
Atlanta, Georgia

President and CEO,
Marcinko Business Associates, Inc.,
Norcross, Georgia

with 196 illustrations

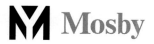
Mosby

St. Louis Baltimore Boston Carlsbad Chicago Naples New York Philadelphia Portland
London Madrid Mexico City Singapore Sydney Tokyo Toronto Wiesbaden

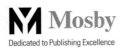
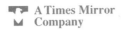

A Times Mirror
Company

Vice President and Publisher: Don E. Ladig
Editor: Jennifer Roche
Developmental Editor: Sandra J. Parker
Project Manager: Mark Spann
Production Editor: Steve Hetager
Book Design Manager: Judi Lang
Manufacturing Supervisor: Karen Boehme

Printed in the United States of America
Composition by Graphic World, Inc.
Printing/binding by Maple-Vail Press

Mosby–Year Book, Inc.
11830 Westline Industrial Drive
St. Louis, MO 63146

ISBN 0-8016-7018-7

97 98 99 00 01 / 9 8 7 6 5 4 3 2 1

Contributors

Frederick J. Bartolomei, D.P.M.
Staff Podiatrist,
Edge Memorial Hospital,
Troy, Alabama

Alan R. Catanzariti, D.P.M.
Director of Residency Training,
The Western Pennsylvania Hospital,
Pittsburgh, Pennsylvania

Rhonda Cope, P.M.A.C.
Certified Podiatric Medical Assistant,
New Hope, Pennsylvania

Thomas M. DeLauro, D.P.M.
Professor,
Division of Medical and Surgical Sciences,
New York College of Podiatric Medicine,
Staten Island, New York

Michael J. DeMarco, D.P.M.
Professor of Anatomy and Physiology,
Jersey City State College,
Jersey City, New Jersey;
Director of External Affairs,
St. Michael's Medical Center,
Newark, New Jersey

Kenrick J. Dennis, D.P.M.
Clinical Assistant Professor,
Health Science Center,
University of Texas,
Houston, Texas

Charles F. Fenton III, D.P.M., J.D.
Staff Podiatrist,
Promina Hospital at Windy Hill,
Marietta, Georgia;
Health law practice,
Atlanta, Georgia

Kaethe P. Ferguson, M.S.
Research Specialist,
Department of Microbiology,
James H. Quillen College of Medicine,
East Tennessee State University,
Johnson City, Tennessee

Hope Rachel Hetico, B.S.N., R.N., C.P.H.Q., M.H.A.
Senior Health Care Consultant,
Foot and Ankle Research Consortium, Inc.,
Norcross, Georgia

Dwight W. Lambe, Jr., Ph.D.
Chairman and Professor,
Department of Microbiology,
James H. Quillen College of Medicine,
East Tennessee State University,
Johnson City, Tennessee

Leonard A. Levy, D.P.M., M.P.H.
Professor of Podiatric Medicine and President,
California College of Podiatric Medicine;
Staff Podiatrist,
Pacific Coast Hospital,
San Francisco, California

Alvario Lopez, M.D.
Department of Infectious Diseases,
Northlake Regional Medical Center,
Tucker, Georgia

David Edward Marcinko, D.P.M., M.B.A.
Founder and Chairman,
Foot and Ankle Research Consortium, Inc.,
Atlanta, Georgia;
President and CEO,
Marcinko Business Associates, Inc.,
Norcross, Georgia

O. Kent Mercado, D.P.M.
Staff Podiatrist,
St. Mary Nazareth Hospital Center,
Chicago, Illinois

Cynthia Mercado-Ciessau, D.P.M.
Staff Podiatrist,
St. Mary Nazareth Hospital Center,
Chicago, Illinois

Nicki Dowdy Nigro, D.P.M., F.A.C.F.A.S., D.A.P.S.
Residency Committee Member,
Extern Director,
Podiatry Hospital of Pittsburgh,
Pittsburgh, Pennsylvania

Jason K. Pearson, D.P.M.
Staff Podiatrist,
Good Samaritan Medical Center,
Johnstown, Pennsylvania

Rachel Pentin-Maki, R.N., M.H.A.
President,
Call RACHEL, Inc.;
Senior Health Care Consultant,
Foot and Ankle Research Consortium, Inc.,
Norcross, Georgia

Rock G. Positano, D.P.M., M.P.H., M.Sc.
Assistant Professor,
Department of Orthopedic Surgery,
Department of Medicine,
New York Hospital/Cornell University Medical
    College,
Lenox Hill Hospital,
New York, New York

Kenneth Y. Rosenthal, D.P.M.
Private Practice,
Falls Church Foot and Ankle Center,
Falls Church, Virginia

David J. Sartoris, M.D.
Professor of Radiology,
University of California;
Chief of Quantitative Bone Densitometry,
UCSD Medical Center, VA Medical Center,
San Diego, California

William P. Scherer, D.P.M., M.S.
Clinical Instructor of Radiology,
Barry University College of Podiatric Medicine,
Miami Shores, Florida

Isidore Steiner, D.P.M., J.D.
Residency Training Committee,
Botsford General Hospital,
Farmington Hills, Michigan

Jon D. Tinkle, D.P.M.
Faculty,
California College of Podiatric Medicine;
Chief of Podiatry,
Davies Medical Center,
San Francisco, California

Kenneth J. Weiss, M.D.
Clinical Professor of Podiatric Medicine,
Pennsylvania College of Podiatric Medicine,
Pittsburgh, Pennsylvania;
Medical Director,
Delaware Valley Research Associates, Inc.,
King of Prussia, Pennsylvania

Elliot T. Udell, D.P.M.
Faculty,
Pennsylvania College of Podiatric Medicine,
Pittsburgh, Pennsylvania;
Staff Podiatrist,
North Shore University Hospital,
Plainview, New York

This book is dedicated to my parents, Cecelia and Edward, brother Eddie, sister Theresa, uncle Stosh, aunt Helen, and all those family members and friends who encouraged me as I grew up in the port city of Baltimore, Maryland. For their professional support, the book is also dedicated to Drs. Peter P. Sidoriak, David C. Scherer, and Paul J. Schapiro, as well as P.K. Shaw, D.L. Lanouette, S.M. Butala-Kurkis, J. Ciegelski, J. Yost, and all the contributing authors, whom I salute for their writing efforts under the constraints of time. Without their assistance, we could not have pursued the elusive goal of producing time-sensitive material which may withstand the test of time. I also acknowledge the editorial aid of Drs. Scott W. Agins, Paul M. Greenberg, and Thomas J. Merrill for their manuscript review assistance.

In addition, this book would not have been possible without the technical wizardry and computer-assisted software engineering (CASE) management acumen of Dr. William P. Scherer of Ft. Lauderdale, Chief Technology Officer, Foot and Ankle Research Consortium, Inc.

Above all, the book is dedicated to my wife Hope and daughter Mackenzie, whose love, intelligence, and patient understanding allowed us to complete this worthwhile endeavor—together.

Forewords

Infections of the Foot: Diagnosis and Management is a tribute to the perseverance and ongoing technical proficiency of the Foot and Ankle Research Consortium, Inc. In this publication, which contains five major sections and eighteen chapters, the always germane subject of infection as it relates to the foot surgeon is explored. Covering the medical basics of cause and prevention, clinical and laboratory diagnosis, infection diversity and differential diagnosis, medical antimicrobial, and surgical management, and protocols, legalities, and regulations as well as prophylaxis, the book speaks predominantly to the pragmatic management of the pedal infectious process.

The volume will find wide application for the seasoned podiatric surgeon, as well as for the medical student, resident, or experienced foot and ankle surgeon. The extensive use of clinical photographs and other illustrations contributes much to the ease of understanding of the textual material.

Dr. Marcinko is to be congratulated for bringing together an outstanding group of diverse authors from the medical professions and for coordinating their individual contributions into a useful, unique, and worthwhile clinical textbook. It is certain to be a valuable addition to all individual and institutional medical libraries.

E. Dalton McGlamry, D.P.M., D.Sc.(Hon.)

When I started podiatric medical school, the number of books written by podiatrists could easily be counted on one hand. In the fall of 1959, when Dr. Henri L. DuVries's classic book, *Surgery of the Foot,* was first published, I remember very well the excitement and admiration that it stirred among the student body and faculty of our own school. At last, we thought, podiatric medicine was getting its own literature. Years later, in 1979, when my own *Atlas of Foot Surgery* was finished, the literature was still sadly lagging behind the tremendous growth that the profession was experiencing. In the last decade, however, podiatric literature has come into its own. There has been an explosion of textbooks in our field, with scores of new titles being published by the very best publishing houses in the medical field.

Perhaps one of the best and most prolific authors of this new generation of educator-authors has been Dr. David Edward Marcinko of the Foot and Ankle Research Consortium, Inc. This book, *Infections of the Foot: Diagnosis and Management,* fills a much needed and important niche in the medical literature. It is well researched, practical, up-to-date, and written in an easy-to-read manner. It truly belongs in the reference library of every student, resident, and surgeon and anyone seriously dealing with the medical problems of the human foot.

Dr. Marcinko has put together a stellar team of authorities and experts, who demonstrate a mastery of their subject matter. In fact, two of the contributors are very close to me. Not only do we practice together, but they are also my son and daughter. This new group of leaders will continue to take our profession to new heights. They make me feel confident of our future as a profession, and, most importantly, they make me feel proud.

Orlando A. Mercado, D.P.M.

1

Preface

The purpose of this book is to provide a clinical resource that encompasses the basic medical principles for the diagnosis and treatment of the infected foot. It is not intended to serve as a comprehensive standard of medical care, since all aspects of medicine are, and will continue to be, individualized to the specific patient and disease process. Similarly, it is not so much a laboratory or theoretically based treatise, as it is a representation of real-time clinical approaches to the selected pathology, with emphasis appropriately placed on bacterial contamination. Important common superficial and deep fungal, parasitic, and viral pathogens of the foot are also reviewed, albeit briefly.

The book will serve as a basic guide for the general diagnostic and treatment practices pertinent to the infected human foot. It has been carefully prepared by a panel of nationally known clinicians, educators, and researchers who are recognized experts in their respective fields. The book is envisioned as a reference for students, residents, practitioners, physicians, and other health care providers who render foot care.

Infections of the Foot: Diagnosis and Management is written without documentation of every statement with a citation from the medical literature, allowing a large amount of information to be condensed into a single and practical volume. A deliberate effort was made to include appropriate bibliographic information at the end of each chapter. The interested reader is then able to easily consult selected volumes. Overlap of material has also been avoided, to eliminate redundancy.

The book is divided into eighteen logically progressive chapters, divided among five sections. Section One, "Prevention and Pathophysiology of Foot Infections," begins with Chapter 1 and its discourse on sterilization, disinfection, and surgical antisepsis, for both patient and physician, as they pertain to the normal and abnormal ecology of the human foot. Chapter 2 details the various types of blood-borne and communicable pathogens, which may potentially affect the entire nation's population. These include the pathogens causing AIDS, hepatitis, syphilis, tuberculosis, and gonorrhea. The intricate details of the new office-based OSHA Standard are discussed in Chapter 3, while the clinically relevant signs and symptoms of the infectious process are discussed with due diligence in Chapter 4. In Chapter 5, the increasingly important role of glycocalyx biofilm, or "slime," in bacterial infections is masterfully presented, and the text is augmented with specially prepared scanning electron microscopic (SEM) illustrations.

Section Two, "Laboratory and Radiographic Diagnostic Modalities," starts with Chapter 6, which reviews basic diagnostic laboratory and cultural methodologies, for both aerobic and anaerobic infections. Chapter 7 provides a richly illustrated pictorial review of the traditional, nuclear, and special interpretative radiographic techniques useful in recognizing the pedal infectious process.

Section Three, "The Spectrum and Clinical Variety of Foot Infections," commences with Chapter 8, which initiates the clinical focus of the textbook by discussing specific infectious disease entities of the pedal integumentary system, including subcutaneous and deep plantar space infections. Chapter 9 presents a dissertation on the special topic of foot ulcerations, while Chapter 10 comments on the wide variety of potential pathogens and complications involved in soft tissue and osseous trauma to the foot. Chapter 11 reviews the difficult and unfortunate topic of bone infections, including pyarthrosis and pediatric and adult osteomyelitis. Chapter 12 continues with an overview of the often overlooked, but catastrophic, topic of major anaerobic foot infections, including diagnostic, chemotherapeutic, and surgical procedures.

Section Four, "Medical and Surgical Treatment of Foot Infections," begins with Chapter 13 and its discussion of oral and parenteral antimicrobial agents of choice, dosage schedules, adverse effects, drug resistance patterns, and the indicators for antibiotic termination. Chapter 14 facilitates entry into the surgical management protocol of foot infections, with special emphasis on decompression, wound healing, and soft tissue coverage. Chapter 15 concludes the section with a review of new treatment modalities useful for the infected lower extremity.

Section Five, "Special Concerns of the Infected Foot," begins with Chapter 16, covering the difficult differentiation that often must be made between osteoarthropathy and osteomyelitis in the insensitive foot. Chapter 17 scrutinizes the psychological considerations involved in treating the infected patient. Chapter 18 rightly concludes the book with a discourse on the medicolegal implications of treating the infected patient.

We hope that *Infections of the Foot: Diagnosis and Management* becomes a valuable reference for all practitioners of the healing arts, regardless of specialty or degree designation.

David Edward Marcinko

Contents

SECTION FOUR
Medical and Surgical Treatment of Foot Infections

SECTION FIVE
Special Concerns of the Infected Foot

Section One

Prevention and Pathophysiology of Foot Infections

Sterilization, Disinfection, Ecology, and Preparation of Pedal Skin

Cynthia Mercado-Ciessau
Leonard A. Levy

Disease is from of old and nothing about it has changed. It is we who change, as we learn to recognize what was formerly imperceptible. Charcot

Sterilization is the destruction of all forms of microbial life, while disinfection is the process by which pathologic microbes are destroyed. These two concepts are important to understand when discussing the normal, pathologic, resident, or transient flora of the pedal skin. Once understood in this context, a logical approach to the gowning, gloving, prepping, and draping process of the surgical patient and operator can be appreciated.

The fabrication of protective equipment and the appropriate use of prophylactic oral and parenteral antibiotics can likewise be formulated. These concepts will be presented and reviewed in this chapter according to this sequential approach.

THE PROCESS OF STABILIZATION

Sterilization is defined as the "destruction of all forms of microbial life, including viruses, bacteria, and spores."[1] A variety of sterilization methods are available, including steam, autoclave, dry heat, gas (ethylene oxide), and liquid or cold sterilization. The steam autoclave is by far the most popular form of sterilization, since it is a simple, reliable, and effective system. The effective steam system setting is 1 atmosphere above atmospheric pressure, at 121° C (250° F). This is equivalent to a pressure of 1 atmosphere (101 kPa, 15 lb/in²) above atmospheric pressure, for at least 20 minutes. The disadvantage of this method is that it cannot be used on materials that are sensitive to moisture or moderate heat. Some newer steam autoclave systems replace the distilled water used with the traditional steam autoclave with methylethylketone, acetone, formaldehyde, and three alcohols. The time, pressure, and temperature settings are the same as for the traditional autoclave.[2]

Dry heat sterilization makes use of an oven. The time pressure is 2 hours at a temperature of 170° C (340° F). Dry heat is advantageous for the sterilization of sharp instruments. The disadvantage is that it cannot be used for plastics, cloth, or paper. Also, special packing containers or foil must be used to cover the individual items.

Gas (ethylene oxide) sterilization is accomplished by means of a mutagenic agent and is a very effective sterilization method for materials that cannot tolerate steam or dry heat. The setting is 450 to 500 mg/L at a temperature of 55° to 60° C. The problem with this method is that ethylene oxide is very toxic and flammable and requires a prolonged exposure time.[3]

Cold (liquid) sterilization is considered a disinfectant procedure and is not very reliable as a sterilization method, except for glutaraldehyde.[3] Several commercial glutaraldehyde preparations are on the market, including Cidex and Cidex-7 (Surgikos, Arlington, Tex.), Acusol (Acuderm, Fort Lauderdale, Fla.), Glutarex (3M Company, St. Paul, Minn.), and Sporicidin (Sporicidin Co., Washington, D.C.). Sporicidin is the newest preparation; it appears to be superior to the other glutaraldehyde preparations because of its faster action on microorganisms.

DISINFECTION AND DISINFECTANTS

With the onset of AIDS and the hepatitis epidemic, the Centers for Disease Control and Prevention (CDC), along with the Occupational Safety and Health Administration (OSHA), devised stringent standards for the protection of the 5.6 million health care workers in the United States. The protocol includes the use of disinfectants that inactivate HIV and hepatitis virus (Fig. 1-1).

Disinfection is defined as "any process, chemical or physical, by which pathogenic agents or disease-producing microbes (but not necessarily all microbial forms) are destroyed."[4] A number of chemical disinfectants have been found to inactivate the HIV; however, they are not always reliable because of their inactivation by blood or other or-

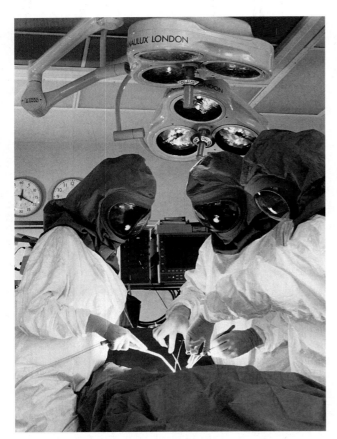

Fig. 1-1 Sophisticated mobile intraoperative air filtration system. *(Courtesy DePuy, Inc., Warsaw, Ind.)*

ganic matter. Consequently, the chemical disinfection of invasive instruments for surgery is not a recommended procedure. Instead, disinfectants should be used to wipe up blood on inanimate objects (fomites), such as table tops and chairs. The World Health Organization (WHO) has determined that the following disinfectants are effective against the AIDS virus: sodium hypochlorite solution (bleach), ethanol (ethyl alcohol), 2-propanol (isopropyl alcohol) 70%, polyvidone iodine (PVI) 2.5%, formaldehyde (formol, formalin) 4%, glutaral (glutaraldehyde) 2%, and hydrogen peroxide 6%.

Sodium hypochlorite

Sodium hypochlorite solution, or liquid bleach, is an excellent inexpensive disinfectant with bactericidal and virucidal activity. A major disadvantage is that bleach is corrosive to nickel, chromium steel, iron, and other oxidizable metals, leading to deterioration of the equipment. The equipment should be soaked for no longer than 30 minutes in diluted bleach.

Ethanol (ethyl alcohol) and 2-propanol (isopropyl alcohol)

Ethanol and 2-propanol are germicidal for vegetative forms of bacteria, mycobacteria, fungi, and viruses after a few minutes of contact. They are not effective against bacterial spores.

Polyvidone iodine

Polyvidone iodine (PVI) is an iodophor that can be used as a disinfectant and antiseptic. Its disinfectant activity is very similar to that of hypochlorite solution, but it is more stable and less corrosive to metal instruments. Equipment may be soaked in a 2.5% solution for 15 minutes.

Formaldehyde

Formaldehyde (formol, formalin) destroys vegetative bacteria, fungi, and viruses in less than 30 minutes and bacterial spores after several hours. The major disadvantage of this solution is the vapor released. It is very toxic and irritating to mucous membranes.

Glutaraldehyde

Glutaraldehyde (Glutarex, 3M Co. St. Paul, Minn., glutaral) destroys vegetative bacteria, fungi, and viruses in less than 30 minutes, while it takes about 10 hours to destroy spores. The problems with this solution are its release of toxic residues and its expense.

Hydrogen peroxide

Hydrogen peroxide (H_2O_2) is a potent disinfectant within 30 minutes, as a result of the release of oxygen. The disadvantage is that it is corrosive to copper, aluminum, zinc, and brass.

INTEGUMENTARY FOOT ECOLOGY

Hippocrates, in 400 BC, noted that wounds could be cleaned with boiling water. Joseph Lister, in 1865, was credited as the father of aseptic technique.[5,6] "Based on Pasteur's discovery and on the germ theory," Lister found that simple hand washing and use of carbolic acid spray reduced the infection rate in his patients dramatically.[7] Carbolic acid was found to be too toxic to the skin, and less noxious agents were later developed.

Current practice requires surgeons to use appropriate degerming agents to reduce the bacterial count on their own skin, as well as the patient's skin. In contrast to surgical instruments, which can be rendered absolutely sterile, living skin can never be completely sterilized of its bacterial colony. One can, however, eliminate bacteria by cleaning in two ways. Initially, vigorously rubbing the hands together produces friction, which removes dirt, transient flora, and some resident bacteria. Then, additional cleansing occurs when soaps or detergents emulsify oil-based bacteria and waste products from the skin.

Bacterial ecology of the feet can be divided into transient flora and resident flora, which are affected in different ways when the feet are scrubbed for surgery. Generally, the specific floral type and quantity of organisms present on the pedal skin will depend upon factors such as temperature, location (e.g., interdigital web spaces), CO_2 concentration, ketone bodies, glucose, pH, moisture, hair follicles, pilosebaceous glands, apocrine and eccrine (lactic acid) sweat glands (salt), and presence or absence of skin lipids. Trauma, from ulcerations and frank lacerations, to superficial skin crevices and microscopic cuts, as well as the systemic or local (e.g., diabetes mellitus or psoriasis) condition(s) of the host, all play a role in the microflora of the skin. Additionally, occlusive or porous footwear play an important role in the presence or absence of specific bacteria on the skin of the human foot.[8]

Resident flora

The resident flora consists of colonizing microorganisms commonly isolated from the dermis and epidermis of the skin and isolated in numbers greater than 10^2 colony-forming units (CFUs)/cm^2 on dry acidic skin, and greater than 10^5 CFUs/cm^2 on wet skin. The dorsal surface contains fewer organisms than the plantar surface, which in turn possesses fewer organisms than the toe web spaces. They are permanent and indigenous to the skin and are not easily removed with washing. They are usually not involved with nosocomial infections, unless invasive procedures introduce them into deeper tissue or the patient is compromised. The resident cutaneous microflora of the wet (lipophilic diphtheroids) and dry pedal skin includes the following organisms, according to Marshall and colleagues,[8] as well as Terleckyji and Abramson.[9]

1. Coagulase-negative staphylococci (CNS) (77% to 100%), such as *Staphylococcus capitis, S. cohnii, S. epidermidis, S. haemolyticus, S. hominis, S. saprophyticus,* and *S. warneri*
2. Aerobic micrococci (35% to 95%), including *Micrococcus luteus, M. varians,* and the aerobic diphtheroids (coryneforms)
3. Anaerobic diphtheroids (92% to 100%), including both lipophilic and nonlipophilic organisms, such as *Brevibacterium epidermidis* (nonfluorescent diphtheroid) and *Corynebacterium minutissimum* (fluorescent diphtheroid), *C. xerosis* (nonfluorescent diphtheroid), and *C. lipophilicus*
4. Yeasts, including *Pityrosporum orbiculare* and *P. ovale*

Transient flora

The transient flora consists of noncolonizing organisms, found on the superficial epidermis, and quantitatively represents less than 0.1% of the normal microflora of the foot. These organisms are isolated in numbers less than 10 (CFU's)/cm^2. Even though this type of flora remains for less than 24 hours and is easily removed by washing; it has been implicated in nosocomial (hospital-acquired) infections. The transient cutaneous bacterial microflora of the human foot includes the following organisms, according to Marshall and colleagues,[8] as well as Terleckyji and Abramson[9]:

1. Gram-positive (0% to 16%) cocci (*S. aureus*, alpha-hemolytic streptococci, group B streptococci, and group D streptococci [enterococci])
2. Gram-positive (12% to 40%) rods (*Clostridium* sp., *Bacillus* sp., and *Propionibacter* sp)
3. Gram-negative (11% to 25%) rods (*Acinetobacter* sp., *Enterobacter* sp., *Escherichia coli, Klebsiella pneumoniae, Moraxella* sp., *Proteus mirabilis, Pseudomonas maltophilia,* and *P. aeruginosa*)
4. Transient cutaneous (6% to 32%) fungal microflora, including *Aspergillus* sp., *Candida albicans* and *C. parapsilosis, Penicillium* sp., *Rhodotorula* sp., *Scopulariopsis* sp., and *Trichophyton* sp.

Opportunistic flora

The microbiological flora of the foot involves a constantly changing environment and may be modified or altered or become disease producing as a result of many factors. For example, in the hospitalized patient, opportunistic skin inhabitants may include *S. aureus, S. epidermidis (S. albus),* and *S. haemolyticus,* as well as *Proteus* sp., *Pseudomonas* sp., or *Candida albicans.* Fecal or urinary fallout, in the elderly or incontinent patient, may also contaminate the pedal skin, with microorganisms such as group D streptococci (enterococci), *E. coli,* and *Klebsiella pneumoniae.*

Coagulase-negative staphylococci (CNS), like the enterococci, are normal human commensals (60% to 90%) and usually represent contamination but not pathogenicity. However, it is now believed that some of these organisms *(S. warneri, S. capitis, S. simulans, S. auricularis, S. xylosus),* and especially *S. epidermidis* and *S. saprophyticus,* may play a more critical role in infected joint implant and fixation devices (<1%). Reasons for this include glycocalyx "slime" biofilm production and antibiotic resistance, but most of these infections are hospital acquired rather than community acquired or postoperative. Many are methicillin resistant, gentamicin resistant, and also not sensitive to the cephalosporins commonly used in surgical prophylaxis ("heterotropic resistance"). Therefore, empiric vancomycin and rifampin are the drugs of choice, if an abundance of CNS organisms are recovered from the site of a potential infection prior to the sensitivity report. Again, this is especially true of hospitalized patients, since almost half of all *S. epidermidis* isolates are methicillin, as well as cephalosporin, resistant.

PROTOCOLS OF SKIN PREPARATION

An antiseptic is defined as any substance used on living tissue to destroy microorganisms, by binding to the stratum corneum; but it does not sterilize the skin. In fact, living, viable epidermis cannot be rendered truly sterile, only surgically clean or decontaminated. Antimicrobial antiseptic scrubs are used for the surgical hand scrub and as a preparative agent for the surgical skin site, to remove superficial flora and debris, and to reduce the risk of wound contamination.

Currently, there are several antimicrobial soaps on the market to reduce the resident and transient flora of the surgeon's hands and the patient's foot. Which specific antimicrobial soap to use is clouded by many uncontrolled studies and confusing testing procedures. The ideal hand scrub should reduce microbes on intact skin, provide nonirritating antimicrobial penetration, be broad spectrum and fast acting, and be an effective detergent. If an antimicrobial soap cannot be used because of allergies, then a liquid nonmedicated soap scrub followed by an application of alcohol-based hand cleanser should be used.[10]

Popular antimicrobial hand scrubs include alcohol, 4% chlorhexidine, povidone-iodine, and 3% hexachlorophene. The less commonly used scrubs include 5% parachlorometaxylenol and triclosan.

The alcohols

The mode of action of alcohols is denaturation of proteins. They have excellent bactericidal activity against gram-positive organisms, gram-negative organisms, the tubercle bacillus, and fungi. However, they have no sporicidal activity. Alcohol's major disadvantage is its drying effects and volatility. There are no data on how alcohol is affected by organic material.

4% Chlorhexidine

Chlorhexidine 4% (Hibiscrub and Hibitane, Stewart Pharmaceuticals, Wilmington, Del.) is a cationic bisbiguanide, in which the mode of action is to disrupt the microbial cell membrane. This antimicrobial has good activity against gram-positive organisms and viruses, with less activity against gram-negative organisms and fungi. Adverse reactions include allergic dermatitis and photosensitivity, although these are rare. Studies show chlorhexidine provides the best immediate and persistent microbial reduction when compared to Betadine and pHisoHex (Winthrop Pharmaceutics, Inc., N.Y.).[11-13]

Povidone-iodine

Povidone-iodine (Betadine Iodophor, 1% to 2% iodine in alcohol) is the most commonly used hand scrub. The mode of action is "cell wall penetration, oxidation and substitution of cell wall contents with free iodine."[10] Povidone-iodine has good activity against gram-positive and gram-negative organisms, tubercle bacillus, fungi, and viruses. It has some activity against spores. Allergic reaction is uncommon.

3% Hexachlorophene

3% hexachlorophene (pHisoHex) is a chlorinated biphenyl in which the mode of action involves disruption of the microbial cell wall. It is bacteriostatic against gram-positive organisms but is less active against gram-negative bacteria, tubercle bacillus, fungi, and viruses. The adverse effects are similar to those of 4% chlorhexidine. Hexachlorophene is contraindicated in pregnant women and infants because of its absorption levels, from the gastrointestinal tract and across the mucous membrane, which can lead to CNS irritability and convulsions. It is also not advisable to use pHisoHex for routine bathing, since acute dermatitis may occur.[11]

A povidone-iodine scrub will decrease the bacterial count faster than chlorhexidine or hexachlorophene for immediate

effect. However, hexachlorophene and chlorhexidine are more effective over a longer period of time in reducing the bacterial count during hand scrubbing.[12]

5% Parachlorometaxylenol

5% Parachlorometaxylenol (PCMX) is a halogen-substituted xylenol, in which the mode of action involves cell wall disruption along with enzyme inactivation. It has good activity against gram-positive organisms, but less activity against gram-negative organisms, tubercle bacillus, fungi, and viruses. PCMX is less effective than chlorhexidine, povidone-iodine, and hexachlorophene in reducing skin microorganisms.[13]

Triclosan

Triclosan (Irgansan DP-300) is a diphenyl ether compound in which the mode of action is disruption of the microbial cell wall. It has good activity against gram-positive organisms and gram-negative organisms, except for *Pseudomonas,* while it has little activity against fungi. Additional studies are still needed to determine the efficacy of triclosan as a hand scrub. Thus overall, chlorhexidine kills the greatest number of microbial organisms, compared to hexachlorophene and povidone-iodine.[14-18]

SURGICAL PREPPING OF THE PATIENT

In the late nineteenth century, Lister first began preoperatively preparing the surgical site with carbolic acid spray. This proved to be a rather toxic method, and over the years different chemical compounds have been used to prepare the skin for surgery. Today the most popular skin preparation is the Betadine scrub-and-paint method (personal communication: Rose Krogh, R.N., St. Mary Nazareth Hospital Center, Chicago, Ill., 1997).

The American College of Surgeons advises that the operative site be scrubbed; however, the methods vary considerably. "The most that can be hoped for is to reduce the bacterial contamination at the surgical site."[19-23] The functions of the antiseptic surgical preparation are to dilute the inoculum present on skin and defat (emulsify) the skin surface of perspiration and oils. Preoperative measures involving the patient include bathing with antiseptics and preoperative shaving. Bathing the night before surgery, with antimicrobial soap, has been suggested to reduce *S. aureus* contamination. However, clinical studies have not substantiated this as an effective means to reduce infection.

Preoperative shaving appears to have been instigated by Gustav Neuber, in Germany, and has remained a ritual through this century; however several authors began to question the effectiveness of shaving the surgical site. Seropian "challenged this dogma of hair removal preoperatively by showing the infection rate of hair removal was 10 times higher than depilatory cream."[24] If preoperative shaving must be done, it should be performed immediately before the surgical procedure. Some suggested alternatives to razor shaving are depilatory creams and electric clippers. Depilatory creams, for hair removal, have given favorable results for several authors, who have confirmed the safety of this technique.

SURGICAL WOUND INFECTIONS

Factors that affect the incidence of postoperative surgical infections include prophylactic antibiosis, the patient's underlying health status, length of operation, and length of stay in the hospital. Additional factors include preoperative shaving and bathing of the patient. Patients who are over 65 years old are six times more likely to develop a postoperative infection. A patient's poor nutritional status, as well as underlying diseases such as sickle cell anemia or diabetes mellitus, and steroid therapy, seem to make the patient more prone to infection. Interestingly, formalities such as "double gloving" to reduce skin bacterial colony counts, or the use of superficial "skin" or dissecting "deep" scalpels, have not been experimentally proven to reduce the rates of postoperative infections.

Early admission, as well as prolonged stay in the hospital, for uncomplicated foot and ankle surgical cases, is now discouraged since there is a causal relationship between the occurrence of nosocomial infection and extra hospital stays. Hughes estimated that "5.5% of hospitalized patients develop a nosocomial foot infection,"[25] while Miller found in-house postoperative infections to range from 2.2% to 5.4%.[26] Martin et al surveyed 151 patients undergoing outpatient foot surgery and found the infection rate to be 1.3%,[27] and Hugar found an infection rate of 1.35% in his freestanding foot surgical center.[28] His study indicates that "all types of foot surgery may increase the risk of infection."

A postoperative infection is defined as a clinical condition caused by the action of a pathogenic microorganism in the surgical site. It is usually manifested by drainage or abscess formation. When an infection occurs, it usually demonstrates the cardinal signs of inflammation, such as redness, edema, and pain. The incubation period lasts from 48 to 72 hours and produces a sharp increase in temperature. The most common causative agents include *S. aureus* and beta-hemolytic streptococci of group A. Enteric gram-negative bacteria are not commonly involved.[29]

Surgical wound classification scheme

With the advent of modern aseptic surgical technique, antibiotic prophylaxis, and advances in clinical nutrition, the overall rate of surgical wound infection has decreased to 4.5%. However, it still accounts for over 40% of all hospital-acquired infections. Perioperative attention should be directed toward reducing the number of potential pathogens, addressing the patient's underlying health status, determining the condition of the wound, and decreasing the duration of the operation; all of which can discourage the growth of opportunistic pathogens.

The American College of Surgeons (ACS) and the National Research Council Study have classified surgical wounds into four categories, according to their potential risk for postoperative infections.

Clean wounds. Surgical wounds are considered clean if they are uninfected, no inflammation is encountered, no break in aseptic technique occurs, and no hollow organs are opened. In addition, if surgery is elective and wounds are primarily closed, a closed drainage system may be employed. Clean wounds have an infection risk of 1% to 5%.[30] Antibiotic prophylaxis is rarely given unless there is a higher risk of infection, such as in joint implant. *Staphylococcus* or *Streptococcus* species are usually the pathogens involved.

Clean-contaminated wounds. These are surgical wounds in which a hollow organ is entered with little or no spillage. They are considered potentially contaminated. These wounds generally result from operations involving the respiratory, alimentary, or genitourinary tracts. They have an infection risk of 8% to 11%.

Prophylaxis is used only for high-risk patients or procedures.

Contaminated wounds. Surgical wounds are considered contaminated if there is a preexisting infection, a major break in aseptic technique, or gross spillage from the gastrointestinal tract, or if an acute inflammation without pus formation is encountered. Traumatic wounds less than 4 hours old are included in this group. Contaminated wounds have an infection risk of 16% to 25%. Most patients require antibiotic prophylaxis, and delayed wound closure is common, unless the wound is believed to have been converted to a clean one prior to closure.

Dirty and infected wounds. Surgical wounds are considered dirty or infected if pus is encountered at the time of the surgery.

PROPHYLACTIC ANTIBIOTICS

In the United States clean surgery accounts for approximately 70% of all surgical cases, with a 1% to 5% infection rate.[30] Unpublished findings by Swiss, German, and other Western European authorities suggest a reduction of 10% to 12% in postoperative morbidity in patients who have received antibiotic prophylaxis (personal communication: Dr. Kai Olms, Bad Schwartau, Germany, 1997). Obviously, the most effective means to treat an infection is to prevent contamination in the first place. Interestingly, antibiotics have been used since 1932 and their role is still controversial. This is because early studies showed that the use of prophylactic antibiotics led to an increase in resistant organisms. The problem was lack of controlled studies, which led to "overdosage and faulty timing of the administration of the IV antibiotic, ranging from several hours to several days postoperatively."[25] These conflicting reports were not resolved until Burke's definitive 1961 study, in which he inoculated experimental lesions, in guinea pigs, with *S. aureus.*[30] He found that the antibiotics suppressed

Staphylococcus growth, when administered "from the moment the bacteria gains access to the tissue, and [the effect] is over in three hours." This is called the "effective" or "definitive period." He defined this period as the time when the developing staphylococcal lesions may be suppressed by the addition of antibiotics."[30] A delay in the administration of the antibiotics, after the crucial 3-hour period, failed to reduce the size of the control lesion.

Additionally, it must be recalled that prophylactic antibiotics are not totally benign and side effects can, and do, occur. Usually these entail hypersensitive cutaneous reactions such as flush, flare, wheel, rash, or hive formation. A superinfection from organisms not sensitive to the specific drug may also occur, and life-threatening anaphylactic shock may be the ultimate complication to consider. Prophylactic antibiotics are generally not used in AIDS patients for fear of sterilizing normal gut flora, allowing overgrowth potential of more resistant organisms.

Since Burke's study, several other studies have substantiated the importance of administering the IV antibiotic at the appropriate time to be effective. For example, Polk and Griffiths,[31] and Chodak and Plaut,[32] established that giving IV antibiotics 30 to 60 minutes before the surgical incision "results in the drug reaching therapeutic levels in the tissues" in adequate time to permit coverage of 100 minutes against *S. aureus* infection.

Prophylactic antibiotic agents of choice

Since their introduction in the early 1960s, cephalosporins have been the most widely used prophylactic intravenous antibiotic in the hospital setting. This is due to the drugs' effectiveness against *S. aureus* and *S. epidermidis,* the most common pathogens in postoperative wound infections. However, the indiscriminate use of these antibiotics has led to the development of resistant organisms. The most commonly used cephalosporins are cefazolin, cephalothin, and cephapirin. There is no conclusive evidence that any one of these antibiotics is the best choice for prophylaxis; nevertheless cefazolin (Ancef, Smith, Kline & French Laboratories, Philadelphia, Pa.) is usually preferred. It is often the agent of choice because it is able to achieve the longest bone level penetration, has good antistaphylococcal activity, rarely causes adverse reactions, and is cost effective. Cefazolin is usually administered as a 1-g intravenous bolus, 15 to 30 minutes prior to surgery. This will provide 100 minutes of protection to the tissue. If the procedure is more than 100 minutes long, the initial bolus may be doubled from 1 to 2 g, or an additional intraoperative dose may be given. This will provide a longer duration of coverage.[33-35] Cefamandole (Mandol, Parke-Davis, Morris Plains, N.J.) is a second-generation cephalosporin, which may also be used for prophylaxis. It has slightly better coverage over gram-negative microorganisms, but it has no added advantage over first-generation cephalosporins.[36-37]

If the patient is allergic to cephalosporins, the two alternatives are erythromycin and vancomycin. Erythromycin is probably the safest and most effective agent; however, an adverse effect is phlebitis at the IV site. Therefore, the lactobionate form is usually recommended. The usual prophylactic dosage is 500 mg to 1 g IVPB given 60 minutes prior to surgery. Vancomycin does offer some promise as a prophylactic antibiotic because of its excellent coverage for methicillin-resistant *S. aureus* (MRSA) infections, which are also resistant to cephalosporins. It is actually less toxic than previously thought, yet ototoxicity and nephrotoxicity are rare adverse effects. Peak and trough levels, formerly mandatory, are now less rigorously monitored. Vancomycin is also the likely drug of choice, in most formularies, for patients with penicillin or beta-lactam sensitivities. However, overuse and possible drug resistance are a concern. The recommended prophylactic dosage is 500 mg IVPB over a 30-minute period prior to surgery.[38-40] Rifampin may be a helpful adjunct.

The semisynthetic penicillins (oxacillin, methicillin, and nafcillin) are not commonly used for surgical prophylaxis, because of the increased numbers of penicillinase-resistant organisms.[41,42]

The aminoglycosides, lincomycin, and clindamycin are generally too toxic and narrow in spectrum for prophylactic use.[43,44] In order for any prophylactic antibiotic to be effective, it should have low toxicity to the patient, be administered 1 hour before surgery, and be continued for only a short period of time after the surgery.

Indications for use of prophylactic antibiotics

There are a number of pedal indications for the use of prophylactic antibiosis (Table 1-1). Antibiotic prophylaxis in limb amputations is still disputed. Very little has been written on this topic. Some previous studies have indicated that

---

TABLE 1-1 Indications for podiatric antibiotic prophylaxis

1. Implantation of foreign material
   a. Prostheses (implants)
   b. Extensive external fixation devices (Ilizarov clamp)
   c. Internal fixation devices.
2. Systemic diseases interfering with the natural mechanism of host defense
   a. Diabetes mellitus
      (1) Lower-extremity amputations
   b. Rheumatic heart disease
   c. Peripheral vascular disease
   d. Poor nutritional status
      (1) Cirrhosis of the liver
   e. Malabsorption syndromes
   f. Corticosteroid therapy
   g. Miscellaneous: leukemia, hemolytic anemia, sickle cell anemia, agammaglobulinemia
3. Acute trauma
4. Other indications
   a. Over 70 years old
   b. Previous surgery at surgical site
   c. Prolonged surgical time.

From: Till K: Indications and use of prophylactic antibiotics in podiatric surgery, *J Foot Surgery* 23: 166, 1984.

prophylactic antibiotics may be useful for lower-extremity amputations.[45-48] Claforan (Hoechst-Roussel Pharmaceuticals, Somerville, N.J.), or cefotaxime, a third-generation cephalosporin, may be beneficial for diabetic amputations since these usually involve polymicrobial-related infections. The suggested dosage is 1 to 2 g, IV, every 8 to 12 hours.

Prophylactic oral and topical agents and antibiotic wound lavage

Oral antibiotic administration has been documented to be ineffective for prophylaxis in foot surgical procedures. Oral agents are poorly absorbed, and several doses are required to attain sufficient bone level concentrations. Studies have shown that oral antibiotics fail to reduce postoperative infection rates, and actually lead to an increased incidence of resistant organisms.

The first topical antibiotics to be used in surgical wounds were gramicidin and tyrocidin, which were developed by René J. DuBois at the Rockefeller Institute. Unfortunately, surgeons soon found these antibiotics to be too toxic, and they were discontinued.[48] Many clinical and experimental studies have been done to determine whether irrigation of surgical wounds with antibiotics is effective in reducing postoperative wound infections. The data from these studies are inconclusive. Local wound irrigation has been found to be beneficial in "washing out fat, detritus, and blood clots which may act as a foreign body nidus and encourage bacterial growth."[48] Some other benefits include low systemic toxicity and lack of hypersensitivity or inflammation.

The commonly used antibiotic flushes are Betadine and Kantrex (Squibb-Navo, Inc., Princeton, N.J.). Betadine prepared as a 50:50 mixture with saline solution is recommended because it is broad spectrum and has low systemic toxicity. Betadine irrigation should not be used with implant surgery, since foreign body reactions may result around the implant as a result of the iodine ions reacting with the surface implant charges. Kanamycin (Kantrex) also has low systemic toxicity. It is bactericidal against gram-positive and gram-negative organisms, except *Streptococcus* and *Pseudomonas*. Kanamycin flush solution is mixed by the addition of 1 g kanamycin to 500 ml of saline solution.

In summary, indiscriminate use of prophylactic antibiotics is discouraged because it can lead to the development of resistant organisms, as well as the high medical costs to the patient. Yet, if used in selective cases, prophylactic antibiotics have an important role in foot and ankle surgery.

CONCLUSION

The definitions and processes of sterilization and disinfection, for both medical instruments and the human integument, were presented in this chapter. The perspective of the chapter was within the context of the normal resident, transient, and modified pathologic microbiological flora of the pedal skin. The use of oral and parenteral prophylactic antibiotics was also reviewed from this same perspective. It is hoped that this knowledge will be useful to the practitioner in the practical aspects of foot surgery.

REFERENCES

1. Ayliffe A: Surgical scrub and disinfection guideline for prevention of surgical wound infection, *Infect Control* 5:23-27, 1984.
2. Seeban EJ: Sterile technique and prevention of wound infection during office surgery, *J Dermatol Surg Oncol* 14:1364-1368, 1988.
3. *Methods of sterilization and disinfection,* OSHA Information Manual, APMA, pp. 2-11, 1993.
4. Coleman D: An overview of disinfectants and their proper use, *Podiatry Today* 12:59-60, 1992.
5. Lister J: On antiseptic principles in the practice of surgery, *Br Med J* 2:246, 1867.
6. Nyhaus L: Wound healing (Proceedings of the Brown University Symposium on the Biology of Skin). Boston, 1963, Little, Brown.
7. Gilliam D: Comparison of one step iodophor skin preparation v. traditional preparation in total joint surgery, *Clin Orthop Related Res* 250:258-260, 1990.
8. Marshall J, Lemming JP, Cunliffe WJ: The cutaneous microbiology of normal feet, *J Appl Bacteriol* 62:139, 1987.
9. Terleckyji B, Abramson C: Microbial ecology of the foot and ankle. In Abramson C, McCarthy DJ, Rupp MJ: *Infectious diseases of the lower extremity,* Baltimore, 1991, Williams & Wilkins.
10. Larson E: APIC guideline for infection control: practice guideline for use of topical antibacterial agents, *Am J Infect Control* 16:253-266, 1988.
11. Aly R: Comparative evaluation of chlorhexidine gluconate (Hibiclens) and povidone-iodine (E-Z scrub) sponge/brushes for presurgical hand scrubbing, *Curr Ther Res* 34:740-745, 1983.
12. Ulrich J: Clinical study comparing Hibistat (0.5% chlorhexidine gluconate in 70% isopropyl alcohol) and Betadine surgical scrub (7.5% povidone-iodine) for efficacy against experimental contamination of human skin, *Curr Ther Res* 31:27-30, 1982.
13. Lowbury EJ: Use of chlorhexidine detergent (Hibiscrub) and other methods of skin disinfection, *Br Med J* 3:510-515, 1975.
14. Pererira L: The effect of surgical handwashing routines on microbial counts of operating room nurses, *Am J Infect Control* 18:354-364, 1990.
15. Dineen P: An evaluation of the duration of the surgical scrub, *Surg Gynecol Obstet* 129:1181-1185, 1969.
16. Tucci VJ: Studies of surgical scrub, *Surg Gynecol Obstet* 145:415-416, 1977.
17. Peterson AF: Comparative evaluation of surgical scrub preparation, *Surg Gynecol Obstet* 146:63-65, 1978.
18. Gall P: Reassessment of the surgical scrub, *Surg Gynecol Obstet* 147:215-218, 1978.
19. Garibaldi R: Comparison of nonwoven and woven gown and drape fabric to prevent intraoperative wound contamination and postoperative infection, *Am J Surg* 152:500-509, 1989.
20. Altemeier W: Manual on control of surgical infections, Philadelphia, 1984, JB Lippincott, pp. 91-106.
21. Hambraeus A: The influence of different foot wear on floor contamination, *Scand J Infect Dis* 11:243-246, 1979.
22. Coop G: Foot wear practices and operating room contamination, *Nurs Res* 36:366-369, 1987.
23. Ritter MA: The antimicrobial effectiveness of the operative site preparative agents, *Am J Surg* 62A:826, 1980.
24. Seropian RE: Wound infection after preoperative depilatory vs. razor preparation, *Am J Surg* 121:251, 1971.
25. Hughes J: Section II: Nosocomial infection: prevention and epidemiological control, *Am J Infect Control* 22:99-103, 1994.
26. Miller W: Postoperative wound infection in foot and ankle surgery, *J Foot Surg*, 1983, pp 102-104.

27. Martin WJ, Mandracchia VJ, Beckett DE: The incidence of postoperative infection in outpatient podiatric surgery, *J Am Podiatr Assoc* 74:89, 1984.

28. Hugar D: Identification of postoperative infection in a free standing ambulatory surgery center, *J Am Podiatr Assoc* 29:265-267, 1986.

29. Burke J: Preventing bacterial infection by coordinating antibiotic and host activity: a time dependent relationship, *South Med J* 70(S):24-26, 1977.

30. Burke J: Effective period of preventive antibiotic action in experimental incisions and dermal lesions, *Surgery* 50:161-168, 1961.

31. Polk D, Griffiths D: Single dose antibiotic prophylaxis in gastrointestinal surgery, *Lancet* 2:325, 1976.

32. Chodak GW, Plaut M: The use of systemic antibiotics for prophylaxis in surgery, *Arch Surg* 112:326-333, 1977.

33. Barza M: Drug therapy reviews, antimicrobial spectrum, pharmacology and therapeutic use of antibiotics. III: Cephalosporins, *Am J Hosp Pharm* 34:621-629, 1977.

34. Pavel A: Prophylactic antibiotics in elective orthopedic surgery: a prospective study of 1,591 cases, *South Med J* 70:50-55, 1977.

35. Cunha BA: Antimicrobial prophylaxis in orthopedic and cardiovascular surgery, *Clin Ther* 2:211, 1979.

36. Rosenfeld M: Chemoprophylaxis with cefoxitin and cephalothin in orthopedic surgery: a comparison of antimicrobial agents and chemotherapy, *J Bone Joint Surg* 5:826, 1981.

37. Burke J: Preventing bacterial infection by coordinating antibiotic and host activity: a time dependent relationship, *South Med J* 70:24-26, 1977.

38. Till K: Indications and uses of prophylactic antibiosis in podiatric surgery, *J Foot Surg* 23:166-172, 1984.

39. Linton R: The prophylactic use of the antibiotics in clean surgery, *Surg Gynecol Obstet*, 1961, pp 218-220.

40. Friis H: Penicillin G v. cefuroxime for prophylaxis in lower limb amputation, *Acta Orthop Scand* 58:668, 1987.

41. Hares M: Failure of metronidazole/penicillin oral prophylaxis to prevent amputation stump infection, *Lancet* 10:1028-1029, 1980.

42. Huizinga WK: Prevention of wound sepsis in amputation by perioperative antibiotic cover with an amoxicillin clavulanic acid combination, *South Med J* 63:71-73, 1983.

43. Moller BN: Antibiotics prophylaxis in lower limb amputation, *Acta Orthop Scand* 56:327-329, 1985.

44. Sonne-Holm S: Prophylactic antibiotics in amputation of the lower extremity for ischemia, *JBS:* 67:800-803, 1985.

45. Norlin R: Short-term cefotaxime prophylaxis reduces the failure rate in lower limb amputations, *Acta Orthop Scand* 61:460-462, 1990.

46. Estersohn H: The local use of antibiotics to prevent wound infection, *J Bone Joint Surg* 69:127-130, 1979.

47. Scherr D: Prophylactic use of topical antibiotic irrigation in uninfected surgical wounds, *J Bone Joint Surg*, vol 54A.

48. Lord J: Intraoperative antibiotic wound lavage: an attempt to eliminate postoperative infection in arterial and clean general surgical procedures, *Ann Surg* 185:634-641, 1977.

ADDITIONAL READINGS

English AJ: Tracing needs of infection control professionals in long term care facilities in Virginia, *Am J Infect Control* 23:73, 1995.

Guideline for isolation precautions in hospitals (Control Practices Advisory Committee). *Am J Infect Control* 24:24, 1996.

Pearson A, Becker L, Almaraz J: Departmental role and scope in infection control: use of a template that meets Joint Commission requirements, *Am J Infect Control* 24:53, 1996.

Rutala WA: APIC Guidelines for Selection and Use of Disinfectants. (1994, 1995 and 1996 Guidelines Committee), *Am J Infect Control* 24:313, 1996.

Zefar AB, Butler DJ, Reese LA: Use of 0.3% triclosan (Bacti-stat-R) to eradicate an outbreak of methicillin-resistant *S. aureus, Am J Infect Control* 23:200, 1995.

2

Blood-Borne and Communicable Pathogens

Jon D. Tinkle
Rhonda Cope

It is the mind which is really alive and sees things, yet it hardly sees anything, without preliminary instruction. Charcot

A good working knowledge of all aspects of blood-borne pathogens is essential now more than ever. This knowledge is imperative not only to the life of the patient, but to the treating physician as well. AIDS and tuberculosis are going to change every life on this planet. It is our duty to treat these patients as we would treat any other patients, with compassion, understanding, and, above all, a firm knowledge of the diseases we are treating.

ACQUIRED IMMUNODEFICIENCY SYNDROME (AIDS)

Epidemics date as far back as 430 BC. In the fourteenth century, 75 million people, a third of the world population died as a result of the bubonic plague ("black death"), caused by *Pasteurella pestis*. AIDS deaths will approach this number worldwide if a cure or vaccine is not found soon. It is already the number one killer of young adults age 20 to 49 in one third of major U.S. cities. The number of AIDS-related deaths in the United States has already surpassed fatalities of the Vietnam War. By the year 2000, the number of HIV-infected people in the United States will fast approach the number with diabetes mellitus. We are now entering the second decade of the AIDS epidemic. Most physicians did not even have HIV in their vocabularies in their medical schools or residencies. As foot specialists, we must learn as much as we can about the disease and join the medical community in recognizing and treating AIDS-related manifestations of the lower extremity.

Historical review

In 1981, 26 cases of Kaposi's sarcoma (KS) and 5 cases of *Pneumocystis carinii* pneumonia (PCP) were reported in young, homosexual men in California and New York. The term AIDS (acquired immune deficiency syndrome) was given to the disease in 1982, and in 1983 the etiologic agent lymphadenopathy-associated virus (LAV) was discovered by

Luc Montagnier. Robert Gallo had found the same virus and labeled it human T-cell leukemia virus III (HTLV III) in 1983. In 1984, Jay Levy and colleagues published findings on their isolate, naming it AIDS-associated retrovirus (ARV). They were all the same virus and eventually given one name, HIV (human immunodeficiency virus).

In 1985, a second type of HIV was discovered in Africa, and it was isolated in the United States in 1987. This new strain was labeled HIV-2 and the old HIV-1. The two are similar, except HIV-2 in general progresses at a much slower rate and patients live longer even after developing AIDS as defined by the Centers for Disease Control and Prevention (CDC). The virus is genetically related to the simian immunodeficiency virus (SIV) rather than HIV-1. It does cross react with the HIV-1 serologic test in 80% of patients. If a patient has symptoms of AIDS but remains negative, the polymerase chain reaction test is specific for HIV-2. By April 1992, only 32 cases of HIV-2 had been reported in the United States.[1,2] The next update is due in the fall of 1997.

Epidemiology

The latest estimates of the number of HIV-infected people are between 2 and 3 million in the United States and 18 million worldwide. Currently, 1 in 250 Americans is infected with HIV. In 1988, the World Health Organization (WHO) predicted a cumulative total of 15 to 20 million adult HIV infections worldwide by the year 2000. This number was surpassed by mid-1997. The current projection is 35 to 125 million. There are four major trends:

1. Geography. Ten years ago, the pandemic was concentrated in cities and towns. The virus is following migration into the countryside. In the future, there will be little or no difference between rural and urban areas.
2. Male/female ratios. Worldwide, men have accounted for two thirds of all HIV infections. By the year 2000, more than half of the new cases will be women. In 1988, women accounted for 9% of the U.S. AIDS

population. In 1992, this increased to 11.5%, and in 1996 represented more than 78,000 women. Worldwide this increase will be accompanied by millions more children being born with HIV and youngsters becoming orphans to HIV-infected mothers.

3. Transmission. In the United States, the best known types of transmission have been blood and body fluid exchange among homosexual men or IV drug users. In Africa, HIV is almost exclusive to the heterosexual population. From 1985 to 1994, the percent of heterosexual transmissions tripled in the United States. In 1994, the World Health Organization (WHO) stated that 75% of worldwide HIV transmission was heterosexual. By the year 2000, this will be approximately 90%.

4. HIV to AIDS. Because the average time for conversion from HIV infection to AIDS is approximately 10 years, the number of AIDS cases will increase significantly into a "second pandemic."

Retrovirus replication

Retroviruses were first described by Ellerman and Bang, in 1908. There are three subgroups: Oncoviruses generally cause neoplastic disorders. Spumaviruses can cause persistent infection. Lentiviruses, to which HIV belongs, are associated with chronic, lifelong infections producing pneumonia, neurologic disorders, arthritis, anemia, or wasting syndromes.

The virus is composed of a viral core containing RNA, a nucleoprotein, and reverse transcriptase. This is surrounded by an envelope with multiple projections, each containing a glycoprotein, gp 120, responsible for binding to a host receptor site, most frequently CD4+. After the binding process, the viral cell is anchored, fused, and injected into the host cell.

The reverse transcriptase then converts the viral RNA into DNA inside the cell. The viral DNA (the provirus) is then spliced into the host DNA, and the cell is permanently infected. The provirus may now become latent and not reproduce its genes. Once activated, it can order the cell to reproduce RNA. This RNA may become viral protein, which is assembled and released as a virion from the cell surface. The provirus can also cause a rapid replication, which can rupture and destroy the cell, releasing the virions in large numbers. Because T cells are often the target of the virus, their numbers decrease as they are ruptured[3] (Table 2-1).

The surfaces of T4 cells are laden with the HIV-inviting CD4+ molecules. These cells play an important role in the disease process because of their production of lymphokines, which are responsible for:

1. Macrophage activation, which kills intracellular bacteria and tumor cells
2. B-cell proliferation, which is responsible for plasma cell antibody production
3. CD8 cytotoxic T-cell maturation, which leads to destruction of virally infected cells and tumor cells

TABLE 2-1   Cells infected by HIV
T-cells
B lymphocytes
Macrophages
Dendritic cells
Langerhans cells
Bone marrow precursor cells
Central Nervous System Cells
Glial cells
Astrocytes
Oligodendrocytes
Capillary endothelium
Other Cells
Kupffer's cells
Bowel epithelial cells
Colon carcinoma cell lines

4. T-cell and B-cell memory clones, which provide a rapid defense against reinfections

CDC definition of AIDS

In 1986, the CDC published a classification system for HIV and a case definition for AIDS. To be defined as an AIDS case, a patient must have laboratory evidence of HIV infection and any one or more of the indicator diseases, such as Kaposi's sarcoma, candidiasis, cryptococcosis, toxoplasmosis, lymphoma, or *Pneumocystis carinii* pneumonia. In the absence of laboratory evidence, the patient must have at least one of the indicator diseases plus have no other cause of immunodeficiency, including systemic steroids, certain lymphomas and other immune-depressing cancers, or a genetic immunodeficiency syndrome. The definition was expanded in 1993 to include HIV-infected adults and adolescents who have less than 200 CD4+ T-lymphocytes/mm^3 and pulmonary tuberculosis, invasive cervical cancer, or recurrent pneumonia.[4]

Laboratory diagnosis

HIV testing is important not only in detecting the disease but also in staging the disease and determining therapy. Sensitivity refers to the proportion of individuals who have a positive test for antibodies in an infected population. Specificity refers to the proportion of individuals with a positive test in an uninfected population. The ELISA (enzyme-linked immunosorbent assay) is the standard test now used. It is inexpensive and highly sensitive. The Western blot assay is more specific and more expensive but is useful in ruling out false positives. The Western blot can identify specific viral proteins, such as p24 and gp120. A latex agglutination test can also identify the gp120, is inexpensive, and takes about 5 minutes.

Viral culture is the "gold standard" for determining HIV infection, although it is technically difficult and expensive. PCR (polymerase chain reaction) detects genetic sequences of HIV in infected cells through magnification. The PCR is sensitive and can detect the HIV virus before replication and before antibodies appear in the blood. The HIV-1 core antigen test is useful in detecting core antigen, which increases with disease progression. Serum antibodies to p24 antigen decrease with disease progression as serum antibodies to p24 increase.

Testing has become accurate in screening blood for transfusions. Studies estimate that the chance of becoming infected with HIV from a transfusion ranges from 1 in 38,000 to 1 in 300,000. The largest study was conducted by the American Red Cross, in which roughly 1 in 225,000 units of blood was capable of transmitting the virus.

There have been cases of AIDS-type diseases reported recently in which the patients have remained negative. First reported at the VIII International AIDS Conference, the syndrome is called idiopathic CD4+ T-lymphocytopenia (ICL). In 1993, an investigation concluded that 47 cases met the criteria for ICL. The investigation was unable to find a transmissible agent and concluded that the syndrome was exceptionally rare and could not be transmitted from patient to patient.[5]

AIDS treatments

Vaccines will be developed slowly because of many obstacles, the most difficult being the ability of the retrovirus to integrate and disappear within the cell and then replicate the cell. Another problem is the ability of the virus to continuously mutate and become resistant to new treatments. The current treatments now revolve around antiviral agents that try to attack the replication process at different stages, most commonly by inhibiting reverse transcriptase. However, because of the emergence of drug-resistant viruses, the HIV replicative life cycle must be attacked at different stages to reduce side effects and minimize the development of drug-resistant HIV variants.

To date, nucleoside analogs such as azidothymidine (AZT, zidovudine, Retrovir) have been the most commonly used antiviral agents. Synthesized nearly 30 years ago and shown to be effective against retroviruses or in vitro, no medical application had emerged before AIDS. AZT was approved in 1987 initially for patients with a history of cytologically confirmed PCP or a decrease in CD4+ T-cells to below 200/mm.[3] AZT serves as a chain-terminating inhibitor of HIV reverse transcriptase. It can produce significant bone marrow suppression, which can lead to megaloblastic anemia. Fortunately, AZT lacks severe cardiac, renal, or hepatic toxicity.

In April 1993, the largest randomized, double-blind AZT study was reported to *The Lancet.* The study determined that early use of AZT in the asymptomatic patient was of no value. This will have great bearing on future treatments. In recent years, other nucleoside analogs, such as dideoxyinosine (ddI) and dideoxycytidine (ddC), have been added to the armory of antivirals. Each has a different level of toxicity, including severe peripheral neuropathy. In 1996 a third

nucleoside analog joined the fight, 3'-deoxythymidin-2'-ene (d4T). Each works against replication of the reverse transcriptase. Combination and alternating therapies are also being used by adding such treatments as interferon and other agents.

A future possibility of a cure, in the late 1990s or beyond, may lie within gene therapy. This concept involves adding programmed DNA, which will be designed to fight disease or perform specific functions, into the cells of patients with AIDS. The DNA may be able to enter the cell and replicate by transport from another, nonharmful virus. It is important to understand the effects and adverse reactions of the medications that the patient with HIV or AIDS may be using. Many of the medications may be new on the market and may have important side effects. A patient with full-blown AIDS could easily be taking as many as 10 to 15 different prescriptions each day.[6]

Clinical disease course

The Centers for Disease Control and Prevention has classified HIV into four groups and various subgroups (Table 2-2) according to the seroconversion status and introduction of HIV-related diseases. In the early 1980s, scientists believed that 30% to 50% of people infected with HIV would go on to develop AIDS. Current estimates now predict 100% of HIV-infected individuals will develop AIDS within 32 years of seroconversion. The average time from seroconversion to full-blown AIDS is approximately 10.8 years.

The average life span after the diagnosis of AIDS is 2 years for males and 12 to 18 months for females. Little is still known about why some individuals develop AIDS faster and whether there is the possibility of a cofactor. Patients who were diagnosed and placed on AZT, who were between ages 20 and 39, or who had KS as one of the first clinical signs of AIDS had the longest survival time according to a survey by the San Francisco Department of Public Health.[7]

 TABLE 2-2   Classification of HIV infection

Group I—Acute Infection

The acute infection begins with flu-like symptoms in 7% to 50% of the patients. The patients remain HIV negative for approximately 2 to 6 weeks. Symptoms may include anorexia, nausea, vomiting, headache, photophobia, diarrhea, or a transient erythematous eruption on the trunk and arms that may last 3 to 4 days. Approximately 75% of those with this syndrome complain of pharyngitis and lymphadenopathy.

Group II—Asymptomatic Infection

There is an absence of signs or symptoms of the HIV infection. These patients may be subclassified according to blood counts.

Group III—Persistent Generalized Lymphadenopathy

Lymph nodes of 1 cm or greater at two or more extra-inguinal sites for more than 3 months in the absence of other condition or disease other than HIV. Again, there may be similar subgroups as above.

Group IV—Other Diseases

This group has many subgroups and includes many of the opportunistic or secondary infectious diseases associated with HIV.

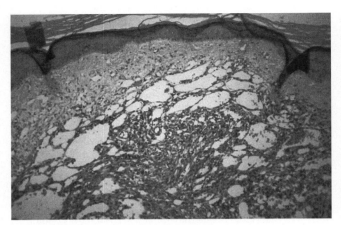

Fig. 2-1 Kaposi's sarcoma. Malignant spindle cells are present.

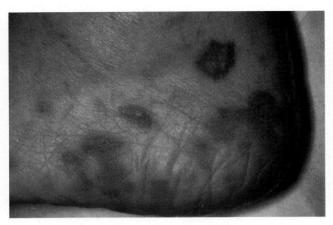

Fig. 2-2 Kaposi's sarcoma of the heel.

The most common systemic diseases associated with AIDS are discussed below.

Kaposi's sarcoma (KS). Kaposi's sarcoma was first documented by Moritz Kaposi in 1872, in a report titled "Idiopathic Multiple Pigmented Sarcoma of the Skin." The neoplasm is a slow-growing vascular lesion of endothelial origin (Fig. 2-1). The first cases occurred in elderly men of the Mediterranean area who were of Eastern European Jewish ancestry. Beginning in the 1960s, the tumors were seen in immunosuppressed renal transplant patients.

In the fall of 1979, the first documented cases of KS were reported in young homosexuals in California and New York. In this new discovery of KS, the lesion was found to be more disseminated and aggressive. The prevalence of this new KS is an epidemic. Compared to classical KS, these lesions are more varied in configuration, develop more rapidly and more symmetrically, and are accompanied by other systemic infections.

The etiology of KS is a complete mystery. Theories include a viral infection of the herpes or papiloma family. Another theory includes a genetic factor. The possibility of a recreational drug or sexual behavior cofactor is high; 95% of all cases of AIDS-related KS have been in homosexual men, and the incidence of KS has dropped from 44% of homosexuals with AIDS in 1981 to 20% in 1987. The lesions are often difficult to diagnose, as they can be red, blue, or brown and may be warty, papular, nodular, macular, or ulcerative (Fig. 2-2). Many other lesions may look similar (Table 2-3), so a biopsy is always indicated (Figs. 2-3 and 2-4). The foot is involved in 20% to 30% of cases. One study involving 212 patients reported that patients presenting with KS alone and CD4+ counts greater than 300/mm^3 had the best prognosis. The survival from onset of the sarcoma was 32 months. The patients with KS alone but CD4+ counts less than 300/mm^3 had a mean survival of 24 months. Patients who had constitutional symptoms at the time of KS had a mean survival of 14 months. Those patients who developed opportunistic infections within 3 months of diagnosis of KS had a mean survival of 7 months.

TABLE 2-3   Differential diagnosis of Kaposi's sarcoma (KS)

Melanoma
Basal cell carcinoma
Squamous cell carcinoma
Dermatofibroma
Glomus tumor
Pyogenic granuloma
Angiokeratoma
Hemangioma
Neurofibroma
Cutaneous lesions, systemic metastases
MAI
Pityriasis rosea
Sarcoidosis
Lichen planus
Insect bite
Diabetic dermopathy
Sarcoidosis
Urticaria pigmentosa
Ecchymoses
Venous stasis
Angioendotheliomatosis

KS is the most common cancer of the AIDS patient. Treatments include radiation therapy, cryotherapy, electrocauterization, intralesional injections of bleomycin or alpha-interferon, and radical excision (Figs. 2-5, 2-6, and 2-7). Rapidly progressive, disseminated Kaposi's sarcoma may be treated with systemic chemotherapy such as bleomycin, alpha-interferon, or vincristine, or in combination. One recent clinical trial injecting 52 cutaneous lesions with vinblastine (VB) reported an 88% complete or partial response following one injection.[8]

Lymphoma. A lymphoma is a cancer of the lymphadenoid cell line; types include non-Hodgkin's lymphoma, immunoblastic lymphoma, and CNS lymphoma. The chance of developing a lymphoma increases with a history of KS,

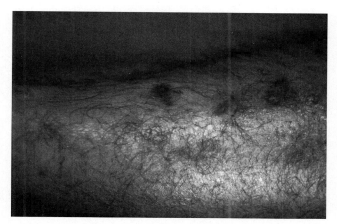

Fig. 2-3 Multiple ant bites with allergic reaction and moderate infection in a 30-year-old AIDS patient.

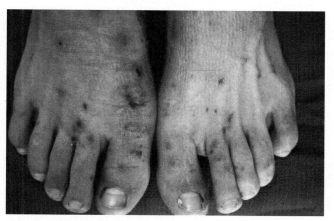

Fig. 2-4 Sjögren's syndrome and diabetic dermopathy in a 45-year-old AIDS patient. The patient later had a complete skin slough.

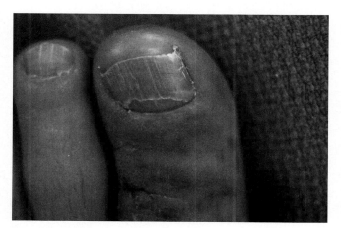

Fig. 2-5 Kaposi's sarcoma in a 48-year-old male. The initial lesion appeared similar to a classic verruca.

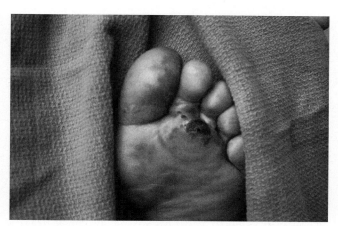

Fig. 2-6 Same patient, 3 months later, with radiation burn on the plantar aspect after 3 weeks of radiation therapy. The patient developed osteomyelitis in 2 more weeks and was treated with intravenous antibiotics.

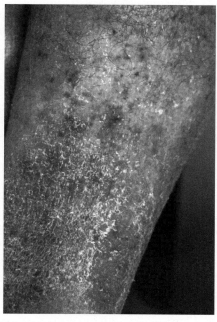

Fig. 2-7 Same patient 6 months after the first lesion. Final resolution was a below-knee amputation, with death 2 days later.

and it occurs in approximately 2% to 5% of the AIDS population. Symptoms include weakness, paralysis, aphasia, seizures, and headache. Diagnosis is by CT scan, lumbar puncture, biopsy, and bone marrow biopsy. Treatments include chemotherapy or radiation therapy, which may cause nausea, vomiting, alopecia, and a significant white blood cell decrease.[9]

***Pneumocystis carinii* pneumonia (PCP).** The most opportunistic infection in people with AIDS, PCP is caused by a protozoan commonly found in over half the population not infected with AIDS. There are no risks of contracting PCP from an AIDS patient, as the compromised immune system is responsible for the disease progression. Early signs include shortness of breath, dry hacking cough, chest pain, fevers, and difficulty walking up stairs. Diagnosis can be made by a combination of chest x-ray, pulmonary function tests, arterial blood gases, sputum induction, and bronchoscopy. Treatment is with trimethoprim-sulfamethoxazole. Aerosol pentamidine and dapsone may be used prophylactically.[10]

Toxoplasmosis. Toxoplasmosis is caused by *Toxoplasma gondii,* another protozoan commonly found in the general population and activated with severe immune suppression. This disease state is most frequently encountered in Florida and most commonly in Haitians. The organism is acquired by eating raw or uncooked meat or through exposure to flies or cat feces. In AIDS patients, the disease most often results in brain infections, leading to seizures, confusion, dizziness, headaches, fever, or weakness. Diagnosis can be made with a CAT scan and more definitively with a brain biopsy. Treatments include a combination of pyrimethamine and sulfadiazine, both of which may cause a white blood cell decrease. Clindamycin is an alternative. Once diagnosed, most patients are maintained on these drugs indefinitely.

Primary AIDS encephalopathy ("AIDS dementia"). The HIV virus can directly infect the brain and spinal cord cells, impairing the patient's mental and coordinating functions. Symptoms may include confusion, leg or foot weakness, tremors, or loss of coordination. There is no treatment for encephalopathy, although some patients may take systemic steroids to decrease cranial pressure. Massage and physical therapy are helpful for muscle tone. Confusion in these patients makes it difficult for them to take responsibility for the administration of medications or keeping appointments.[11]

***Mycobacterium avium-intracellulare* (MAI) infection.** MAI is a mycobacterium, similar to the one that causes tuberculosis (TB), that is present in most healthy individuals. Activated by a depressed immune system, MAI can enter the bloodstream and become highly disseminated. Symptoms may include fever, fatigue, wasting syndrome, swollen glands, sweats, diarrhea, and even skin lesions (Fig. 2-8). It is not spread person to person. Treatment is difficult, as MAI is highly resistant to anti-TB drugs. Combination anti-TB drugs are given in severe cases, sometimes involving up to six different prescriptions.

Cytomegalovirus (CMV) infection. CMV is a member of the herpesvirus family. Nearly all patients with AIDS have had a previous infection with CMV. Again, antibodies are commonly found in healthy individuals, but the pathogen is exacerbated by the HIV infection. The most common conditions resulting from CMV infection in AIDS patients include pneumonia, colitis, encephalitis, and blinding retinitis. There is no proven treatment, although DHPG and foscarnet have been shown to inhibit the disease, resulting in less severe symptoms.

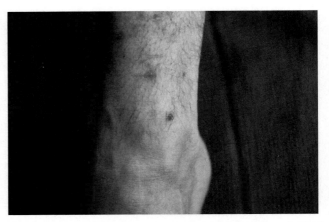

Fig. 2-8 Atypical presentation of MAI in a 27-year-old AIDS patient, looking very much like KS but with culture and biopsy indicative of the mycobacterium.

Pedal manifestations of AIDS

Vascular manifestations. The vascular system of the HIV-infected patient may closely resemble that of a patient with diabetes mellitus. Pulses may be weak from peripheral vascular disease. Hyperalgesic pseudothrombophlebitis with red indurated cords or lower-extremity swelling has been reported. Most patients with this syndrome will often have fever with painful lower extremities. Deep-vein thrombosis must be ruled out, since anticoagulant therapy is not the treatment of choice in pseudothrombophlebitis. This syndrome has been characterized as a phlebitis secondary to Kaposi's sarcoma of proximal lymph nodes. Telangiectasias are not uncommon and may appear early in the disease process. They are often associated with mild diffuse erythema in the same distribution. Lower-extremity edema may appear secondary to various etiologies, such as malabsorption, liver disease, increased protein catabolism, or hypoalbuminemia. Vasculitis may present as diffuse purpura with shiny, cool skin (Fig. 2-9). Telangiectasias and phlebitis are often related to *Pneumocystis carinii* pneumonia. Thrombocytopenic purpura may present as petechiae and may be secondary to recreational drug use, viral antigens, or CMV infection. Treatments may include pentoxifylline (Trental), which has proven advantages in HIV-infected patients. Support hose have been found to be effective not only in patients with peripheral vascular disease but also in those with severe neuropathies.[12]

Neurologic manifestations. The nervous system pathologies of HIV are numerous and complex. Ten percent of patients with AIDS will initially present with neurologic symptoms, and 60% will eventually develop some type of neurologic disease. In one pathologic autopsy study, 90% of the cadavers showed disease-related neuropathic abnormalities. The etiology of neurologic disorders may be a combination of HIV infection, opportunistic infections, neoplastic disorders, and cerebrovascular complications, or

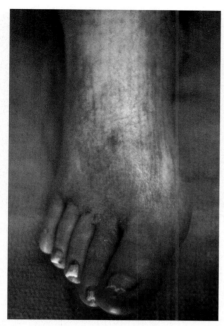

Fig. 2-9 Vasculitis in a 48-year-old AIDS patient who responded well to physical therapy and Trental.

a side effect of therapeutic drugs. The most common cause of neurologic dysfunction is subacute encephalitis secondary to HIV.

Aseptic meningitis and myopathies are also considered to be secondary to the HIV infection. Neoplasms such as lymphoma and KS may present with focal defects, but the prognosis is generally poor. Cerebral infarcts have been reported in 12% to 20% of AIDS patients. The etiology is unclear, but hypercoagulable states have been suspected. When pathogens are involved in CNS pathologies, nonviral infections such as TB, MAI, toxoplasmosis, *Candida*, and *Cryptococcus* are generally responsible. Viral opportunistic agents such as papovavirus can cause ataxia, unsteadiness, or hemiparesis. Infection with Herpesvirus, CMV, or varicella-zoster virus may present as meningitis, encephalitis, and myelitis. Herpes zoster radiculitis may occur with both motor and sensory symptoms and is normally associated with a characteristic dermatomal rash. The prognosis in viral CNS infections is poor, with an average survival of 2 months.

Most important to the lower extremities are peripheral neuropathies, symptoms of which may occur in 50% of patients with AIDS. Four HIV-related peripheral nervous system complications should be distinguishable to the physician:

1. Distal symmetrical sensory peripheral neuropathy: the most common involvement in AIDS patients. The sensory functions are affected more than motor functions. Signs are hypoesthesia, paresthesia, sensory ataxia, weakness, and hypoactive deep tendon reflexes. AZT, Elavil, or nonsteroidal antiinflammatory

drugs (NSAIDs) can be effective. An ankle-foot orthosis may be necessary for footdrop.

2. Inflammatory demyelinating polyradiculoneuropathy: normally occurs in HIV patients without AIDS. Motor symptoms are more severe than sensory. There are similarities to Guillain-Barré syndrome. Weakness may be more prominent distally and tendon reflexes hypoactive. Treatment is through plasmapheresis.
3. Mononeuropathy multiplex: the hallmark is rapid development of sensory and/or motor loss, which is generally asymmetric. Occurs mostly in HIV positive patients without AIDS.
4. Progressive polyradiculopathy: motor function is affected more than sensory, beginning with leg weakness distally and progressing proximally over several weeks. Urinary retention is common. Mostly seen in AIDS patients, but has been reported in CMV or herpes simplex infections.

Complicating the diagnosis of the symptoms above is the fact that many of the medications used in treating HIV and AIDS have CNS symptoms. Also, it is not unusual for a patient with AIDS to develop diabetes mellitus when there is a family history of diabetes. The neuropathic diseases of diabetes may be exacerbated (Figs. 2-10 and 2-11). Patients on low-dose antiemetics may present with extrapyramidal motor symptoms. Chemotherapy may be associated with myelopathy or peripheral neuropathy, and antiviral therapies often cause myoclonus, dysphasia, and delirium.[13]

Dermatologic manifestations. Dermatophytic infections in the toenails are common and generally coincide with a decreasing T cell count, usually below 100 cells/mm³.[14] Some of the more common presentations in HIV patients include a proximal white subungual onychomycosis (Fig. 2-12). There also may be chalky white involvement of the outer nail, normally caused by *Tricophyton rubrum* (in the immunocompetent patient, this is more often caused by *T. mentagrophytes*). Dompmartin, in a report on 62 HIV patients with onychomycosis, found 58% cultures of *T. rubrum*, 11.3% *Candida*, 9.7% *T. mentagrophytes*, and 4.8% *Epidermophyton floccosum*; 88.7% presented with the proximal white subungual onychomycosis. The toenail mycoses seem to spread rapidly and symmetrically, and may involve the periungual regions. *Candida albicans* is another common infection of the HIV patient, presenting in the perineum region and nails and in the oral cavity as thrush. There is high incidence of *Candida* paronychia or hypertrophic nail bed (Fig. 2-13). These fungal infections are highly resistant to oral antifungals and have a high relapse rate if treatment is successful but stopped.[15,16]

Ingrown toenails are extremely common in the HIV patient (Fig. 2-14). In a study of 100 HIV patients presenting to our podiatry clinic, 13 patients accounted for 27 ingrown and infected nails.[16] *Staphylococcus aureus* and beta-hemolytic streptococci are the two most suspected pathogens. All of the above ingrown nails were treated with partial

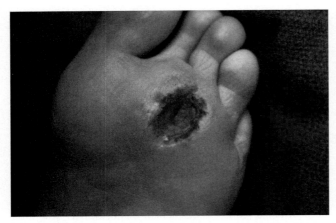

Fig. 2-10 A 24-year-old HIV-positive patient with diabetes mellitus. The nonhealing ulcer did not respond to any conservative treatment and finally healed after a metatarsal head resection.

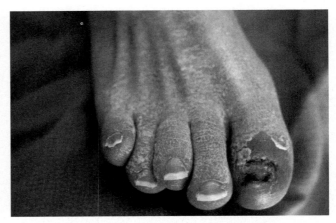

Fig. 2-13 Combination staphylococcal and *Candida* infection in a 29-year-old AIDS patient. The patient was placed on amoxicillin and ketoconazole with excellent healing. Also notice psoriatic-appearing lesions of the skin, which responded well to topical steroids.

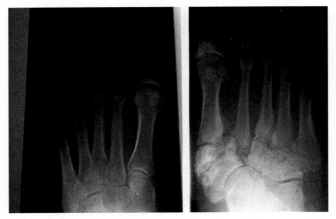

Fig. 2-11 A 32-year-old AIDS patient with diabetes mellitus and severe Charcot changes. He was treated at a clinic for 6 months with intravenous antibiotics under the diagnosis of chronic osteomyelitis.

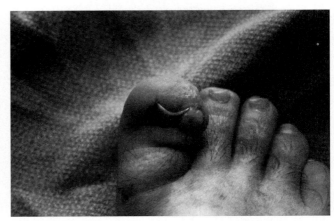

Fig. 2-14 Patient treated successfully with intravenous antibiotics for 6 weeks. The patient died 3 months after the bone scan.

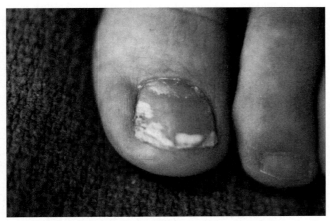

Fig. 2-12 Typical proximal white subungual onychomycosis in a 35-year-old AIDS patient. The discoloration will usually migrate distally.

phenol and alcohol procedures, with only one recurring infection, the patient with *Candida* paronychia. Crusted scabies has also been documented in HIV patients, causing a hypertrophic nail bed and plate. Treatment includes debridement and topical permethrin cream. Numerous viral or neoplastic diseases may also be seen. Herpetic whitlow, papillomavirus infection, squamous cell, metastatic lesions, and KS must all be ruled out. Psoriatic nails can mimic onychomycosis but require different treatment modalities. A new finding, slowly being documented, is yellow nail syndrome in HIV patients (Fig. 2-15). In one report, symptoms included yellowing of the nails, cross ridging, clubbing, onycholysis, and shedding. No bacterial or fungal agent has been found to be causative. This disorder seems to correlate with PCP. Another anomaly is nail shedding of unknown origin. As many as three to five nails may shed spontaneously.[16]

Neoplastic manifestations. Kaposi's sarcoma has already been discussed. Lymphomas may affect the skin, including both Hodgkin's and, more commonly, non-Hodgkin's B-cell lymphoma. The lesions may appear as nodules or papules. Basal and squamous cell carcinomas have been reported in AIDS patients. Squamous cell carcinomas generally affect the oral and anal or rectal regions. Basal cell carcinomas must be excised because of the possibility of metastases.[17] It is not known if there is an increase in malignant melanomas; however, the severity may be increased.[18]

Bacterial manifestations. Bacterial infections are common in AIDS patients. Both staphylococcal and streptococcal cutaneous infections occur. *Staphylococcus* infection has manifested as cellulitis, abscesses, pyomyositis, impetigo, and itchy folliculitis, and within paronychia. Mycobacterial infections, such as with *Mycobacterium avium-intracellulare* and *M. marium,* have been reported.

Fungal manifestations. Candidiasis, most often presenting as oral thrush, has been isolated in the feet, associated with nail dystrophies and nail infections and as interdigital tinea. This opportunistic infection is often the first symptom of HIV infection. If both oral and lower-extremity infections are noted, ketoconazole is the drug of choice. If infection is found only on the feet, topical creams may help, although the fungus is often refractory to treatment. Tinea cruris, tinea pedis, and tinea versicolor have all been reported in AIDS patients. Tinea versicolor may be extensive, with thickened skin and patchy distribution. *T. rubrum* is often isolated in tinea pedis, as well as *T. mentagrophytes.*

Cryptococcus infection has been reported as a herpetiform lesion or may resemble molluscum contagiosum. Early identification may be lifesaving, facilitating the administration of the appropriate antibiotics. Histoplasmosis may appear as nonspecific lesions. One patient presented with papular lesions on the sides of the palms and feet, with central keratotic plugs. Cultures grew *Histoplasma*. Other cases have presented as folliculitis, pustules, or ulcers. Sporotrichosis has also been reported, appearing as papules, nodules, or ulcers. Amphotericin B is the treatment of choice.

Viral manifestations. Molluscum contagiosum is caused by a poxvirus and appears as shiny, pearly, white papules, usually over the facial areas in HIV patients. Herpes simplex may appear as chronic leg ulcers but more commonly as perianal ulcers. Classically, they may appear as vesicular lesions with an erythematous base. Herpes zoster may be an early manifestation; lesions are usually along dermatomes in the HIV patient.

Plantar warts have been the second most common dermatologic presentation seen in our clinic. They generally tend to be of the mosaic type and are highly resistant to all forms of treatment, such as laser hyfercation, fluorouracil (Efudex), cryotherapy, and excision (Fig. 2-16). The recurrence rate is about 35%.[19]

Papulosquamous disorders. Seborrheic dermatitis mostly involves the face, scalp, chest, groin, and genitals. It presents as scaling or hyperkeratosis. Psoriasis has often been reported as occurring with onset of AIDS or becoming much more severe at the same time. Nails and bone may also be involved (Fig. 2-17). Psoriasis may be a first diagnosis in HIV infection and generally has a poor prognosis. Methotrexate and ultraviolet light are both immunosuppressive therapies and therefore are often contraindicated in treatment.

Ichthyosis, xerosis, and erythroderma, especially of the lower extremity, have all been documented in AIDS. Pityriasis rosea has also been noted. Acute exanthemata may be associated with the acute stage of HIV infection. This condition may appear several weeks before seroconversion. The rash may present as asymptomatic, fine, symmetric, erythematous morbilliform eruptions on the trunk or arms. Duration may be from 3 days to 2 weeks. Xerosis causes papular eruptions seen on the head, neck, trunk, and extremities. They appear as plateau-like violaceous lichenoid papules on the hands. Granuloma annulare produces disseminated papular eruptions previously reported on the

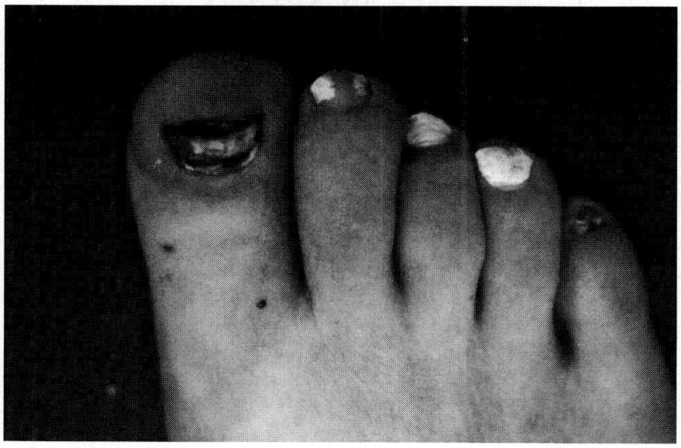

Fig. 2-15 Yellow nail syndrome in a 29-year-old AIDS patient. The patient began the yellow discoloration shortly after developing PCP.

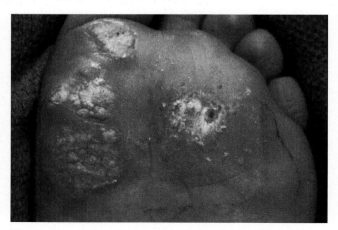

Fig. 2-16 A common presentation of mosaic-type warts in a 35-year-old HIV-positive male. Treatment was successful with laser after condition did not respond to acid treatments.

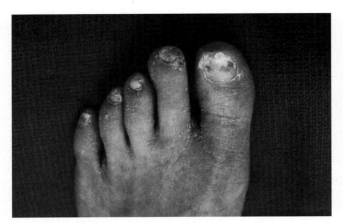

Fig. 2-17 Psoriasis in a 32-year-old AIDS patient. The skin condition covered nearly 25% of the body. The feet responded well to topical steroid therapy.

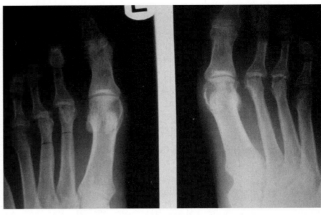

Fig. 2-18 HIV-related arthritis in a 36-year-old AIDS patient. The second and third metacarpophalangeal joints had crippling degeneration. Treatment included arthroplasties and joint-destructive procedures, with excellent results.

feet. They are composed mostly of T-suppression cytotoxic cells. Ulcers of the lower extremities have been diagnosed as resulting from pyoderma gangrenosum. Urticaria and pruritus correlate with the HIV infection.[20]

The arthritides. Rheumatic manifestations of HIV are increasing as the number of infected individuals and their survival rates increase. In one report, 71.3% of 101 patients described some type of arthritis past or present. The most commonly seen is arthralgia, especially during the acute phase. As many as one third of all HIV patients may experience this intermittent joint pain. Most arthritic conditions are oligoarticular, some are polyarticular, and a few are monoarticular. The majority of patients complain of pain in the knees, with shoulders and small joints being the next most common locations. This pain can be severe and may require intravenous narcotics.

Another common articular syndrome is arthritis caused by HIV infection directly (Fig. 2-18). The average length is approximately 31 days. Symptoms normally occur in stages III or IV. HLA-B27 antigen is not found, and the etiology is unclear. Reiter's syndrome, although often incomplete, was the first rheumatic syndrome associated with HIV. The symptoms may precede, occur with, or, most commonly, follow the HIV infection. The majority of patients, 60% to 90%, will test positive for the HLA-B27 antigen. The patients present with severe, persistent oligoarticular arthritis primarily affecting the ankles and knees.

A similar manifestation is a painful articular syndrome characterized by sharp articular pain of short duration (2 to 24 hours). The pain is severe and may require the use of intravenous narcotics in a majority of cases. Psoriatic arthritis is another inflammatory disease, which may present as polyarticular and asymmetric. Nail involvement is common, with a high correlation with skin and joint involvement. Treatment is difficult, as most antipsoriatic drugs are immunosuppressants.

Myalgias are frequent and may appear anywhere along the course of the HIV infection. Muscle enzymes are generally elevated. The etiology is unclear. The incidence of septic arthritis is surprisingly low. Some organisms found in HIV patients with septic arthritis include *Cryptococcus neoformans, Sporothrix schenckii,* and pyogenic organisms.

There are other connective tissue disorders, such as Sjögren's syndrome, necrotizing vasculitis, and possibly other arthritides, involved with the HIV infection. Treatment ranges from NSAIDs to low-dose steroids. Keep in mind that some treatments may cause further immunodepression. Bone tumors may also be present and must be ruled out from other musculoskeletal diseases[21] (Fig. 2-19).

Bone infections. Osteomyelitis secondary to Kaposi's sarcoma is not uncommon (Figs. 2-20 and 2-21). KS may directly infiltrate the bone, carrying along *Staphylococcus* or other pathogens, or osteomyelitis may develop secondary to the treatment of the KS. The standard of treatment is much like that in any other osteomyelitis infection. In three cases recently seen, one patient had osteomyelitis secondary to radiation therapy for KS. The infection began at the second metatarsal area and rapidly spread proximally, leading to a final below-knee amputation. Two other cases were from direct infiltration from the KS with a *Staphylococcus* infection, one leading to a hallux amputation and the other treated with IV antibiotics. All three patients died of other complications within 6 months.[22]

Bacillary angiomatosis is a newly recognized systemic bacterial disease seen in HIV patients. The disease begins with cutaneous vascular lesions containing the bacteria, with about one third leading to symptomatic osteolytic lesions. The bone lesions show increased uptake using both technetium-99m methylene diphosphonate and gallium scans. Diagnosis is well correlated with a positive skin biopsy from a specimen overlying a bone lesion. A bone biopsy is definitive. The bacteria that cause bacillary angiomatosis cannot be cultured, but can be identified using a polymerase chain reaction or visualized using Warthin-Starry staining.[23] The prognosis is excellent with antibiotic treatment alone, erythromycin being the drug of choice.[24]

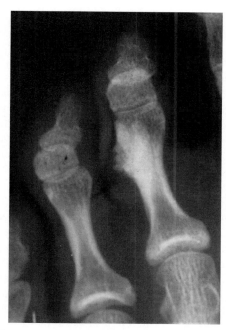

Fig. 2-19 An unusual bone tumor of the proximal phalanx with acute onset and mild pain. Pathology was inconsistent with any known tumor. Treatment was successful with a resection arthroplasty, and there had been no recurrence after 2 years.

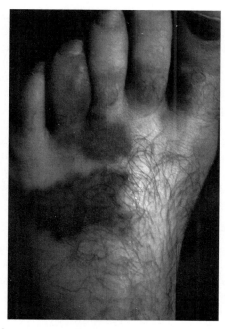

Fig. 2-20 Chronic KS in a 39-year-old male with full-blown AIDS. The patient was treated with chemotherapy over a 2-month period and later developed osteomyelitis.

Surgery and the HIV-infected patient

Knowledge of universal precautions is imperative for the patient and the physician. The use of goggles, the use of a mask with the highest protection against viruses in fumes, and not recapping needles are all common knowledge to the physician in this era. With the HIV patient, certain aspects

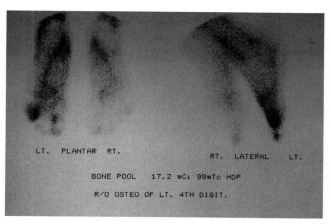

Fig. 2-21 Bone scan of the same patient with osteomyelitis secondary to KS. Treated successfully with intravenous antibiotics for 6 weeks. The patient died 3 months after the bone scan.

must be considered. For example, patients receiving chemotherapy may have severely decreased white blood cell counts. Patients with active PCP may require greater quantities of oxygen. Many patients may be using systemic steroids.[25] Patients using AZT may show bone marrow suppression (megaloblastic anemia), and those taking ddI may have severe pancreatitis.

Postexposure prophylaxis

Although the risk of exposure to HIV through occupational accidents is low, (0.3% from a percutaneous injury), there are variables as to the exact risks. These include the patient's viral load, amount of fluid transmitted, gauge of the needle, and site of exposure.

Although there are only limited data on its effectiveness, postexposure prophylaxis should be considered if the risks appear to be high for transmission. One should consider combination therapy using medications not used by the source of exposure. This could help reduce a virus that has already built a resistance.[26] More studies are needed in this area.

Recent trends

Recently new medications have become available to decrease the activity of HIV. These include the class of protease inhibitors and the nonnucleoside reverse transcriptase inhibitors. It is of great importance to the physician to understand the new medications and their interactions with other medications.[27,28]

Protease inhibitors. The protease inhibitors attempt to stop HIV-infected cells from making new copies of the virus. The three presently on the market are saquinavir (Invirase), ritonavir (Norvir), and indinavir (Crixivan). Nelfinavir (Viramune) and vertex (141W94) should be available soon. Protease inhibitors are usually utilized in combination therapies with the other classes of medications.[29]

When taking saquinavir, one must not take the antibiotics rifampin and rifabutin. Both drugs reduce the amount of saquinavir in the body.[27]

Patients taking Norvir should eliminate the following: Demerol, Darvon, Enkaid, Rythmol, Mycobutin, Vascor, Seldane, Wellbutrin, Xanax, Tranxene, Valium, ProSom, Dalmane, Versed, Halcion, Ambien, Feldene, Cordarone, Tambocor, quinidine, Hismanal, Propulsid, and Clozaril.[27]

Patients who are taking Crixivan should avoid: Seldane, Hismanal, cisapride, triazolam, midazolam, and Rifadin.[27]

Another possibility in trial includes targeting the retroviral-type zinc ring structures found in the HIV-1 nucleocapsid protein.

Viral load testing. Viral load tests measure HIV RNA. One test presently used is the polymerase chain reaction Amplicor HIV-1 Monitor test (PCR test). This test has enabled health care professionals to monitor the health of the patient and the effects of the antiviral medications. The test is able to detect copies of HIV RNA per milliliter of plasma. It can detect 200 RNA copies at the low end and 1,000,000 at the upper. Another viral load test available is the branched DNA (bDNA) test. This test produces a chemical reaction with the HIV RNA to give off measurable light. The results of this test can be reported as HIV RNA equivalents per milliliter of plasma. The range of this test is 10,000 to 1,600,000 eq/ml. The bDNA test is not as sensitive as the PCR, but is more precise over time. It is important to understand which test is being used and to remain with that same test.[29]

Conclusion

The practitioner rendering foot care may see the first and often subtle signs of HIV infection. As the number of AIDS patients increases and the patients live longer, we will see more severe manifestations and more chronic opportunistic diseases. We may even see new and undocumented medical presentations of the virus or associated secondary diseases. Knowledge of these pathologies alone is not enough to provide the patient with the best professional care. The entire disease process and the multiple, changing treatments must be understood and correlated to the examination and treatment by the foot specialist.

TUBERCULOSIS

The worldwide epidemic of HIV infection has resulted in a major secondary epidemic of tuberculosis (TB). As the case rates of AIDS increased, the 20-year-old decline in tuberculosis was reversed by 1986. Over the last 5 years, we have seen an average annual increase of 6% in tuberculosis cases, concentrated mostly in the HIV population. The areas of high HIV infection have shown the greatest increases in tuberculosis. Tuberculosis was the leading cause of death in the early 1900s. Over 80% of the U.S. population was infected with TB before the age of 20. In 1906, TB was the cause of death in 200 per 100,000 people, dropping to 1.5 per 100,000 in 1980. Today, there are an estimated 10 million people with the latent stage of tuberculosis infection.

Etiology

Tuberculosis is a necrotizing bacterial infection normally affecting the lungs, although the kidneys, bones, lymph nodes, or meninges may be vulnerable. The disease may cause symptoms shortly after infection or may remain dormant for months or decades. The tubercle bacilli are aerobes and prefer the lungs for the oxygen content. The species that most commonly affect humans are *Mycobacterium tuberculosis* and *M. bovis*. *M. avium-intracellulare* and *M. kansasii* can also affect the lungs. Transmission is by inhalation of airborne bacilli droplets.

Clinical features

Early symptoms include fever, malaise, night sweats, headache, cough, and abdominal pain. Complications may include cavitation of the lungs, hemoptysis, pleurisy, pneumonia, and gastrointestinal symptoms. Hematogenous spread of TB to the ends of long bones is most common in children because of the high oxygen content of the epiphyseal plates. TB spondylitis (Pott's disease) can be seen in childhood or delayed with spread from lymph nodes to the vertebrae.

Tuberculosis can affect the bone as tubercular osteomyelitis, which is always hematogenous in origin. It is most common in children, in whom the metaphysis is most commonly involved. In young adults, the epiphyseal area is most commonly involved. Osteolytic activity is involved without proliferation of new bone. The calcaneus and phalanges are common areas affected. The digits will present with fusiform swelling, a condition that has been named "tubercular dactylitis." The bone will appear as if there is diffuse osteoporosis secondary to intense hyperemia.

About 84% of the people who suffer from tuberculosis osteomyelitis show severe joint involvement, while 16% show a true osseous involvement. Cartilage is resistant to tuberculosis destruction, and therefore the epiphyseal plate is not destroyed. In general, tuberculosis osteitis is characterized by pronounced demineralization of the involved bone and adjacent structures, bone destruction, mineral-reactive sclerosis, and lack of sequestra.

Diagnosis

Diagnosis is through the tuberculin sensitivity test. Tuberculin is a protein derivative of the broth in which tubercle bacilli are grown. 0.1 ml of the tuberculin solution is injected below the skin in the forearm, and the site is read 48 to 72 hours later. If the diameter of a resulting area of erythema and induration is 10 mm or greater, the test is positive, doubtful at 5 to 10 mm, and negative if less than 5 mm. Hypersensitivity has a strong correlation with living tubercle bacilli. The larger the skin reaction, the greater the chance of an active infection. An absolute identification is from a culture of tissue or body fluids, especially sputum.

Treatment

The initial treatment for tuberculosis includes isoniazid (300 mg/day), rifampin (600 mg/day), and pyrazinamide (20 to

30 mg/kg/day). There are increasing cases of multiple drug–resistant tuberculosis. Ethambutol (15 to 25 mg/kg/day) is added to the above combination in these cases. The four-drug regimen is continued for 2 months. If the tuberculosis is isoniazid sensitive, isoniazid and rifampin are continued for an additional 6 to 12 months.

HEPATITIS

Types of hepatitis

Hepatitis A (HAV) may also be known as infectious, short-incubation, or MS-1 hepatitis. The RNA-type virus is spread by feces, saliva, and contaminated food or water. HAV does not progress to chronic hepatitis, a carrier state, or cirrhosis, decreasing the danger to the practitioner. Detection is by blood screening for the anti-HAV antibody. There are no vaccines available. Treatment is generally supportive, with recovery within 6 to 10 weeks.

Hepatitis B (HBV) may be referred to as serum, long-incubation, or MS-2 hepatitis. The incidence is approximately 300,000 new cases each year. Five to eight percent of cases progress to chronic hepatitis, which is responsible for around 6500 deaths per year. Transmission of this DNA virus is from exposure to infected blood or body fluids and by maternal-fetal transmission.

Hepatitis B (HBV) virus has antigen markers that help identify the status of the disease. The surface antigen (HBsAg) (Australia antigen) is found in serum and helps identify an acute infection. The antigen is not found in the recovery stage, and antibodies to HBsAg are rarely found in chronic carriers. The hepatitis B core antigen (HBcAg) is located in the core of the virus and normally not found in serum. However, anti-HBcAg may be present in the serum during and after acute infection. The hepatitis B envelope antigen (HBeAg) is found in the serum and usually is an indicator of chronic disease. Antibodies to HBeAg appear after the disappearance of HBeAg. Their appearance in HBsAg-positive serum indicates low infectivity. Treatment for chronic hepatitis includes interferon alfa-2b.

One type of arthritis not often mentioned is associated with HBV. Characteristics of hepatitis-associated musculoskeletal diseases are similar to those of HIV infection. Arthralgias have occurred in approximately 50% of hepatitis B–infected persons. The manifestations tend to be acute, monoarticular or oligoarticular, and self-limited.

Hepatitis C (formerly non-A, non-B hepatitis) accounts for more than 90% of the cases of hepatitis that develop after transfusion. One estimate is that 5% to 10% of transfusion patients may develop HCV. As many as 50% will develop chronic hepatitis. An apparent RNA virus, serologic testing may show a moderate amount of false positives. Acute and chronic stages can be separated by the levels of alanine aminotransferase (ALT). Acute stages are characterized by high levels of serum ALT, and patients may experience nausea, vomiting, or low-grade fever. High levels of ALT lasting longer than 6 months indicate chronic HCV. Transmission is through blood products and community acquisition.

Hepatitis D (delta virus) requires a co-infection with hepatitis B virus. It occurs mostly in Italy, the Middle East, and parts of Africa and South America. It is the most severe form of viral hepatitis and frequently progresses to chronic active hepatitis or death. Transmission is through sexual contact and contaminated blood. Mortality is 2% to 20%. Blood tests are available to serum antigens and antibody, although no treatment or vaccine has been found.

Hepatitis E (HEV) is a waterborne virus found mostly in developing countries. The disease is acute and self-limiting, and does not progress to chronic hepatitis. Mortality is high in pregnant women, with a 10% death rate. No treatment or vaccine is available.

Exposure to HBV and HCV

The risks associated with percutaneous exposure to HBV range from 5% to 43%. All health care workers should be immunized with the hepatitis B vaccine. The risk of exposure to HCV from a needle-stick injury has not been determined, although estimates are at 2.7%. A vaccine for hepatitis A should be approved in the near future. Recombovax-HV and Heptavax-B are available for health care workers with risks of exposure and those who have been recently exposed. Any exposure should be addressed within 7 days after injury. Hepatitis B immunoglobulin (HBIG) is injected intramuscularly twice, at 1-month intervals.

GONOCOCCAL INFECTIONS

Gonorrhea is the most common reported communicable disease in the United States. The infection is of columnar and transitional epithelium, caused by *Neisseria gonorrhoeae*. Local complications include endometriosis, salpingitis, peritonitis, bartholinitis, periurethral abscess, and epididymitis. Systemic manifestations include arthritis, dermatitis, endocarditis, meningitis, myopericarditis, and hepatitis.

Etiology and epidemiology

Humans are the only natural hosts for *N. gonorrhoeae*. The disease has been on the rise, with approximately 3 to 4 million cases each year. Eighty-five percent of all cases have been in patients under age 30. As in AIDS, the single most important factor in the spreading of *N. gonorrhoeae* is that the carriers are normally asymptomatic or ignore early signs. In 1976, a beta-lactamase–producing strain of *N. gonorrhoeae* emerged that was completely resistant to penicillin and ampicillin. As the numbers of this strain increase, the specific diagnosis is increasingly important.

Clinical manifestations

Gonococcal infections must be identified as to the site of inoculation, duration of infection, and the presence or absence of local or systemic spread of the organism. In the male, the incubation period is normally 2 to 17 days, and

90% of those who develop urethral gonococcal infection develop urethral discharge. Other areas infected in the male include anorectal and phalangeal. In the female, acute uncomplicated gonorrhea causes dysuria, frequent urination, increased vaginal discharge, abnormal menstrual bleeding, or anorectal pain. The areas most involved in the female include endocervix, urethra, anal canal, and pharynx, in decreasing order.

Most important to the foot and ankle specialist is disseminated gonococcal infection. The majority of men and women with gonococcemia have no symptoms of urogenital, anorectal, or pharyngeal infection. Gonococcemia is characterized by fever, polyarthralgias, and papular, petechial, pustular, hemorrhagic, or necrotic skin lesions. These lesions may appear in numbers and usually on the lower extremities. The initial joint involvement is usually limited to tenosynovitis involving several joints asymmetrically. The wrists, fingers, knees, and ankles are the most commonly involved.

Septic arthritis may cause pain and swelling in one or more joints, with accumulation of purulent synovial fluid. This may lead to progressive joint destruction if treatment is delayed. Septic arthritis may begin without any other signs or symptoms of gonococcemia. Joint aspiration is imperative. Repeated joint aspiration or closed irrigation of the joint with sterile saline may reduce inflammation of the joint and decrease the amount of active infection, thus decreasing the chance of joint erosion. Rarely do incision and drainage need to be performed. Immobilization of the joint may decrease pain and decrease effusions.

Laboratory diagnosis

The Gram stain of urethral or endocervical exudate is considered diagnostic for gonorrhea when typical gram-negative diplococci are seen within leukocytes. It is equivocal if only extracellular or atypical gram-negative diplococci are seen and negative if no gram-negative diplococci are seen. Standard blood culture broth medium containing 3% to 10% carbon dioxide should be used in culturing synovial fluid. For pus from skin lesions, Gram stain or immunofluorescent staining should be ordered.

Treatment

The drugs most commonly used for treatment of gonorrhea include penicillin G, ampicillin, amoxicillin, tetracycline hydrochloride, spectinomycin, and flouroquinolones. Oral penicillin is not recommended. For uncomplicated gonococcal infection in heterosexual adults, the treatment of choice is 3.0 g amoxicillin in a single oral dose with 1.0 g probenecid by mouth, followed by 0.5 g tetracycline given orally four times a day for 7 days (or a single dose may be used).

SYPHILIS (LUES)

In 1905, Schaudinn and Hoffman discovered the cause of syphilis, *Treponema pallidum*. However, syphilis was first described as early as the fifteenth century in Europe and Asia. Syphilis is a chronic and systemic infection that is usually sexually transmitted. It can be divided into four stages: primary, secondary, latent, and late.

Etiology and epidemiology

Treponema pallidum is a spiral hyphen-shaped microorganism that propels itself by spinning around on its longitudinal axis. Humans are the only known natural hosts. Nearly all cases of known syphilis are acquired through sexual contract, although it is possible to contract the disease by contact with contaminated fomites, in utero, or by blood transfusion. Infant deaths and cases of syphilitic psychosis have fallen by 99% since 1940. The peak age group for infection is 20 to 24, and the male/female ratio 3.2 to 1. Homosexual and bisexual males make up approximately 50% of all cases.

Stages of syphilis

Primary syphilis begins with a single painless papule, which rapidly becomes eroded and sometimes indurated. The lesion appears at the site of inoculation after an incubation period of approximately 3 weeks. This primary lesion persists for 2 to 6 weeks and spontaneously heals. Regional lymphadenopathy accompanies the lesion 1 week after onset of the chancre.

Secondary syphilis, seen 6 weeks after healing of the chancre, manifests as mucocutaneous lesions, generalized nontender lymphadenopathy, and round, discrete, pale red, bilateral, and symmetrical macules 5 to 10 cm in diameter, usually appearing on the lower extremities. These may lead to an eroded, pink, highly infectious lesion called condyloma lata. Other symptoms include fever, weight loss, malaise, anorexia, and headache. Gastrointestinal involvement, nephropathy, arthritis, and periostitis may also be seen. Secondary syphilis may last from 2 to 6 weeks.

Latent syphilis is diagnosed when there is a positive treponemal antibody test, a normal cerebrospinal fluid examination, and no clinical signs of syphilis. Early latent syphilis involves the first 2 years after infection, as relapse of mucocutaneous lesions may occur. Late latent syphilis begins 2 years after infection and has resistance to reinfection.

Late syphilis involves progressive inflammatory disease of the aorta and central nervous system. There may be asymptomatic neurosyphilis, in which there are no clinical signs of nerve damage although there is an abnormal cerebrospinal fluid study and positive Venereal Disease Research Laboratory (VDRL) test. Symptomatic neurosyphilis may present as general paresis, tabes dorsalis, and meningovascular disease. These manifestations normally appear 10 years or more after infection.

Other late syphilis symptoms include ataxia, a wide-based gait and foot slap, paresthesias, bladder disturbances, impotence, areflexia, loss of position, and loss of deep pain and temperature sensations. Charcot's joints may result, with perforating ulcers due to loss of pain sensations.

Chronic osteomyelitis can also occur with acquired syphilis, with the long bones and skull most commonly involved. Dense sclerosis is the outstanding feature. The earliest changes are periosteal reaction and later new bone formation outside the cortices. The formation of gummata in sclerotic bone is irregular on the external surface. There may be large destructive areas, but the usual foci are small and scattered.

Diagnosis

Any suspicious lesion should be evaluated using dark-field examination. Serologic tests include rapid plasma reagin (RPR), which is the most commonly used today, and the VDRL, which can give a quantitative titer of serum antibodies. The standard antitreponemal antibody test is the fluorescent treponemal antibody-absorption test (FTA-ABS). This is more specific than the above tests. An estimated 20% to 40% of reagin tests give false positives, which can be excluded with follow-up FTA-ABS or other antibody sensitive tests.

Treatment

For most stages of syphilis, the treatment of choice is benzathine penicillin, 2.4 million units divided and given intramuscularly in two separate areas. For late neurosyphilis and congenital syphilis, the drug of choice is aqueous procaine penicillin, 600,000 units daily for 10 to 15 days.

CONCLUSION

This chapter has reviewed the practical aspects of important blood-borne communicable diseases, such as AIDS, tuberculosis, hepatitis, gonorrhea, and lues. Clinicians, regardless of specialty, should not only possess a firm knowledge of these disorders but also treat all patients with respect and dignity.

REFERENCES

1. Lifson A: Progression and clinical outcome of infection due to HIV, *Clin Infect Dis* 14:966, 1992.
2. Jaffe H: AIDS: epidemiologic features, *J Am Acad Dermatol* 22:1167, 1990.
3. Rabson A: HIV virology: implications for the pathogenesis of HIV infection, *J Am Acad Dermatol* 22:1196, 1990.
4. Abrams D: Clinical manifestations of HIV infection, *J Am Acad Dermatol* 22:1217, 1990.
5. Friedman-Kien A: What we now know—and must do—about HIV disease and AIDS, *J Am Acad Dermatol* 22:1163, 1990.
6. Mitsuya H: Antiviral therapy against HIV infection, *J Am Acad Dermatol* 22:1282, 1990.
7. Maxey L: *AIDS medical guide,* ed 2, San Francisco, 1988, AIDS Foundation.
8. Haverkos H: The changing incidence of KS among patients with AIDS, *J Am Acad Dermatol* 22:1250, 1990.
9. Myskowski P: Lymphoma and other HIV associated positive patients, *J Am Acad Dermatol* 22:1253, 1990.
10. Gordon S: Seroconversion, staging and survival: natural history of HIV infection, *J Am Podiatr Med Assoc* 80:9, 1990.
11. Gabuzada D: Neurologic disorders associated with HIV infections, *J Am Acad Dermatol* 22:1232, 1990.
12. Abramson C: Podiatric implications of acquired immunodeficiency syndrome, *J Am Podiatr Med Assoc* 76:124, 1986.
13. Levy R: Neurologic complications of HIV infection, *Am Fam Physician* 41:517, 1991.
14. Burns S: Podiatric manifestations of AIDS, *J Am Podiatr Med Assoc* 80:15, 1990.
15. Daniel C: The spectrum of nail disease in patients with human immunodeficiency syndrome, *J Am Acad Dermatol* 27:93, 1992.
16. Dompmartin D: Onychomycosis and AIDS, *Int J Dermatol* 29:337, 1990.
17. Fisher B: Cutaneous manifestations of the acquired immunodeficiency syndrome, *Int J Dermatol* 26:615, 1987.
18. Davis G: Treatment of chronic hepatitis C with recombinant interferon alfa, *N Engl J Med* 321:1501, 1989.
19. Bolognesi D: Vaccine development for HIV infection, *J Am Acad Dermatol* 22:1295, 1990.
20. Sadick N: Papulosquamous dermatoses of AIDS, *J Am Acad Dermatol* 22:1270, 1990.
21. Kaye B: Rheumatologic manifestations of infection with HIV, *Ann Intern Med* 111:158, 1989.
22. Steinbach L: Human immunodeficiency virus infection: musculoskeletal manifestations, *Radiology* 186:833, 1993.
23. Baron A: Osteolytic lesions and bacillary angiomatosis in HIV infection: radiographic differentiation from AIDS related KS, *Radiology* 177:77, 1990.
24. Pedowitz W: Foot and ankle signs and symptoms in HIV positive patients, *J Musculoskeletal Med* 22:1196, 1990.
25. Reveille J: Human immunodeficiency virus associated psoriasis, psoriatic arthritis and Reiter's syndrome: a disease continuum, *Arthritis Rheum* 33:1574, 1990.
26. Carpenter CCJ, Fischal MA, Hammer S, Hirsch MS, Jacobsen DM, Katzenstein DA, Montaner JSG, Richman D, Saag M, Achooley R, Thompson M, Vella S, Yeni P, Volberding P: Antiretroviral therapy for HIV infection in 1996, *JAMA* 276:146-154, 1996.
27. Gallant J: Protease inhibitors: a practical guide, *Hopkins HIV Report* 8(2):1-3, July 1996.
28. Deeks S, Smith M, Holodniy M, Kahn J: HIV-1 protease inhibitors: a review for clinicians, *JAMA* 277:145-153, 1997.
29. Paxton WB: Understanding HIV-1 viral load, *Positively Aware,* Sept-Oct 1995, pp. 10-11.

ADDITIONAL READINGS

Goldrick BA: Tuberculosis: old nemesis, new problems, *Am J Infect Control* 24:223, 1996.

Ramphal-Naley L, Kirkhorn S, Zelterman D: Tuberculosis in physicians, *Am J Infect Control* 24:243, 1996.

Sinkowitz RL, Fridkin SK, Manangan L: Status of tuberculosis infection control programs at United States Hospitals (1989-1992), *Am J Infect Control* 24:226, 1996.

3

The OSHA Standard and Requirements for the Physician

Charles F. Fenton III

*I also maintain that clear knowledge of natural science must be acquired,
in the first instance, through mastery of medicine alone.* Hippocrates

In 1992, the Occupational Safety and Health Administration (OSHA) Bloodborne Pathogen Standard became the law of the land. All employers must follow the Standard if their employees are at risk of occupational exposure to body fluids, including blood. The primary purpose of the Standard is to limit the risk that an employee, as well as a practitioner, will contract the AIDS virus, hepatitis B, or other communicable diseases in the work place. The Standard has the secondary effect of protecting the public, both from primary inoculation while at the employer's premises and from secondary exposure by contact with an employee outside the premises (by prevention of infection of the employee in the first place).

The Standard provides for stiff fines, which can reach $70,000 and provide an incentive to rigidly comply with the Standard. Remember, an OSHA inspector's job is easier if he or she inspects several physicians' offices within a large medical complex, than if he has to inspect less pleasing surroundings, such as a chicken processing plant, for other OSHA violations. Physicians in large complexes in metropolitan areas may be most at risk for inspection. The threat of inspection and the size of potential fines may be incentives for unincorporated solo practitioners or partnerships to consider incorporation, in order to benefit from the so-called "corporate veil." Remember, as a solo practitioner, you (and all of your assets) are the employer. However, when you are incorporated, the corporation is the employer, and you may be able to shield personal assets. Prudence dictates a legal evaluation of each specific circumstance.

RATIONALE FOR THE STANDARD

The purpose of the Standard is to protect people in the United States who have exposure to infections that can be transmitted by blood or body fluids. The Standard is intended to reduce the national morbidity and mortality associated with such diseases. A secondary effect will reduce the health care costs of the nation. By implementation of the standards, not only will employees be afforded a greater measure of protection, but patients will also benefit. Finally, by preventing the transmission to physicians, patients, and employees, the Standard will prevent the domino effect of their transmitting the disease to others, both at and away from the work place.

For example, it is estimated that 30% of spouses or sexual partners of patients with acute hepatitis will acquire the disease. Not only is the spouse at risk, but studies have also shown that 40% to 60% of household contacts of chronic carriers acquire the disease.

Although AIDS is the most feared of these blood-borne diseases, it is not the one that causes the greatest morbidity. Hepatitis B is spread to more health care workers each year than is the human immunodeficiency virus (HIV). In addition to AIDS and hepatitis B, numerous other, more remote illnesses can be transmitted by body fluids.

These include non-A, non-B hepatitis, syphilis, malaria, babesiosis, brucellosis, leptospirosis, arboviral infections (including Colorado tick fever), *Borrelia* (relapsing fever agent), the virus causing Creutzfeldt-Jakob disease, human T-lymphotrophic virus type I, and the viral hemorrhagic fever agent. In support of this, OSHA cites one incident in which a health care worker developed a syphilitic chancre following a needle-stick accident. There are also reported cases of syphilis transmission by transfusion and by needle stick with tattooing instruments. OSHA also cites two cases in which malaria was transmitted by transfusion and needle stick. Although transmission of these infectious agents is rare, it does occur, and the Standard will provide additional precautions against it. Finally, 2% (3400 cases out of 170,000 cases) of non-A, non-B hepatitis have occurred in health care workers.

By far, however, the Standard is meant to reduce the transmission to health care workers of the hepatitis B virus (HBV). OSHA describes HBV as the major infectious blood-borne occupational hazard to health care workers. The Centers for Disease Control and Prevention (CDC) estimates that there are approximately 8700 infections of HBV in health care workers each year. Of these, 8700 infections, 2100 cases become clinically apparent, 440 cases require hospitalization, and 200 people die. Those are 200 deaths that OSHA hopes to prevent each year. In about 33% of HBV infections, the individual is asymptomatic. Consequently, the infected individual can spread the disease to others without even being aware that he or she is a carrier. Most cases of HBV are acute and self-limiting. However, about 1% to 2% of the cases of HBV develop into fulminant hepatitis, which is 85% fatal. Approximately 6% to 10% of patients infected with HBV develop chronic hepatitis and become carriers for life. Chronic carriers may be asymptomatic and may not be aware of their status. In chronic carriers, the HBV DNA can become incorporated into the liver cells, which can lead to the development of primary hepatocellular carcinoma.

The percentages of people in the general population (patient pool) with antibodies indicative of past or present HBV infection are as follows: 3% to 4% for whites, 13% to 14% for blacks, and 50% for foreign-born Asians. Among these, 0.2% of whites, 0.7% of blacks and 13% of foreign-born Asians are chronic carriers. Health care workers are more likely to be infected than the above statistics indicate. For example, testing conducted in relation to blood donations reveals that physicians and dentists are 4 to 10 times more likely to have HBV antibodies than the general population.

The risk of contracting HBV infection from a single needle-stick accident, when the needle had been used on a patient who has positive HBV antigens, is great. One milliliter of blood from a patient who has positive HBV antigens contains 100 million infectious virus particles. Studies have shown that 7% to 30% of health care workers who had a needle-stick injury from such patients became infected, if they did not receive postexposure prophylaxis. In 1988, the CDC reported that there were 280,000 HBV infections in the United States. Of these, 8700 (3%) were in health care workers.

The HBV virus can be transmitted in many ways. Open lesions on the hand or elsewhere, or even dermatitis, may provide a portal of entry for the virus. The virus can be spread from inanimate objects or environmental surfaces that have been contaminated with blood containing the virus. Studies have shown that the HBV virus can survive up to 1 week dried at room temperature on environmental surfaces. Fewer than 20% of health care workers developing on-the-job infections report a discrete needle-stick incident.

Although the hepatitis B virus is more contagious, the HIV is 100% lethal. The CDC estimates that between 1 million and 1.5 million people in the United States are infected with the HIV. As of July 1991, 186,895 cases of AIDS had been reported. Of those, 63.5% of the adult patients and 52.4% of the pediatric patients had already died.

More than 100,000 new cases were reported in 1993, with an equal number projected for 1994. As of September 1996, there were 650 confirmed cases of health care workers being infected with HIV secondary to occupational exposure. These were cases of occupational exposure in patients with no other risk factors. The studies also show that 4.8% of the reported cases of AIDS were among health care workers. This 4.8% is proportionate to the percentage of the labor force engaged in health care.

The HIV is spread via body fluids. Infection often occurs by sexual transmission or by the use of contaminated needles by IV drug users. The virus can also be spread through open lesions in the skin or through the mucosa when exposed to infected body fluids. Studies show that AIDS is not spread by casual contact. To date, there have been no reported cases of infection of household members of AIDS patients who had no risk factors. In addition, other studies show that HIV is not spread by mosquitos or other animals.

Different studies show an average seroconversion rate of 4.8 per 1000 (0.48%) following a needle-stick injury with a known HIV-contaminated needle. As can be seen, the overall seroconversion rate is very low. However, it still takes only one needle-stick injury to spread the virus in that small percentage of cases, with devastating consequences. The single largest cause of needle-stick injuries has been shown to be recapping of the needle, when workers missed the cover and stabbed themselves. The rate of needle-stick accidents for disposable syringes is 6.9 needle sticks per 100,000 needles.

It takes approximately 6 months for most infected people to have antibody levels against HIV rise to a level where they are detectable through serologic testing. Therefore, even routine preoperative testing will not inform surgeons of a risk, nor will it eliminate the risk of exposure. OSHA admits that it is unable to calculate the risk that health care workers exposed to blood will acquire HIV solely as a result of occupational exposure.

OSHA estimates that over 500,000 establishments and 5.6 million employees will be affected by the Standard. Of these establishments, 122,104 are physicians' offices. Also affected are dental and podiatry offices, nursing homes, hospitals, medical and dental laboratories, hospices, hemodialysis units, drug rehabilitation units, governmental clinics, blood, tissue, and plasma centers, residential care centers, mortuaries, research laboratories, linen services, medical equipment centers, law enforcement agencies, fire and rescue agencies, correctional facilities, schools, and waste removal services. As can be seen, a wide range of facilities is affected by the Standard.

OSHA believes that the total cost of compliance will be approximately $327,000,000 per year. Of this amount, the vaccine for hepatitis B alone will account for $107 million. The burden on physicians' offices is estimated to be $143,990,528.00. OSHA feels that "a large part of the compliance costs will be passed to consumers and third party payers" (56 *Fed. Reg.* 64004,64041, 1991). It is obvious that OSHA has not heard of physician payment reform, limiting charges, capitation, cost containment, or cries for national health insurance. The calculations denote that compliance costs were to be 0.16% of revenues and 2.6% of profits (i.e., the doctor's salary). Although this may appear to be a hefty cost to bear, like all of the other recent and near-future changes in health care, it is but one of the costs of being in the health care business.

DEFINITIONS

Certain words and phrases are specifically defined by the Standard. Being familiar with these definitions may mean the difference between compliance and noncompliance, and hence a fine, in the case of an OSHA inspection. Some of these definitions are included here:

1. "Blood" means human blood, human blood components, and products made from human blood.
2. "Bloodborne pathogens" means pathogenic microorganisms that are present in human blood and cause disease in humans. These pathogens include, but are not limited to, hepatitis B virus (HBV) and human immunodeficiency virus (HIV).
3. "Contaminated" means the presence, or the reasonably anticipated presence, of blood or other potentially infectious materials on an item or surface.
4. "Decontamination" means the use of physical or chemical means to remove inactive, or destroy blood-borne pathogens on a surface or item to the point that they are no longer capable of transmitting infectious particles. The surface or item is rendered safe for handling, use, or disposal.
5. "Other potentially infectious materials" include the following human body fluids: semen, vaginal secretions, cerebrospinal fluid, synovial fluid, pleural fluid, amniotic fluid, saliva in dental procedures, any body fluid that is visibly contaminated with blood, and all body fluids in situations where it is difficult or impossible to differentiate between body fluids. Any unfixed tissue or organ (other than intact skin) from a human (living or dead) is also included.
6. "Parenteral" means piercing the mucous membranes or skin barrier through such events as needle sticks, human bites, cuts, and abrasions.
7. "Sterilize" means the use of a physical or chemical procedure to destroy all microbial life, including highly resistant bacterial endospores.

Other words and phrases are identified below, and it is important to be familiar with them. If OSHA conducts an inspection, the meanings of these words and phrases, and not their usual connotations, will determine whether the office is in compliance.

EXPOSURE CONTROL PLAN

One of the main requirements of the Standard is that each office must have a written Exposure Control Plan (ECP). If a practice has multiple locations, then each location must have its own plan and it must be on location. This may pose a problem for the physician who makes house calls, has many satellite clinics, or practices in the office of another practitioner. But each employer must have a plan at each location.

A practitioner who practices at nursing homes should ensure that each nursing home has a written plan. It would even be a good idea to request that a nursing home provide a letter stating that there is a valid Exposure Control Plan in place.

The purpose of the plan is to eliminate or minimize employee exposure. Specific items in the ECP must include engineering controls, housekeeping requirements, personal protective equipment, vaccination, record keeping, and training. The plan must be available to employees and OSHA inspectors. It should be available to the employees to ensure that the plan is followed by everyone and to ensure consistency. Also, the OSHA compliance officers will be able to familiarize themselves with the employer's identification of those tasks, procedures, and job classifications with occupational exposure. The plan must also be updated annually or whenever new procedures that affect occupational exposure, are implemented.

The Standard requires that the plan determine "occupational exposure" potential for each and every employee. Occupational exposure is defined as reasonably anticipated skin, eye, mucous membrane, or parenteral contact with blood or other potentially infectious materials that may result from the performance of an employee's duties. To satisfy exposure determination requirements, the employer should make a list of (1) all job classifications in which all employees in those jobs have occupational exposure, (2) all job classifications in which some employees have occupational exposure, and (3) all tasks and procedures or groups of closely related tasks and procedures in which occupational exposure occurs and that are performed by employees subject to "occupational exposure." The list should consider exposure determination without regard to the use of personal protective equipment.

OSHA has chosen to make the Standard as general as possible because of the wide array of scenarios that can be encountered in the various establishments covered by the Standard. Therefore, it is very important that your plan be specifically tailored to your office or clinic.

There are many commercially available plans on the market. However, if you purchase one, be sure to take the time to individualize the program to your office.

METHODS OF COMPLIANCE

The employer may comply with the plan by adopting the following procedures:

1. Observing universal precautions
2. Implementing engineering and work practice controls
3. Using personal protective equipment
4. Implementing proper housekeeping measures
5. Providing hepatitis vaccination

6. Communication of hazards to employees
7. Keeping proper records

Each of these areas will be discussed in more detail below.

Universal precautions

"Universal precautions" is an approach to infection control whereby all human blood and certain human body fluids are treated as if known to be infected by HIV, HBV, or other blood-borne pathogens. Universal precautions should be observed to prevent contact with blood or other potentially infectious materials. Under circumstances in which differentiation between body fluid types is difficult or impossible, all body fluids should be considered potentially infectious.

Engineering and work practice controls

Engineering and work practice controls consist of methods, such as shields and sharps disposal containers, to isolate or remove blood-borne pathogen hazards from the work place. These practices should be used to eliminate or minimize employee exposure. However, when occupational exposure remains after institution of these controls, personal protective equipment should be employed, as described below.

Engineering controls serve to reduce employee exposure by removing the hazard or isolating the employee from the hazard. Once implemented, engineering controls permanently protect the employee. It is the employer's responsibility to implement and maintain engineering controls. Engineering controls should be examined and maintained or replaced on a regular schedule to ensure their effectiveness; conducting only an annual review of them is inappropriate under the Standard.

Unlike engineering controls, which permanently protect the employee, work practice controls depend upon the behavior of the employee to reduce exposure. Even with properly implemented work practice controls, exposure can still occur. For example, OSHA admits that 60% of needle-stick injuries will be unaffected by these controls.

Engineering and work practice controls consist of (1) proper hand washing facilities and practices, (2) proper treatment of sharp instruments, (3) proper separation of food from contamination, (4) certain procedures in the treatment of contamination, (5) sterilization, and (6) care of equipment.

Proper hand washing facilities. The Standard requires that hand washing facilities be readily available to employees. "Hand washing facilities" means facilities that provide adequate supplies of running potable water, antiseptic soap, and single-use disposable towels or hot air drying machines. The facilities should be located where the employee will have easy access to them. This will ensure that the employee will be likely to use the facilities and will minimize the time that contamination remains in contact with the employee.

In those instances, such as nursing home visits, in which the provision of hand washing facilities is not feasible, an appropriate antiseptic hand cleanser (such as an alcohol-based rinse or an antiseptic foam), in conjunction with clean cloth or paper towels or antiseptic towelettes, should be provided. When antiseptic hand cleansers or towelettes are used, the hands should be washed with soap and running water as soon afterward as feasible.

Not only must the employer provide the hand washing facilities, but he must also ensure that employees in fact do wash their hands immediately or as soon as feasible following contact with blood or other potentially infectious materials. An employee should also wash his or her hands immediately after removal of gloves or other personal protective equipment. It is the employer's responsibility to ensure that hand washing occurs, and OSHA feels that hand washing should be strictly enforced by the employer.

Proper treatment of sharp instruments. The Standard requires that contaminated needles and other contaminated sharp instruments (sharps) not be bent, recapped, or removed. "Contaminated sharps" means any contaminated object that can penetrate the skin, including, but not limited to, needles, scalpels, broken glass, broken capillary tubes, and exposed ends of dental wires. Also, shearing or breaking of contaminated needles is prohibited. Contaminated needles and other contaminated sharps should not be recapped or removed from syringes unless the employer can demonstrate that no alternative is feasible or that such action is required by a specific medical procedure (e.g., those instances, such as during surgery, when recapping is necessary because of the need to give multiple injections from the same syringe). If needles are recapped, it should be done through the use of a one-handed technique. Two-handed needle recapping is strictly prohibited by the Standard.

Recapping of needles can be a very dangerous procedure, and it is during recapping that most skin punctures occur. There have been many fines levied by OSHA when it has found recapped needles in the office or within the sharps container.

Immediately, or as soon as possible after use, contaminated reusable sharps should be discarded and placed in appropriate containers until properly reprocessed. Containers should be (1) puncture resistant, (2) labeled or color coded, and (3) leakproof on the sides and bottom. Finally, the container should be at the site of the use of the sharp. This will limit the risk of injury during the time the sharp would otherwise have been transported from the site of use to the site of disposal. The sharps container should be maintained upright throughout use, not be allowed to be overfilled, and replaced routinely. When containers of contaminated sharps are moved from the area of use, the containers should be closed immediately prior to removal or replacement, to prevent spillage or protrusion of contents during handling. The container should be placed in a secondary container if leakage is possible. Reusable containers should not be opened, emptied, or cleaned manually or in any other manner that would expose employees to the risk of percutaneous injury. There are programs available, whereby for an extra cost, a physician can purchase turnkey sharps containers.

The physician purchases the container and then, when it is full, ships the container back to the distributor for proper disposal.

Proper separation from food contamination. Activities such as eating, drinking, smoking, applying cosmetics or lip balm, and handling contact lenses are prohibited in work areas where there is a reasonable likelihood of occupational exposure. However, hand cream application is allowable, provided the hands are thoroughly washed before application, because hand creams may be necessary to counter chapping or dryness caused by the powder of disposable gloves. However, the use of petroleum-based. lubricants is prohibited because such lubricants can degrade the gloves and hence render them unable to provide protection.

Furthermore, food and drink should not be kept in refrigerators, freezers, shelves, or cabinets or on counter tops or bench tops where blood or other potentially infectious materials are present. The rationale is to prevent accidental exposure from contamination of food by blood or other materials. This requirement would also dictate that food not be prepared, dishes cleaned, or cosmetics applied or used (including use of toothpaste) at a site or sink used to clean instruments and other contaminated items.

Miscellaneous procedures in treatment of contamination. All procedures involving blood or other potentially infectious materials should be performed in such a manner as to minimize splashing, spraying, spattering, and the generation of droplets of these substances. This in particular pertains to minimizing the aerosol created by the use of power surgical instrumentation, lasers, or electrocautery devices. This is important because aerosolization can create droplets that can last for a few seconds to several days. These inspirable aerosols have been shown to contain hemoglobin. Studies have shown that laser plumes during verruca surgery contain papilloma virion particles.

At this time, OSHA lacks adequate information concerning the ability to control aerosols in the ambient atmosphere. OSHA considers the worst-case scenario to be the production of a single infective virion within aerosols suspended in the office air. This would require the unacceptable requirement of respiratory protection for all personnel within the facility. Once such information becomes available and technology produces engineering controls adequate to control aerosols, OSHA is likely to promulgate additional regulations in this area.

Specimens of blood or other potentially infectious materials should be placed in a container that prevents leakage during handling. This would also apply to culture specimens and unfixed pathology specimens (e.g., verrucae). This requirement often does not apply to specimens that are fixed in formalin. The container for transport should be labeled or color-coded and closed prior to being transported. One exception is that when a facility utilizes "universal precautions" in the handling of all specimens, the labeling or color-coding of specimens is not necessary, provided that the

containers are recognizable as containing specimens. However, this exemption only applies while such specimens and containers remain within the facility. Labeling or color-coding is required when they leave the facility.

If a night pick-up box is employed by the office, it should be labeled on the outside as containing biohazardous material. This will warn the lab courier and may inhibit any curious member of the general public. If contamination of the outside of the primary container occurs, the primary container should then be placed within a second container which prevents leakage during handling. These secondary containers should be labeled or color-coded according to the requirements of this standard. If the specimen could puncture the primary container, then the primary container should be placed within a secondary container that is puncture-resistant in addition to the above characteristics.

Sterilization. All items are required to be sterilized between patient uses when they have become contaminated. Proper procedure involves cleaning the instruments with an instrument cleaner and water, followed by complete rinsing. All contaminated items should be cleaned in a separate area that is away from the treatment areas or other cleans areas. The item can then be autoclaved. Sterilization can be accomplished by several methods, such as steam autoclave, dry heat sterilizer, chemical vapor such as ethylene oxide, or cold (liquid) sterilization. Hot "bead" sterilizers are considered inadequate under the Standard.

Care of equipment. Equipment (e.g., autoclave, surgical saw) that may become contaminated with blood or other potentially infectious materials should be examined prior to servicing or shipping and should be decontaminated as necessary, unless the employer can demonstrate that decontamination of such equipment or portions of such equipment is not feasible. A readily observable label should be attached to the equipment, stating which portions remain contaminated. The employer must ensure that this information is conveyed to all affected employees, the servicing representative, and/or the manufacturer prior to handling so that appropriate precautions will be taken by them. This requirement would also apply to used blades sent for resharpening. The shipping box containing any blades sent out for sharpening should be labeled "decontaminated." Although it appears at this time that resharpening of decontaminated used blades is allowable, this may change in the future.

Personal protective equipment

The Standard provides that when the potential for occupational exposure exists, the employer should provide personal protective equipment, at no cost to the employee. Personal protective equipment should be utilized when engineering controls and work practices are insufficient to eliminate all occupational exposure. The Standard allows the employer to determine which personal protective equipment is required based upon the type of exposure and the quantity of contaminated substance that would be reasonably anticipated under the circumstances.

Personal protective equipment (PPE) is specialized clothing or equipment worn by an employee for protection against hazard. General work clothes (i.e., uniforms, pants, scrub suits, shirts, or blouses) not intended to function as protection against a hazard are not considered to be personal protective equipment. Appropriate personal protective equipment includes, but is not limited to, items such as gloves, gowns, laboratory coats, face shields or masks and eye protection, mouthpieces, resuscitation bags, pocket masks, and their ventilation devices.

Personal protective equipment will be considered appropriate only if it does not permit blood or other potentially infectious materials to pass through to or reach the employee's work clothes, street clothes, undergarments, skin, eyes, mouth, or other mucous membranes under normal conditions of use and for the duration of time that the protective equipment is being used. The employer should ensure that appropriate personal protective equipment in the appropriate sizes is readily accessible at the work site or is issued to employees. The determination of whether an item is to be considered personal protective equipment, and hence the responsibility of the employer to purchase and maintain it, depends upon the use to which the item is devoted. If the item is used as a barrier to exposure, then it is personal protective equipment. For example, if a lab coat is required solely as a uniform, then it is not personal protective equipment. However, if the same lab coat is used to prevent the employee's skin or street clothes from being soiled with blood or other contamination, then it is personal protective equipment and hence the responsibility of the employer.

Gloves must be worn when it can be reasonably anticipated that the employee may have hand contact with blood, other potentially infectious materials, mucous membranes, or nonintact skin or may handle or touch contaminated items or surfaces. Disposable examination gloves should be kept in each treatment room and at each site where contaminated instruments and equipment are kept. Disposable (single-use) gloves such as surgical or examination gloves shall be replaced as soon as practical when contaminated or as soon as feasible if torn or punctured or when their ability to function as a barrier is compromised. The gloves must be removed when contaminated to prevent spreading of contamination to fomites such as telephones and door handles. The Standard does not require that disposable gloves be changed between patients. OSHA is only concerned with patient-to-employee contamination, not patient-to-patient contamination. However, removal of gloves between patients is a sagacious practice. Finally, disposable (single-use) gloves should not be washed or decontaminated for reuse.

Hypoallergenic gloves, glove liners, powderless gloves, or other similar alternatives should be readily accessible to employees who are allergic to the gloves normally provided. Utility gloves (gloves used in cleaning, not gloves used for patient exams) may be decontaminated for reuse if the integrity of the glove is not compromised. However, they must be discarded if they are cracked, peeling, torn, or punctured, or exhibit other signs of deterioration or when their ability to function as a barrier is compromised. All gloves must be provided in appropriate sizes. Gloves must fit each and every employee; they must "fit like a glove" so that the employees will be able to conduct their work and so that they will in fact wear the gloves. The Standard allows either latex or vinyl gloves to be used. However, plastic-film food gloves (what OSHA calls "baggie gloves") are not appropriate under the Standard. These gloves do not fit properly and are not strong enough to provide adequate protection.

Masks in combination with eye protection devices, such as goggles or glasses with solid side shields, or chin-length face shields, must be worn whenever splashes, spray, spatter, or droplets of blood or other potentially infectious materials may be generated and eye, nose, or mouth contamination can be reasonably anticipated. The goggles or glasses must have side shields. However, mesh or perforated side shields are not adequate under the Standard. If such protective eye wear is used in lieu of a face shield, then a mask must be used to protect the mouth and nose. Protective eye wear need not be impact resistant unless projectiles (such as bone or toenail spicules) can be anticipated.

Appropriate protective clothing such as, but not limited to, gowns, aprons, lab coats, clinic jackets, or similar outer garments shall be worn in occupational exposure situations. The type and characteristics will depend upon the task and degree of exposure anticipated. As a general rule, any garment should be resistant to leak-through of any fluids or blood spilled onto the garment. The Standard does not distinguish between "fluid-resistant" and "fluid-proof." The requirement is only that fluid should not leak through personal protective equipment to employee clothing or skin. Finally, surgical caps or hoods and/or shoe covers or boots shall be worn in instances when gross contamination can reasonably be anticipated (e.g., autopsies, foot surgery). Head and foot protection is required because a study of 102 surgical operations revealed 16 instances of foot contamination and 14 cases of head area contamination.

If a garment is penetrated by blood or other potentially infectious materials, the garment should be removed immediately or as soon as feasible. Additionally, all personal protective equipment should be removed prior to leaving the work area. When personal protective equipment is removed, it shall be placed in an appropriately designated area or container for storage, washing, decontamination, or disposal. The employer must provide the personal protective equipment to the employee at no charge. The employer must also clean, launder, and dispose of personal protective equipment at no cost to the employee. The Standard does not permit the employee to wash his or her own personal protective equipment at his or her home, because proper handling of the contaminated laundry could not be insured and there would be a risk of further contamination. Therefore, the employer must arrange for laundering by outside services. The employer must also repair or replace personal protective equipment as needed to maintain its effectiveness, at no cost to the employee. The employer should ensure that the employee uses appropriate personal protective equipment unless the employer shows that the employee temporarily and briefly declined to use personal protective equipment when, under rare and extraordinary circumstances (such as unanticipated emergency lifesaving procedures), it was the employee's professional judgment that in the specific instance its use would have prevented the delivery of health care or public safety services or would have posed an increased hazard to the safety of the worker or coworker. When the employee makes this judgment, the circumstances must be investigated and documented in order to determine whether changes can be instituted to prevent such occurrences in the future.

The Standard, however, does not allow avoiding the use of personal protective equipment because the patient is considered a "low risk" by the employer or the employee, the glasses get fogged, the patient would get scared, the patient is a child, or the gloves dull tactile sensation.

Housekeeping measures

Employers must ensure that the work site is maintained in a clean and sanitary condition. Housekeeping measures pertain to (1) contaminated work surfaces, (2) regulated waste, and (3) contaminated laundry. All equipment and environmental and working surfaces should be cleaned and decontaminated after contact with blood or other potentially infectious materials. Therefore, the employer shall determine and implement an appropriate *written* schedule for cleaning and method of decontamination. The cleaning and decontamination schedule should be based on (1) the location within the facility, (2) the type of surface to be cleaned, (3) the type of soil present (gross contamination vs. mild splatter), and (4) the tasks or procedures being performed in the area.

Contaminated work surfaces. Contaminated work surfaces should be decontaminated with an appropriate disinfectant (1) after completion of procedures, (2) immediately or as soon as feasible when surfaces are overtly contaminated, (3) after any spill of blood or other potentially infectious materials, and (4) at the end of the work shift if the surface may have been contaminated since the last cleaning. Protective coverings, such as plastic wrap, aluminum foil, or impervious-back absorbent paper used to cover equipment and environmental surfaces, should be removed and replaced as soon as feasible when they become overtly contaminated during the work shift. Of note is that the Standard does not require the use of such protective coverings. Rather, protective coverings are but one way to protect equipment when it might otherwise be difficult to decontaminate such equipment.

Furthermore, all bins, pails, cans and similar receptacles intended for reuse that have a reasonable likelihood of becoming contaminated with blood or other potentially

infectious materials should be inspected, cleaned, and decontaminated on a regular basis. Such items should be cleaned and decontaminated immediately or as soon as feasible upon visible contamination. Broken glassware that may be contaminated should not be picked up directly with the hands. Rather, such items should be cleaned using mechanical means, such as brush and dust pan, tongs, or forceps. The use of vacuums is strictly prohibited in the cleaning of such spills, because the vacuum exhaust can spread contamination.

Reusable sharps that are contaminated with blood or other potentially infectious materials should not be stored or processed in a manner that requires employees to reach by hand into the containers where these sharps have been placed. Transfer forceps should be available and used whenever reusable sharps are kept in such a container.

Proper cleaning must be done with agents that will destroy HBV and HIV. Examples of disinfectants include 2% glutaraldehyde, iodophors, chlorine compounds, sodium hypochlorite, and phenolics. When using these compounds, be sure to read the directions to determine the proper dilution ratio and to determine the safety of use on various surfaces. Diluted solutions (1:10 to 1:100) of sodium hypochlorite (household bleach) are particularly effective in killing HBV on surfaces. However, bleach should not be used on aluminum or oxidizable metals (such as stainless steel, carbide steel, brass, and copper), as these items may be subject to corrosion. Remember to include these chemicals in the OSHA Hazard Communication Program. Also, this program may require that utility gloves be worn when these substances are handled.

Regulated waste. Proper housekeeping includes the proper handling of regulated waste. "Regulated waste" means (1) liquid or semiliquid blood or other potentially infectious materials, (2) contaminated items that would release blood or other potentially infectious materials in a liquid or semiliquid state if compressed, (3) items that are caked with dried blood or other potentially infectious materials and are capable of releasing these materials during handling, (4) contaminated sharps, and (5) pathologic and microbiologic wastes containing blood or other potentially infectious materials. Regulated waste should be placed in containers that are closable and constructed to contain all contents and prevent leakage of fluids during handling.

Regulated waste containers should be labeled or color-coded and closed prior to removal, to prevent spillage or protrusion of contents during handling. If outside contamination of the regulated waste container occurs, it shall be placed in a second container. The second container should be closable and constructed to contain all contents to prevent leakage of fluids during handling. The secondary container should be labeled or color-coded and closed prior to removal, to prevent spillage or protrusion of contents during handling.

Disposal of all regulated waste shall be in accordance with applicable regulations of the United States, states and territories, and political subdivisions of states and territories.

This requirement is very vague; it does not tell physicians how they should handle such waste. The OSHA regulations set minimum requirements and leave their implementation in this area to other jurisdictions and agencies. Therefore, physicians should verify the requirements of their own states regarding handling of regulated waste. For example, the state of Georgia has specific requirements for the handling and disposal of medical waste. Essentially, all medical waste must be removed in separate containers by a licensed disposer. This requires that all medical waste be kept in a separate box and removed at specific intervals. Generators of medical waste who produce less than 100 pounds per month are exempt from the statute. Such generators are allowed to dispose of medical waste in municipal solid waste landfills, as other waste is disposed of (Georgia Department of Human Resources Rules & Regulations for Solid Waste Management, Chapter 391-3-4.14(7)(b)). This exception would exempt most physicians' offices.

In addition, the Environmental Protection Agency (EPA) has promulgated the Medical Waste Tracking Act (40 CFR 259). This act sets strict standards for the treatment of medical waste in Connecticut, New York, New Jersey, Puerto Rico, and Rhode Island. The EPA may enact similar regulations on a nationwide basis, and then the OSHA Standard would require that the employer conform to these regulations.

OSHA admits that there are no cases yet of HBV or HIV infection associated with the collection, transportation, and final disposal of regulated waste, but it sees a possibility for such exposure. OSHA remarks that those in an office who dispose of regulated waste often overlook persons later in the chain (e.g., the janitor) and that precautions are therefore necessary. The biggest risk to this group is needle-stick injuries from needles improperly packaged when disposed of. It is important to note that an employer is responsible not only for his or her own employees, but also for other workers who are on the premises where the employer controls the hazard. This would apply specifically to a janitor who is supplied by an outside contractor; the practitioner is as liable in regard to this person as to his or her own employees.

Contaminated laundry. "Contaminated laundry" means laundry that has been soiled with blood or other potentially infectious materials or may contain sharps. Contaminated laundry includes any linens or clothes, including personal protective equipment, that may have become soiled with any body fluids. The Standard requires that contaminated laundry be handled as little as possible and with a minimum of agitation. Contaminated laundry should be bagged or containerized at the location where it was used and should not be sorted or rinsed in the location of use. Contaminated laundry shall be placed and transported in bags or containers that are labeled or color-coded. When a facility utilizes universal precautions in the handling of all soiled laundry, alternative labeling or color-coding is sufficient if it permits all employees to recognize the containers as requiring compliance with universal precau-

tions. Whenever contaminated laundry is wet and presents a reasonable likelihood of soak-through or leakage from the bag or container, the laundry shall be placed and transported in bags or containers that prevent soak-through and/or leakage of fluids to the exterior. The employer should ensure that employees who have contact with contaminated laundry wear protective gloves and other appropriate personal protective equipment. When a facility ships contaminated laundry off-site to a facility that does not utilize universal precautions in the handling of all laundry, the facility generating the contaminated laundry must place such laundry in bags or containers that are labeled or color coded.

Hepatitis B vaccination and postexposure evaluation

OSHA considers the hepatitis B vaccination requirement to be the most important part of the program to control the risk of acquiring HBV. The rationale is that all of the other safety measures will not eliminate the possibility that an exposure incident, such as a needle-stick injury, could occur. The requirement for hepatitis vaccination includes (1) vaccination of employees with occupational exposure, (2) documentation of all employees who decline vaccination, and (3) follow-up of any "exposure incident."

Vaccination of all employees with occupational exposure. The current vaccines are administered in the deltoid muscle over a 6-month period. The vaccination series provides immunity for up to 9 years in 85% to 97% of recipients. OSHA estimates that, if all health care workers were vaccinated, then over the period of the average health care worker's career (45 years), approximately 250,000 HBV infections and 6100 deaths would be prevented.

The employer must make available the hepatitis B vaccine and vaccination series to all employees who have occupational exposure, and must provide postexposure evaluation and follow-up to all employees who have had exposure incidents. All medical evaluations and procedures, including the hepatitis B vaccination and vaccination series, and postexposure evaluation and follow-up, including prophylaxis, are to be made available at no cost to the employee. They should be made available to the employee at a reasonable time and place. Furthermore, they are to be performed by or under the supervision of a licensed physician or other health care professional. The employer should ensure that the health care professional responsible for the employee's hepatitis B vaccination is provided a copy of this regulation. All laboratory tests are to be conducted by an accredited laboratory at no cost to the employee.

After employees have received the training required by the Standard and within 10 working days of initial assignment, hepatitis B vaccination should be made available to all employees who have occupational exposure, unless an employee has previously received the complete hepatitis B vaccination series and antibody testing has shown that the employee is immune, or unless the vaccine is contraindicated for medical reasons. The employer shall not make participation in a pre-screening program a prerequisite for receiving hepatitis B vaccination. If a routine booster dose(s) of hepatitis B vaccine is recommended by the U.S. Public Health Service at a future date, such booster dose(s) should be made available.

Documentation of all employees who decline vaccination. If an employee initially declines hepatitis B vaccination but at a later date while still covered under the Standard decides to accept the vaccination, the employer shall make available hepatitis B vaccination at that time. The employer should ensure that employees who decline to accept hepatitis B vaccination offered by the employer sign the statement below:

> I understand that due to my occupational exposure to blood or other potentially infectious materials I may be at risk of acquiring hepatitis B virus (HBV) infection. I have been given the opportunity to be vaccinated with hepatitis B vaccine, at no charge to myself. However, I decline hepatitis B vaccination at this time. I understand that by declining this vaccine, I continue to be at risk of acquiring hepatitis B, a serious disease. If in the future I continue to have occupational exposure to blood or other potentially infectious materials and I want to be vaccinated with hepatitis B vaccine, I can receive the vaccination series at no charge to me.

Follow-up of any "exposure incident." The Standard requires adherence to a follow-up procedure for any exposure incident. An "exposure incident" means a specific eye, mouth, other mucous membrane, nonintact skin, or parenteral contact with blood or other potentially infectious materials that results from the performance of an employee's duties. It is important to note that the exposure of the intact skin of a health care worker to a patient's blood is not considered an "exposure incident" for purposes of this plan, but is indicative of inadequate personal protection and warrants follow-up and correction.

After a report of an exposure incident, the employer should make immediately available to the exposed employee a confidential medical evaluation and follow-up, including at least the following elements:

1. Documentation of the route(s) of exposure and the circumstances under which the exposure incident occurred
2. Identification and documentation of the source individual, unless the employer can establish that identification is infeasible or prohibited by state or local law

A "source" individual" is any individual, living or dead, whose blood or other potentially infectious materials may be a source of occupational exposure to an employee. Examples include, but are not limited to, hospital and clinic patients; clients in institutions for the developmentally disabled; trauma victims; clients of drug and alcohol treatment facilities; residents of hospices and nursing homes; human remains; and individuals who donate or sell blood or blood components.

The source individual's blood shall be tested as soon as feasible, and after consent is obtained from the source individual, in order to determine HBV and HIV infectivity. If the patient refuses consent, the employer shall establish that legally required consent cannot be obtained. When the source individual's consent is not required by law, the source individual's blood, if available, shall be tested and the results documented. When the source individual is already known to be infected with HBV or HIV, testing for the source individual's known HBV or HIV status need not be repeated. Results of the source individual's testing shall be made available to the exposed employee, and the employee shall be informed of applicable laws and regulations concerning disclosure of the identity and infectious status of the source individual. The exposed employee's blood shall be collected as soon as feasible and tested after consent of the employee is obtained.

If the employee consents to baseline blood collection, but does not give consent at that time for HIV serologic testing, the sample shall be preserved for at least 90 days. If, within 90 days of the exposure incident, the employee elects to have the baseline sample tested, such testing shall be done as soon as feasible. The employee is also entitled to postexposure prophylaxis, when medically indicated, as recommended by the U.S. Public Health Service, counseling, and evaluation of reported illnesses.

The employer shall ensure that the health care professional evaluating an employee after an exposure incident is provided a copy of this regulation, a description of the exposed employee's duties as they relate to the exposure incident, documentation of the route(s) of exposure and circumstances under which exposure occurred, results of the source individual's blood testing, if available, and all medical records relevant to the appropriate treatment of the employee, including vaccination status, that are the employer's responsibility to maintain.

The employer shall obtain and provide the employee with a copy of the evaluating health care professional's written opinion within 15 days of the completion of the evaluation.

The health care professional's written opinion in regard to hepatitis B vaccination shall be limited to whether hepatitis B vaccination is indicated for an employee, and if the employee has received such vaccination. The health care professional's written opinion in regard to postexposure evaluation and follow-up shall be limited to the following information:

1. The employee has been informed of the results of the evaluation.
2. The employee has been told about any medical conditions resulting from exposure to blood or other potentially infectious materials that require further evaluation or treatment.

All other findings or diagnoses shall remain confidential and shall not be included in the written report. Medical records required by this standard shall be maintained.

Communication of hazard to employees

Communication of hazards to employees includes (1) use of warning labels and, (2) training of employees.

Use of warning labels. Warning labels must be affixed to containers of regulated waste, refrigerators and freezers containing blood or other potentially infectious material, and other containers used to store, transport, or ship blood or other potentially infectious materials. Labels required by this section must include the international BIOHAZARD legend.

These labels shall be fluorescent orange or orange-red or predominantly so, with lettering or symbols in a contrasting color. Labels should be affixed as closely as feasible to the container by string, wire, adhesive, or other method that prevents their loss or unintentional removal. Red bags or red containers may be substituted for labels. Labels required for contaminated equipment shall also state which portions of the equipment remain contaminated. Regulated waste that has been decontaminated need not be labeled or color-coded.

Training of employees. Employers must ensure that all employees with occupational exposure participate in a training program, which must be provided at no cost to the employee and during working hours. Training shall be provided at the time of initial assignment to tasks in which occupational exposure may take place or within 90 days after the effective date of the Standard and at least annually thereafter. Employers must provide additional training when changes such as modification of tasks or procedures or institution of new tasks or procedures affect the employee's occupational exposure. The additional training may be limited to addressing the new exposures created. All training should be appropriate in content and vocabulary to educational level, literacy, and language of the employee.

The training program should contain at a minimum the following elements:

1. An accessible copy of the regulatory text of the Standard and an explanation of its contents
2. A general explanation of the epidemiology and symptoms of blood-borne diseases
3. An explanation of the modes of transmission of blood-borne pathogens
4. An explanation of the employer's Exposure Control Plan and the means by which the employee can obtain a copy of the written plan
5. An explanation of the appropriate methods for recognizing tasks and other activities that may involve exposure to blood and other potentially infectious materials
6. An explanation of the use and limitations of methods that will prevent or reduce exposure, including appropriate engineering controls, work practices, and personal protective equipment
7. Information on the types, proper use, location, removal, handling, decontamination, and disposal of personal protective equipment
8. An explanation of the basis for selection of personal protective equipment

9. Information on the hepatitis B vaccine, including information on its efficacy, safety, and method of administration, the benefits of being vaccinated, and that the vaccine and vaccination will be offered free of charge
10. Information on the appropriate actions to take and persons to contact in an emergency involving blood or other potentially infectious materials
11. An explanation of the procedure to follow if an exposure incident occurs, including the method of reporting the incident and the medical follow-up that will be made available
12. Information on the postexposure evaluation and follow-up that the employer is required to provide for the employee after an exposure incident
13. An explanation of the signs and labeling and/or color coding required by the Standard
14. An opportunity for interactive questions and answers with the person conducting the training session

The person conducting the training should be knowledgeable in the subject matter covered by the elements contained in the training program as it relates to the physician's office. This means that the physician or a nurse may conduct the training, or the training can be performed at a seminar.

Record keeping

The employer must establish and maintain an accurate record for each employee with occupational exposure. This record shall include (1) the name and social security number of the employee, (2) a copy of the employee's hepatitis B vaccination status, including the dates of all the hepatitis B vaccinations and any medical records relevant to the employee's ability to receive vaccination as required, (3) a copy of all results of examinations, medical testing, and follow-up procedures, (4) the employer's copy of the health care professional's written opinion, and (5) a copy of the information provided to the health care professional.

The employer should keep the employee's medical records confidential. The records are not to be disclosed or reported to any person, within or outside the work place, without the employee's express written consent. These records must be maintained for at least the duration of employment plus 30 years. Medical records should be provided upon request, for examination and copying, to the subject employee, to anyone having written consent of the subject employee, or to OSHA.

Training records should include (1) the dates of the training sessions, (2) the contents or a summary of the training sessions, (3) the names and qualifications of persons conducting the training, and (4) the names and job titles of all persons attending the training sessions. These records should be maintained for 3 years from the date on which the training occurred.

If the employer ceases to do business and there is no successor employer to receive and retain the records for the prescribed period, the employer shall notify OSHA at least

3 months prior to their disposal and transmit them to OSHA, if required by OSHA to do so.

The following will be of assistance in developing forms that can be employed in establishing the plan for a facility.

1. Employee hepatitis B vaccination form:
   a. Employee name
   b. Accepted or declined vaccination
   c. Date of inoculation #1
   d. Date of inoculation #2
   e. Date of inoculation #3
   f. Name of administering health care professional
2. Personal protective equipment survey:
   a. Name of personal protective equipment (PPE)
   b. Site of PPE
   c. Date reviewed
   d. Date of next scheduled review
   e. What type of exposure does PPE protect against?
   f. Does PPE provide adequate protection?
   g. Additional PPE required?
3. Exposure incident investigation form:
   a. Date of incident
   b. Time of incident
   c. Location of incident
   d. Potentially infectious material (type and source)
   e. Circumstances of incident
   f. How incident was caused
   g. Personal protective equipment being employed at time
   h. Post-incident actions taken
   i. Recommendation for future avoidance
4. Cleaning schedule:
   a. Area involved
   b. Schedule of cleaning
   c. Disinfectant employed
   d. Special instructions
5. Postexposure evaluation and follow-up checklist:
   a. Employee provided with information concerning the incident
   b. Identity of source individual
   c. Date source individual's blood was tested or consent was refused
   d. Results of test and results given to employee
   e. Exposed employee's blood collected and tested
   f. Results of employee's blood test
   g. Appointment made with health care professional
   h. Documentation forwarded to health care professional
      (1) Blood-borne pathogen standard
      (2) Description of employee's duties
      (3) Description of exposure incident, including route of exposure
      (4) Result of source individual's blood testing
      (5) Employee's medical records
6. Engineering controls questionnaire:
   a. Engineering control
   b. Does device provide exposure protection?
   c. What type of exposure protection does device provide?
   d. Are additional engineering controls needed?
7. Exposure determination
   a. Job classification
   b. Tasks and procedures in which occupational exposure is reasonably anticipated to occur
   c. Required personal protective equipment
   d. Required engineering controls
   e. Additional protection recommendations
8. Barrier requirements
   a. Task
   b. Personnel performing task
   c. Barrier required
9. Work practice controls checklist:
   a. Hand washing facilities
   b. Work area/food restrictions
   c. Immediate first aid available for blood exposure
   d. Handling reusable contaminated equipment
   e. Preparing and transporting contaminated equipment
   f. Procedures to minimize spilling and splashing
   g. Personal protective equipment
   h. Proper sharps handling and disposal
10. Employee training record:
    a. Date
    b. Employees present
    c. Topics covered
    d. Conducted by (name of instructor)

The forms outlined above should be used only as a guide. Remember, the Standard requires that each plan be individualized to each facility.

TORT AND WORKER'S COMPENSATION

An unanswered question, to date, is to what extent the Standard will fuel tort and/or Worker's Compensation liability. The OSHA enabling statute does not authorize a civil course of action for violation of an OSHA regulation. However, violation of an OSHA regulation may be used as evidence of employer negligence. The presence of a statute like this places a duty on the employer to follow the Standard. Any dereliction of duty that causes any employee injury (HBV or HIV infection) may result in liability. Some jurisdictions hold that violation of a regulation may be negligence per se (negligence in and of itself) if (1) the person injured is within the class of persons to be protected (i.e., employees) and (2) the injury that occurred was one that the regulation sought to prevent. However, the employee must still prove that the employer's violation of the statute caused the injury.

Depending upon the infection and the outcome, the damages can vary significantly. An employer who disregards the Standard and has an employee contract HIV may find himself or herself in a potentially destructive economic situation. Since the employee would have firsthand knowledge of the Standard and any noncompliance, negligence of the employer in not adhering to the Standard could be easily proved.

Failure to adhere to the Standard, then, may subject an employer not only to possible OSHA sanctions and fines but also to civil action by employees. However, OSHA believes that the probability of a successful outcome of litigation is low. It bases this contention upon the fact that since there would be no definite data concerning hazards, it would be difficult to show employer negligence.

CONCLUSION

The OSHA Bloodborne Pathogen Standard is now the law of the land. Any employer whose employees are subject to occupational exposure to blood or other contamination is required to conform to the Standard. The cost of conforming to the standard is just an additional item of overhead in conducting the practice of medicine. The future portends additional cost containment steps in health care combined with the possibility of additional health care regulation, including the potential for additional OSHA requirements. Such future requirements will probably address the air quality within some medical specialists' offices. The requirements might include measures for equipment to extract dust or vapors from the ambient atmosphere.

ACKNOWLEDGMENT

This chapter has made use of the *Federal Register*.

ADDITIONAL READINGS

Alpert LI: OSHA: new player in the battle against AIDS, *Med Lab Observer* 22:49, 1992.

Company sponsors AMA training program on OSHA regulations, *AIDS Weekly*, Jan 13, 1992, p. 13.

Federal agencies not getting safety devices to workers, *AIDS Alert* 7:54, 1992.

Ferguson TJ: Needle-stick injuries among health care professionals, *West J Med* 156:409, 1992.

Ginzburg HM: Occupational exposure to bloodborne pathogens: the new OSHA regulation, *AIDS Patient Care* 5:4, 1992.

Glantz LH, Mariner WK, Annas GJ: Risky business: setting public health policy for HIV-infected health care professionals, *Milbank Q* 70:43, 1992.

Goldsmith MF: OSHA bloodborne pathogens standard aims to limit occupational transmission (Medical News & Perspectives), *JAMA* 267:2853, 1992.

Heeg JM, Coleman DA, Driscoll DW: Hepatitis kills, *RN* 55:60, 1992.

Jones L: Lawmaker says new OSHA rules don't offer enough protection, *Am Med News* 35:8, 1992.

Lab groups criticize OSHA rules for AIDS, hepatitis B protection, *Med Lab Observer* 21:11, 1992.

Longer gloves, forearm covers recommended for lab workers, *AIDS Alert* 7:88, 1992.

Maasarani D: Infectious disease control could be costly to employers, *Business & Health* 10:21, 1992.

Makulowich GS: The OSHA standard and the unions: president calls for hepatitis B vaccine and more AIDS education, *AIDS Patient Care* 3:14, 1992.

Miller KE, Krol RA, Losh DP: Universal precautions in the family physician's office, *J Fam Pract* 35:163, 1992.

Mitka M: How to deal with requirements of OSHA safety rules, *Am Med News* 35:23, 1992.

Murphy BS, Barlow WE, Hatch D: OSHA issues final rule on bloodborne pathogens, *Personnel J* 71:24, 1992.

Valenti WM: Infection control: HIV and home healthcare. II: Risk to the caregiver, *Am J Infect Control* 23:78, 1995.

4

Recognition and Pathophysiology of Foot Infections

David Edward Marcinko
Rachel Pentin-Maki

More mistakes are made from want of a proper examination, than for any other reason.   J.H. Russell

Organized medicine has made many specialized and innovative advances in the past decade, especially within the realm of foot and ankle surgery. In this era of managed medical care, the technical expertise of the foot specialist has had a major impact on traditional medicine and the insurance industrial complex. For example, Weiner and colleagues, in 1987, reported in the *American Journal of Public Health* that the average procedural charge submitted by an orthopedist was 17% higher than that of a foot specialist. In addition, the orthopedic surgeon was five times more likely to perform a procedure on an inpatient basis, admitted patients to the hospital had longer stays, and, although podiatrists performed a greater number of procedures per surgical episode, their overall charges were 30% lower.[1] The cost effectiveness of this philosophy has not gone unnoticed by the government and lay community, as the respect, scope, and dominance of the well-trained foot specialist are brought to the forefront of today's health care climate. This increasing recognition, however, has brought with it the additional responsibility of dealing with the eventuality of soft tissue and bone infections, regardless of etiology. The treatment of these infections has been a dilemma that has plagued all surgeons for years, and is a major cause of morbidity in the footsore public. The subject of postoperative foot infections, for example, has been studied extensively by Bouchard, who in 1977 presented the results of his 3½-year retrospective survey of nosocomial infections at a community hospital. He concluded that *Staphylococcus aureus, Proteus, Escherichia coli, Pseudomonas,* and group D streptococci were common causative agents.[2] Similarly, Martin et al reported a 1.3% podiatric infection rate in outpatient surgery, which falls well within the mathematically predictable and acceptable range of 1% to 5% for clean surgery.[3] Both reports emphasized the significance of increased hospital costs and prolonged recovery time. Furthermore, a freestanding ambulatory surgical center in Atlanta recently reported two postoperative infections out of 1252 cases over a 4-year period (personal communication: Dr. Winfield E. Butlin, 1997). It is unfortunate, but almost axiomatic, that such infections are fertile ground for legal entanglements.

Therefore, because the infectious process seems to have such a profound influence on the clinical practice of any physician rendering foot care, the purpose of this chapter is to review the basic identification and pathophysiologic processes necessary for the successful management of this difficult situation. Since severe infections often require hospitalization, the correct use of hospital personnel, facilities, and protocol will also be discussed. Thus, by utilizing this information, we believe that the causal relationship between infections and litigation can be controlled or stymied. More importantly, patient treatment and welfare can be enhanced.

CLINICAL RECOGNITION OF THE INFECTED FOOT

Community-acquired or postoperative foot infections occur through either the direct extension route or trauma. Hematogenous infections, on the other hand, are secondary to bacteremia (from skin or respiratory tract) and more commonly occur in children (8 to 18 years). They usually begin with fever, chills, leukocytosis, pain, redness, swelling, and lost function. A child with joint pain and hyperpyrexia is almost considered to have hematogenous osteomyelitis or joint sepsis until proven otherwise. Postoperative foot infections usually occur 3 to 4 days after surgery and are typically caused by contamination from a break in sterility, excess duration of surgery, or inadequate skin preparation or sterilization. The presence of a good wound culture medium results from ineffective hemostasis or dead space formation, epinephrine or tourniquet use, ischemia and peripheral vascular disease (PVD), poor surgical technique, tissue cautery, hardware or prosthetic implants, or presence of foreign bodies (suture material, wires, or hand-ties). Bacterial resistance and susceptibility depend on several host- or bacteria-specific factors. Under the right circumstances, a mild pathogen can produce a severe infection or a virulent pathogen may produce only a mild infection. These situations are the exception and not the rule, but they do demonstrate the wide spectrum of possibilities in clinical foot infections. Why certain microbes characteristically colonize or infect certain patients ("patient tropism") or tissues ("tissue tropism"), but spare others, is an enigma. For example, although the skin can withstand the assault of 1×10^6 bacteria without producing an infection, the implantation of a foreign body such as suture material, a fixation screw, or an implant device, is said to lower host resistance so that the number of bacteria needed to produce an infection is reduced to 1×10^2. Microorganisms clinging to crevices can then disseminate along tissue planes and may travel proximally—for example, along the extensor or flexor tendon sheaths into the posterior compartment of the leg. Significant lower extremity pathology can then occur.

According to Oloff and colleagues, when the resistance or susceptibility of potential pathogens is described, several terms are used, including: pathogenicity (ability of a microbe to produce infection), virulence (degree of pathogenicity), and invasiveness (ability to spread).[4]

Important host factors include the immune response, which is composed of two basic systems: the humoral (antibody production) system and the cell-mediated system. Lymphocytes are involved in both and consist of short-lived B cells (20%), with Fc and C3d receptors, and the longer-lived T (thymus gland) cells (60% to 80%), with CD8/T8 suppressors and CD4/T4 inducers.

The humoral system is mediated through IgM, IgG, IgA, IgE, and IgD antibodies. For example, absent or abnormal IgG or IgM is associated with an increased incidence of infections, particularly those caused by organisms that are killed by mechanisms requiring complement or opsonins (polysaccharide bacterial capsules), such as *Haemophilus influenzae* and pneumococci. IgM antibodies (6% immunoglobulin) are the first to be released (opsonin) when stimulated by an antigen. IgG antibodies (80% immunoglobulin) enhance phagocytosis and neutralize toxins through four subgroups. IgA antibodies (13% immunoglobulin) are secretory and are reflected in mucosal surfaces. Their role in microbial defense is still not fully understood, since many patients appear to suffer no clinical consequences when titers decrease. IgD antibodies are found on most B cells, and IgE is involved in allergic reactions.

The cell-mediated system is primarily a function of cytotoxic T cells, which produce interleukin-1 (acute reaction), interleukin-2 (growth factor), and interferon (activators). Infections activating this system include yeast, TB, leprosy, and protozoan and *Pneumocystis* contamination. Small T lymphocytes are central to the development of delayed hypersensitivity and intracellular parasitism. Deple-

tion or impairment is associated with "opportunistic" infections due to any variety of bacterial, viral, or fungal elements.

Age is another important host factor in regard to infections. For example, during the first few months of existence, gram-negative enteric rods, *S. aureus,* and group B streptococci are the predominant causes of infections. During childhood the predominant culprit is *H. influenzae,* while viral exanthem diseases become more common in adolescence. Gram-negative bacilli are common in the elderly or debilitated patient.

Other factors that diminish host resistance include obesity, diabetes mellitus, PVD, immunosuppression, other coexisting infections, malnourishment, chronic steroid therapy (Addison's or Cushing's disease), and anemia.

Local manifestations of infection

The critical first step in the treatment of an infection is early recognition and confident diagnosis. Infection is a pathologic process, but its early stage may mimic the more benign inflammatory process. Inflammation is considered a dynamic response to any tissue damage, including infection, reflecting the body's attempt to regain homeostasis. In its first phase, vasoconstriction occurs, followed by vasopermeability, leukocyte migration (diapedesis), and phagocytosis. Indeed, the phagocytic ability of the host, the level of inflammatory response, the route of infection, and the presence of IgG, C3, C5a, and other components can affect the ability of the patient to fight the infection. All these factors help to eliminate organisms, limit infection spread, and remove debris and necrotic tissue to initiate wound healing.

However, it is the intensity of these signs and symptoms of inflammation that hold the key to early diagnosis and management. Of course, other causes of difficulty include hematoma or seroma formation, bandage or cast restriction, and gout precipitated by the trauma of surgery itself. Obviously, these causes must be considered and ruled out in a systematic manner before further investigation is warranted. The most obvious symptom is pain.

A traditional truism in medicine is that acute inflammation follows trauma (surgical or accidental), and the classic signs of inflammation are often difficult to distinguish from those of an infectious process. These signs and symptoms, according to Celsus (30 BC to 38 AD) include pain (dolor), especially out of proportion to the surgery or the likely etiologic event. Tumor or swelling (edema) represents fluid in the intercellular tissue spaces, usually the subcutaneous tissue, which occurs as a result of increased vascular permeability or lymphatic or venous obstruction. If a frank fresh hematoma is suspected, it is treated through wound pressure extravasation, elevation, aspiration, or incision and drainage. Older hematomas are painful and produce abundant scar tissue and fibrosis. They may be less effectively managed with contoured pressure bandages, steroid injections, moist packs, and physical therapy such as cross-fiber massage, therapeutic ultrasound, and range-of-motion exercises. Oral preoperative enzymatic agents are no longer in vogue to control edema, but oral NSAIDs seem helpful in both acute and chronic situations. Rubor (redness) is localized skin color produced by the congestion of capillary flow, which may have a variety of etiologies. It is localized and not necessarily ascending in nature. Heat (calor) is the local sensation of increased temperature, which indicates an increase in metabolic activity in the region. According to Virchow (1858), lost function (functio laesa) occurs because the above processes independently and confluently decrease the movement of the affected body part.

Finally, drainage is the systematic production of fluid or discharges from a wound, sore, or sinus tract. The consistency or appearance of drainage can vary and may offer important diagnostic clues to the nature and content of contamination. For example, serous drainage is clear to slightly cloudy and resembles serum. Purulent drainage is cloudy to dense, consisting of or containing pus. Pus itself is a liquid inflammatory product made up of leukocytes and invariably bacteria. Serosanguinous drainage contains both pus and blood, while seropurulent drainage contains both serum and pus (Fig. 4-1). The odor of a wound may provide other valuable diagnostic clues. For example, anaerobic organisms may smell foul or putrid, *Proteus* sp. contamination may smell "cheesy," and *Pseudomonas* infections may be sweet or "fruity."[4]

Systemic manifestations of infection

Body temperature is an indicator of infection. It is well known that elective surgery should not be performed on a febrile patient. Preoperative fever should be medically evaluated and controlled before the surgery is performed. A normal oral temperature range is 36.5° C (97.7° F) to 37.5° C (99.5° F), while rectal temperatures are about 0.5° C lower than the oral readings. The metabolic rate rises about 15% for each degree Celsius of temperature elevation. Temperature normally decreases from the body core to the periphery, and may fall 2 degrees during a night's sleep. Mercury, liquid crystal, or infrared tympanic membrane thermometers, through the external auditory meatus, are used for accurate readings.

Patterns of fever (pyrexia), according to Miller, include (1) sustained (elevated throughout the day), (2) remittent (elevated temperature that fluctuates but remains high throughout the day), (3) intermittent (fluctuations with temperatures below 37.5° C), (4) relapsing (alternating febrile and afebrile periods), (5) septic (temperature oscillations with chills [muscle contractions] and sweats), (6) febricula (slight elevation), and (7) hyperthermia (elevation greater than 40° C or 105° F).[5] Fever results from the action of endogenous pyrogens and/or endotoxins on the central nervous system. It may be caused by such benign occurrences as menses, exercise, pregnancy, stress, or anxiety neurosis. The principal site of action within the central nervous system is the preoptic nucleus in the anterior hypothalamus, which induces the release of Kupffer cell products and other endogenous

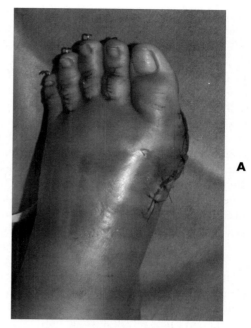

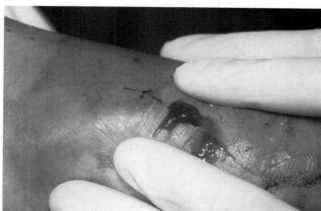

Fig. 4-1 **A,** The cardinal signs of inflammation are seen in this postoperative infection. Appearance of foot 3 days after HAV and digital stabilization surgery. The patient had all the classic signs and symptoms, including constitutional chills, fever, and severe pain. **B,** Drainage was expressed from the wound with only slight manual pressure. *(Courtesy Dr. Brian Holcomb, Atlanta, Ga.)*

pyrogens, such as interleukin-1 and prostaglandin. The metabolites of arachidonic acid, including prostacyclins, thromboxanes, and endoperoxides, also produce fever. Commencement intraoperatively is unusual, although it is normal for patients to have a slight temperature decrease during general anesthesia. This is because anesthesia renders the central hypothalamic thermoregulatory center inactive, and the patient is unable to control loss of body heat by other mechanisms.[5] Fever can also be produced by altering the Na^+/Ca^{++} ratio as regulated by the posterior hypothalmus.

Changes associated with the febrile patient include increases in erythrocyte sedimentation rate (ESR) and haptoglobin, ceruloplasmin, C-reactive protein (CRP), and fibrinogen levels. Decreases occur in serum iron and zinc levels. Any adult patient with a fever of more than 2 to 3 weeks' duration is said to have an FUO (fever of unknown origin). This is usually a result of infection, neoplasm, or collagen vascular disease(s), such as rheumatoid arthritis, systemic lupus erythematosus, and polymyositis. *Mycobacterium tuberculosis, Listeria, Bartonella,* and *Brucella* are historically associated with FUOs, as are various parasites, viruses, chlamydiae, spirochetes, and rickettsiae.

If a fever develops within the first 6 to 8 hours following surgery, the most likely cause is an endocrine imbalance, which may lead to a temporary thyroid crisis ("storm") or adrenocortical insufficiency. Should a fever develop 8 to 10 hours after surgery, a pulmonary malfunction should be entertained as a likely cause. Atelectasis and pneumonitis are the most common lung disorders and, if not properly treated, may lead to bacterial pneumonia. Urinary tract infection (UTI) is one of the most frequently found causes of postoperative fever after the second or third day, especially if a catheter was used. Usual signs and symptoms of UTIs include urgency, frequency, pain, and bacteriuria. After the third postoperative day, infection is the most important and devastating cause of postoperative fever. A spiking temperature is indicative of an infection, along with tachycardia, chills, malaise, lethargy, and lost appetite. Of course, there are other causes of postoperative fever during this time frame, and a prime example is acute thrombophlebitis. The condition may have a rapid onset and begins typically between the third and tenth postoperative days. The patients' calves should be inspected and examined for deep tenderness and a positive calf compression test (Homans' sign).[6] A duplex doppler ultrasound examination may be helpful if clinical suspicions warrant additional testing.

The initial treatment of fever should be directed toward its etiology. This can include simple rehydration when dehydration is a contributing factor. Treatment of the fever with aspirin, acetaminophen, or steroidal or other nonsteroidal antiinflammatory medications is acceptable. Cool sponge baths or compresses are also helpful. A temperature greater than 41° C may produce delirium, one over 42° C may produce unconsciousness or brain damage, and a fever greater than 43° C may induce death.

In summary, in regard to the etiology of postoperative fever, the five W's are evaluated: wind (pulmonary pathology), water (urinary and bowel retention), wound (infection), walk (thrombophlebitis), and wonder drugs (antibiotics and others). When these items are appropriately considered in their respective time frames, this mnemonic can be an effective aid in the total systemic evaluation of the postsurgical patient.

LYMPHANGITIS AND LYMPHADENOPATHY

According to Agoada, the largest anatomic group of lymph nodes is found in the inguinal region and is divided into superficial and deep groups.[7] The smaller and more superficial group is the proximal group, parallel to the inguinal ligament and just inferior to it. The larger and more deep distal group is found along the final part of the great saphenous vein. Each T-shaped group of about 25 individual nodes drains into the external iliac nodes. The deep inguinal lymph nodes are found in the femoral canal and drain into the external iliac lymph nodes. The popliteal lymph nodes are located in the deep part of the popliteal fossa, along the popliteal vessels, and drain into the deep inguinal nodes. The anterior tibial lymph node receives deep lymphatic drainage from the anterior part of the leg.

Lymphatic vessels, like veins, are divided into superficial and deep groups. Superficial vessels originate principally from the skin of the toes, heel, and plantar aspect of the foot and form a plexus that completely surrounds the toes and may be better developed medially, laterally, and plantarly. At the metatarsophalangeal joints (MPJs), the lymphatic channels of adjacent toes may unite, forming major draining vessels. On the top of the foot, superficial vessels may be divided into two collecting systems, medial and lateral. On the bottom of the foot, the superficial vessels are divided into three groups: anterior, medial, and lateral. The deep lymphatic vessels of the foot follow the arterial trunks and are divided into three groups: (1) dorsalis pedis and anterior tibial lymphatics, (2) plantar and posterior tibial lymphatics, and (3) the peroneal lymphatics along with the peroneal artery. Like the posterior tibial lymphatics, they all drain into the popliteal nodes. On the foot proper, the interphalangeal joint vessels drain into the lymphatic system on the top of the foot, while the metatarsophalangeal joint vessels divide into two systems, plantar and dorsal. The plantar lymphatic vessels run with the plantar metatarsal arteries. The dorsal vessels drain into the superficial lymphatic system on the dorsum of the foot. Around the ankle joint, vessels divide into superficial (anterior and posterior channels run with the saphenous veins to drain into the inguinal and popliteal nodes) and deep channels (directed transversely toward the anterior tibial artery). Deep posteromedial lymphatics drain into the posterior tibial lymphatic vessels, while deep posterolateral lymphatics drain into the peroneal lymphatic system.[7]

Kidawa defines lymphangitis as an infection of the lymph vessels, usually caused by group A streptococci, resulting in vasodilation with inpouring of leukocytes for phagocytotic activity.[8] Interestingly, *S. aureus* may have recently surpassed group A streptococci as the most common causative agent.

Other causes of lymphangitis include bacterial (diphtheria, scrofula, leptospiroses, syphilis, chancroid, tularemia, anthrax, glanders), rickettsial (scrub typhus, rickettsialpox, boutonneuse fever), chlamydial (lymphogranuloma venereum), viral (measles, cytomegalovirus, rubella, herpes, lasa or cat-scratch fever), protozoan (Chagas' disease, toxoplasmosis, trypanosomiasis, or kala-azar), mycotic (histoplasmosis, *S. schenckii,* paracoccidioidomycosis), and helminthic (filariasis) contamination.

Lymphangitis represents painful erythematous streaks (millimeters to centimeters wide) under the skin, which extend proximally toward the trunk from the origin of infection, site of contamination, or point of bacterial entry. The associated edema draws on the anchoring filaments, pulling the lymphatic sinusoidal channels open while dilating the end and side openings. This phenomenon, as well as lymphatic wall permeability, facilitates the entry of toxic by-products from the infected site into the lymphatic vessels, provoking an inflammatory reaction. Lymph nodes become tender, visible, red, and prominently hard. They may enlarge up to 3 cm in diameter. Fluctuance suggests pyogenic organisms. Once initiated, the lymphatic transport upstream advances the inflammatory process proximally, noted clinically as red streaking along the longitudinal axis of the leg or thigh with distal cellulitis.

Similarly, acute generalized lymphadenopathy is inflammation and congestion of lymph nodes located, most commonly, at the popliteal and inguinal levels and periodically at other sites in the lower extremities, as well as along the course of the thoracic duct. It is most commonly of bacterial or viral origin.

The diagnosis of lymphadenopathy is made through palpation for possible heat along the lymphatic vessel and pain at the nodes in the popliteal fossa or inguinal area medially. Lymphangiograms are not warranted unless there is persistence of nodal pain or advancing lymphedema in the stage following resolution of infection.

Local treatment of lymphangitis and lymphedema includes warm compresses applied over superficially inflamed lymphatic vessels to facilitate flow. Antibiotics are administered systemically to resolve the etiology of lymphangitis. Systemic treatment, with oral and parenteral antimicrobial agents, may include penicillin, erythromycin, or clindamycin, depending on the etiologic agent. Long-term complications of both conditions include nodal scarring with inability for filtration, leading to chronic lymphatic insufficiency and lymphedema and eventuating in significant distension and disfigurement of the lower extremity.

Finally, lymph node biopsy may be performed when all other diagnostic tests have been exhausted, but the inguinal nodes are usually avoided. When biopsy is performed, it is best to remove the largest lesion in toto, with its capsule intact. The nodes are then bisected for pathologic and bacteriologic examination.

MALAISE, TACHYCARDIA, AND SHOCK

Malaise is a generalized and vague feeling of bodily discomfort, lethargy, and lost appetite, in which the patient simply "feels bad." It may be entirely normal or due to a wound infection producing (1) bacteremia (presence of bacteria in blood), (2) septicemia (bacteremia plus chills and fever), and/or (3) toxemia (clinical state produced by effects of toxins, not bacteria themselves). Blood cultures are diagnostic. These bloodstream infections represent the host's failure to localize the infection.

Tachycardia is excessive heart action, with a pulse rate above 120 beats per minute. The mechanism of cardiovascular disintegration depends on the organism(s) involved, usually gram-negative ones. Septic gram-negative shock is a condition of acute peripheral circulatory failure resulting from abnormalities in circulatory control or circulating fluid loss secondary to severe infection and the release of enterotoxins. It is particularly induced by organisms such as *Pseudomonas aeruginosa, Salmonella typhi, E. coli, Yersinia pestis, Klebsiella, Serratia, Proteus, Enterobacter,* and *Haemophilus.* Specific signs and symptoms of gram-negative rod bacteremia include chills, fever, hypothermia, hyperventilation, mental status alterations, hypotension, bleeding, leukopenia, and major organ failure.

Disseminated intravascular coagulation (DIC) may occur along with renal failure, and is a medical emergency. The physiology of DIC is vascular endothelial damage, resulting in platelet adhesion and activation of the intrinsic coagulation system and Hageman factor XII. The diagnosis of DIC is made through evidence of decreased platelets, fragmented RBCs, Döhle's bodies, and toxic granules. Consumption of factors II, V, and VIII and fibrinogen, is also seen. Common screening tests include partial thromboplastin time, prothrombin time, platelet count, and fibrin split product tests.

Signs and symptoms of septic shock include pallor and clamminess or coolness of the skin, decreased blood pressure and urine output, fever, rapid pulse, decreased respiration, restlessness, anxiety, and unconsciousness. Septic shock is generally a sign of a more serious or systemic infection, rather than a minor or local one. For example, in some cases of gas gangrene, the blood pressure may drop to as low as 40 to 70 mm Hg, with resulting coma and even death.

Treatment of DIC is emergent, with airway maintenance and alveolar ventilation with humidified oxygen and tracheal toilet; preservation of intravascular volume by monitoring urine production, monitoring central venous or pulmonary wedge pressure, and administering fluids; maintenance of electrolyte status with sodium bicarbonate to lessen metabolic acidosis; and protection of cardiac, hematologic, and vasomotor status. Heparin anticoagulation therapy in the treatment of DIC may be useful, as may be the use of corticosteroids. The therapeutic role of granulocyte transfusion and gram-negative antiserum is still being evaluated.

Locally, radical debridement, resection, or even amputation may be needed, along with supportive medical care such as fluid replacement therapy and parenteral antibiotics.

IDENTIFICATION OF FOOT INFECTIONS

Specimen acquisition

The Gram stain and culture data from a suspected wound infection are only as good as the specimen source and type of culture media (solid, slants, or broth) used ("selective or nonselective"). For example, cotton swabs of a wound, ulcer, or sinus tract are contaminated, but not colonized, with bacteria that are not often the real culprit. Findings that suggest a significant or acute foot infection include (1) many organisms, (2) abundance of polymorphonuclear neutrophil leukocytes (PMNLs), and (3) predominance of a single organism. When there are only a few PMNLs or bacteria, or multiple bacterial species exist, one should consider the possibility of either nonpathogenic bacterial colonization (saprophytes) or cross-contamination from a poorly collected specimen. Therefore, when a specimen is obtained, adherence to the following guidelines will maximize diagnostic information[6]:

1. Obtain the specimen most likely to reflect the disease process. Try to obtain at least 1 cm^3 of infected tissue. Pus is not a good specimen to culture, since it contains mostly dead white blood cells. For example, a tissue specimen or a culture from the ascending border of a cellulitis is preferable. A sinus tract swab is more likely to produce benign saprophytic organisms than the true pathogen(s). Also, chronic infections often contain more organisms than acute ones. Swabs are also no substitute for biopsy specimens, fluid, curettements, or surgically removed tissue.

2. Obtain the specimen in a manner that avoids cross-contamination from the patient's own body flora. (Avoid unaffected toe web spaces.) This information may only confuse and obfuscate the offending organism(s).

3. Obtain a specimen of sufficient volume for both microscopic and cultural examination. For example, the recovery of a specimen from a nondraining cellulitis may be achieved by first infiltrating 0.5 ml. of sterile saline (sans preservative) into the advancing border of the surrounding subcutaneous tissue and then aspirating a sample, with a no. 25 needle attached to a syringe, for analysis. Care is taken not to spread the infection through intradermal tissue planes, and the technique remains controversial to many clinicians.

4. If possible, obtain the specimen at least 2 days before initiating antibiotic therapy. Antibiotic therapy based on empiric findings can be started in severe cases, pending clinical signs and symptoms. If possible, discuss the specimen(s) with an infectious disease specialist or laboratory microbiologist. Fungal and mycobacterial evaluation is suggested (Fig. 4-2).

Wound cultures

Wound exudate specimens for aerobic bacterial culture should be placed in a clean sterile container, with a preservative such as sodium bicarbonate. Routine cultures are generally incubated at 37° C and examined after 18 hours. Negative initial cultures are usually examined daily for 1 week. Fungal cultures are held for 3 to 4 weeks, while mycobacterial cultures are incubated for 6 to 10 weeks.[6]

Culture and sensitivities may be deferred in superficial or minor clinical situations, when an organism is not readily or confidently retrieved, especially in an uncompromised host. Mailing of clinical specimens is governed by federal law and is not generally recommended, because of time constraints (Fig. 4-3).

Stool cultures

Stool cultures are routinely evaluated for organisms, such as *S. aureus, Shigella, Salmonella, E. coli, Vibrio,* viruses, and parasites. Not normally primary contaminants of the lower extremity, they still may cause secondary infections in selected patients, as a result of "fecal fallout."

Bacteriologic report results

The bacteriologic report lists the organisms that were found in the specimen sent to the clinical laboratory, with an estimate of their relative numbers, and the antibiotic susceptibility, if requested. The attending physician must then interpret the significance of the results, in terms of the entire clinical presentation, and be familiar with the normal flora and pathogens in the specimen.

Report timing. Most significant pathogens grow to detectable levels in 1 to 3 days, although preliminary reports can often be obtained in 18 to 24 hours. "No-growth" cultures are incubated for varying lengths of time, depending on the expected pathogen. The importance of conferring early with the laboratory when an uncommon pathogen is suspected cannot be overemphasized.

Reported bacterial flora. Generally, all organisms appearing on a specimen are reported in terms of their relative numbers. However, since complete identification of some wound cultures is time consuming and yields very little new information, only potential pathogens are reported if present in sufficient numbers. Thus, differentiation is made between the "normal" flora of contaminated wounds and actual pathogenic wound colonization by disease-producing microbes.

Microbial quantitation. The number of bacteria present in a given specimen is usually reported in descriptive terms such as "rare" (1 to 3 colonies per streakout), "few" (less than 1 to as many as 20 colonies per streakout), "moderate," "abundant," or "TNTC" (too numerous to count). Quantitative bacterial counts, on the other hand, require incubation of a known volume of specimen on or in the agar medium. After inoculation, the bacterial colonies are counted, and a calculation is made to determine the number of organisms per millimeter of the original specimen. However, since the quantitative count determines the number of bacteria at the moment of in vitro planting, the count may not reflect true in vivo conditions of the patient. Additionally, conclusions about the significance of the count must be made. For example, 10^5 or more bacteria per millimeter of a urine sample may indicate an infection, while only a few organisms in a joint fluid aspirant may signify osteomyelitis.

The procedures for final laboratory identification may include clinical testing and subculturing. Preliminary anti-

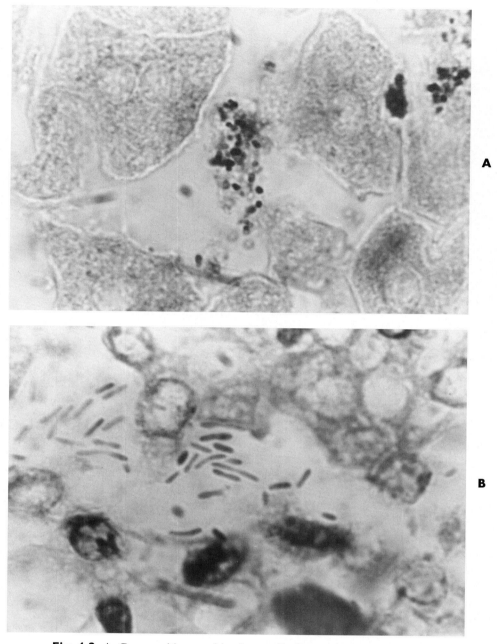

Fig. 4-2 **A,** Gram-positive cocci in clusters. **B,** Gram-negative rods.

biotic susceptibility tests can be initiated in 24 hours. Thus, the species of bacteria suggested by Gram stains and cultural methods may generally lead to an educated empiric guess about the identity of and treatment plan for the invading culprit. On the other hand, slower-growing aerobic or anaerobic organisms may eventually be cultured, with the clinician having a false sense of security in treating on the basis of the initial results. Therefore, clinical response rather than cultural results should guide the physician in the course of care.

Antibiotic sensitivity testing. According to the World Health Organization–International Collaborative Study

(WHO–ICS), using the antibiotic impregnated disc diffusion (Kirby-Bauer) method, sensitivity or resistance zone diameter results are recorded as either "susceptible," intermediate," or "resistant," according to standardized criteria. The last category means that the offending microbe is not totally constrained by the minimum inhibitory concentration (MIC) of the tested antibiotic. The first two categories imply that the microbe may be successfully treated with the recommended MIC for the clinical infection present. When the tube dilution broth method is performed, the minimum bactericidal concentration (MBC) or minimal lethal concentration (MLC), for terminating 99.9% of the organisms, is often

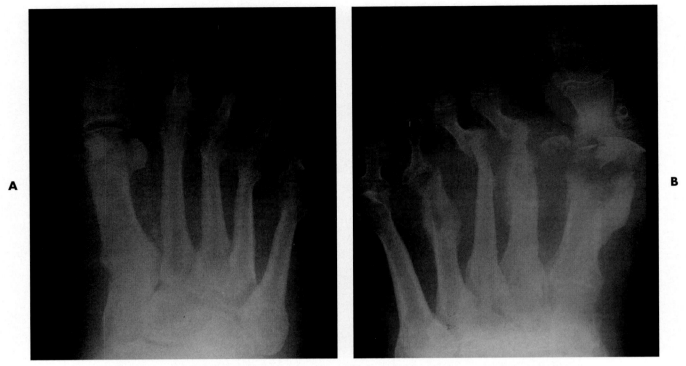

Fig. 4-3 A, Osteomyelitis of the hallux due to coagulase positive *S. aureus.* **B,** Osteomyelitis of the hallux due to an open fracture. *(Courtesy Dr. Cynthia Mercado-Ciessau, Forest Park, Ill.)*

used with traditional MICs. This is especially true of fragile or fastidious bacteria not amenable to MIC reports. Antibiotic tolerance is defined as an MBC:MIC ratio of greater than 32. Serum bactericidal tests and assays, biologic assays, radioenzymatic assays (REAs), radioimmunoassays (RIAs), nonisotopic immunoassays (NIAs), and chromatography are also used to determine antimicrobial activity.

When pathology indicates the need for potentially toxic agents, such as aminoglycosides or vancomycin, antibiotic therapy must be titrated with periodic peak and through therapeutic and toxic blood levels. However, current recommendations tend not to favor the use of peak and trough levels for vancomycin.

COMMON CAUSES OF "NO-GROWTH" CULTURAL RESULTS

Invading microorganisms may fail to appear in culture, and the following may be causes of this phenomenon:

1. Infection was absent, or the specimen was not indicative of infection.
2. The Gram stain was erroneous.
3. The organism was not a specimen cultured from the appropriate site, by prompt routine methods of planting, or with correct incubation length, temperature, and environmental conditions.
4. The specimen was no longer viable because of antibiotics or prior treatment.
5. Human error.

CLASSIFICATION OF BACTERIA

Although bacterial taxonomy cannot be condensed into a few pages, the following is a brief review of common pathogens to refresh the practitioner's memory and to demonstrate where less common organisms fit into the current classification scheme.[6]

Kingdom—Procaryotae
    Division I—Cyanobacteria
    Division II—Bacteria
    A. Sheathed bacteria *(Leptothrix)*
    B. Spirochetes
    C. Spiral/curved bacteria *(Spirillum* and *Campylobacter)*
    D. Gram-positive cocci
       1. Staphylococci and other micrococci (nonpathologic). Staphylococci are gram-positive cocci that occur singly, in pairs, in short chains, or in irregular clusters. Their diameters range from 0.7 to 1.2 µm on blood agar, with hemolysis within 48 hours. Although *S. aureus* typically produces golden yellow (carotenoid) convex colored colonies, and *S. epidermidis (S. albus)* produces white colonies, a coagulase test is used to differentiate taxonomic classes. *S. saprophyticus* is not generally pathologic. More pathogenic strains of *S. aureus* are coagulase positive and may or may not cause hemolysis. Other identifying characteristics include the production of deoxyribonuclease or

catalase, mannitol fermentation, beta hemolysis, and the tellurite reduction reaction (TRR). Further differentiation is made through phage typing, with five lytic and antigenic groups known. Gram-positive cocci growth is inhibited on gram-negative media, such as eosin–methylene blue (EMB) or MacConkey agar. The majority of staphylococcal strains are producers of penicillinase, which destroys the beta-lactam ring of penicillin. Semisynthetic agents, developed in the 1960s, are therefore used (methicillin, oxacillin, cloxacillin, nafcillin). "Methicillin chromosomal resistance" is characteristic of all beta-lactam antibiotics, including cephalosporins, and is defined as an MIC above 20 μg/ml by the broth dilution method. The term "intrinsic resistance" may be a more accurate designation than "methicillin resistant." The following enzymes and toxins are considered important in human infections caused by *Staphylococcus* species:

a. Coagulase: *S. aureus* produces both "bound" and "free" coagulase, able to coagulate human serum. This characteristic is used to differentiate *S. aureus* from *S. epidermidis.*

b. Enterotoxin: produced by most species and capable of causing food poisoning. Some *S. epidermidis* organisms may also produce this substance.

c. Exfoliative toxin: produced by staphylococci phage group II and known to cause "scalded skin syndrome." Interestingly, phage typing is not an absolute identification guide, since the lysis of *S. aureus* may be altered by "wild phages" through transduction or loss of prophage.

d. Leukocidin: extracellular protein that may destroy human white blood cells, especially PMNLs in-vitro.

e. Toxic shock syndrome toxin (TSST-1): produced by *S. aureus*. It is unlikely that it can be produced by *S. epidermidis.*

f. Catalase: H_2O_2 is converted to H_2O and O_2 by the action of this enzyme on all staphylococcal strains.

g. Hyaluronidase: cleaves hyaluronic acids present in the matrix stroma of connective tissue.

h. Alpha, beta, gamma, and delta toxins are produced by *S. aureus.*

2. Streptococci. Streptococci are gram-positive cocci, from the family Streptococcaceae, that tend to appear in pairs and/or chains. Hemolytic properties (Brown classification) have been used for precise identification of these organisms:

a. Alpha (partial) green hemolysis with gray colonies (*S. viridans, S. faecalis, S. liquefaciens, S. salivarius,* and *Aerococcus*)

b. Beta (complete) hemolysis (*S. pyogenes*) (Lancefield groups A [M types], B, C, D, E, F, G, L, M, P, U, and V)

c. Gamma (non) hemolysis (enterococci)

The older Bergey classification also grouped streptococci into a pyogenic group, a viridans group (alpha-hemolytic), an enterococcus group, and a lactic group. Since no single system of classification exists, differentiation depends on many factors, but the Lancefield classification, based on the group-specific cell wall antigen (C-carbohydrate or teichoic acid in groups D or N), is very important. The following streptococcal species are considered important in human infections:

Group A streptococci include almost all the hemolytic streptococci (*S. pyogenes*) that affect humans. Foot infections caused by this group include erysipelas, suppurative infections, cellulitis, impetigo, lymphadenitis, and septicemia.

Group B streptococci (*S. agalactiae*) have been recovered from the cervix and vagina. In the foot, this group may produce septic arthritis, osteomyelitis, pyoderma, and septicemia.

Group C streptococci (*S. equisimilis, S. zooepidemicus,* and *S. dysgalactiae*) and pneumococci (*S. pneumoniae*). Foot infections from this group may be seen as opportunistic infections in compromised hosts.

Group D streptococci contain both hemolytic and nonhemolytic types. These include enterococci (*S. faecalis, S. durans, S. liquefaciens*) and nonenterococci (*S. bovis*), and the oral streptococcus (*S. mutans*) may be implicated in pedal wound infections.

Group E streptococci (*S. uberis*) may be either alpha- or gamma-hemolytic and are usually seen in cows or swine. They are not particularly noted in the foot but may be recovered from the human respiratory system.

Group F streptococci (*S. anginosus*) are commonly found in the throat but may infect blood and pedal wounds.

Group G streptococci (*S. anginosus*) have been isolated from humans and dogs and may be implicated in pedal wound and skin infections.

Group H streptococci (*S. sanguis*) may be seen in the human respiratory tract.

Group K streptococci (partial hemolysis).

Group L and group M streptococci (beta-hemolytic) have been found in dogs and pigs and may contaminate human pedal wound abscesses.

Group N streptococci (*S. lactis* and *S. cremoris*) are found in milk and cream.

Group O streptococci may be either alpha- or beta-hemolytic and have been implicated in tonsillitis and endocarditis.

Group R streptococci have been isolated from patients with meningitis.

3. Pneumococci. Diplococci and pneumococci are important pathogens in the lungs, meninges, and middle ear. They are not common wound contaminants and are infrequently seen on examination. Types 1, 2, 3, 4, 7, 8, 12, and 14 are highly pathogenic.
4. Anaerobic gram-positive cocci. These organisms may be slow growing and difficult to isolate and identify but tend to do well under conditions of reduced oxygen tension. Microaerophilic streptococci are often recovered from wound abscesses.

E. Gram-negative cocci and coccobacilli
   1. *Neisseria* (*N. gonorrhoeae*, *N. meningitidis* [groups A to D and X to Z], *N. lactamicus*, *N. flavescens*, *N. mucosa*, *N. sicca*, and *N. catarrhalis*) are gram-negative diplococci arranged in pairs with adjacent sides flattened. *Neisseria* infections may contain both saprophytic and pathogenic species. They all grow well on Thayer-Martin medium or chocolate agar.
   2. *Acinetobacter* (*Mima* and *Herellea*) and other miscellaneous gram-negative cocci are widely found in nature and are normal inhabitants of the skin. They are not usually pathogenic, except to debilitated patients or those with infected wounds or osteomyelitis. Examples include *A. calcoaceticus* and *A. anitratus*, which are frequently mistaken for *Neisseria* species.
   3. Anaerobic gram-negative cocci (*Veillonella*) are not usually considered primary pathogens in foot infections. *Veillonella* has been found on human skin, and in the respiratory, gastrointestinal, and genitourinary systems.

F. Gram-positive bacilli. These are either sporulating or nonsporulating organisms.
   1. Small (mostly), nonsporulating gram-positive rods
      a. *Corynebacterium* ("diphtheroids"), recently possibly implicated in prosthetic implant sepsis. *Propionibacterium* may be confused with *Actinomyces*. Others include *C. diphtheriae* (Pai's or Loeffler medium) and *C. anthracis*. Appear as gram-positive club-shaped rods with irregular granules with palisade arrangements. Found in the soil and on human skin. Several species are pathogenic (*C. acnes, C. aquaticum, C. enzymicum, C. equi, C. hemolyticum, C. hoagii, C. minutissimum, C. pseudotuberculosis, C. ulcerans, C. vaginale,* and *C. xerosis*).
      b. *Listeria* (perinatal infants and neonates), *Lactobacillus* (*L. acidophilus, L. bifidus, L. brevis,*

L. bulgaricus, L. casei, L. cellobiosus, L. fermentum, and *L. jensenii*), and *Erysipelothrix rhusiopathiae* ("fisherman's disease") and infectious arthritis.
      c. *Nocardia* (aerobic) and *Actinomyces* (anaerobic) resemble fungi, with branching filaments. Some are acid-fast. *N. asteroides* is normal flora of the skin and upper respiratory tract and may produce "sulfur granules" in a Madura foot. *N. brasiliensis* may produce subcutaneous abscesses (mycetomas), while *N. caviae* may cause osteomyelitis, *N. farcinica* may produce suppurating lymph nodes, and *N. transvalensis* has been found in patients with pedal mycetomas in South Africa.
      d. Other anaerobic nonsporulating gram-positive rods
   2. Large, sporulating gram-positive rods
      a. *Bacillus* (*B. subtilis, B. megaterium, B. polymyxa,* and bacillus Calmette-Guérin) are usually saprophytes of soil and water and are common laboratory contaminants. *B. anthracis,* however, is the causative agent of anthrax; *B. cereus* may cause "food poisoning."
      b. *Clostridium.* Gas and foul odor are associated with clostridial contamination. The species most commonly associated with myonecrosis (gas gangrene) are *C. perfringens, C. sporogenes, C. novyi, C. bifermentans, C. sordellii, C. tertium, C. septicum, C. putrificum, C. butyricum, C. fallax, C. regulare,* and *C. paraputrificum.* The toxin of *C. tetani* and *C. botulinum* can appear as "tennis rackets" on culture and is responsible for serious human illnesses. There are more than 150 species.

G. Gram-negative bacilli
   1. *Haemophilus influenzae* (X and V factors with six serologic types [a to f]) and other usually small, gram-negative rods are a common cause of respiratory infections, especially in children. Other species include *H. parainfluenzae, H. aphrophilus, H. paraphrophilus,* and *H. ducreyi. Haemophilus influenzae* grows well on chocolate agar with added CO_2. Other pathogenic agents are *H. aegyptius* (pink eye), *H. aphrophilus, H. parapertussis,* and *H. vaginalis.*
   2. Enterobacteriaceae. These organisms are common facultative gram-negative rods that inhabit the gastrointestinal tract, urinary tract, soil, water, and dairy products; they are difficult cross-contaminants in pedal wound infections.
      a. *Escherichia* (*E. aurescens, E. coli,* and *E. freundii*) and *Shigella* (*S. boydii, S. dysenteriae,* and *S. flexneri*)
      b. *Edwardsiella* ("Bartholomew group"), isolated from diarrheal stools, abscesses, and wound infections

c. *Salmonella (S. choleraesuis, S. derby, S. enteritidis, S. gallinarum, S. oranienburg, S. typhi,* and *S. typhimurium*), *Arizona (A. hinshawii)*, and *Citrobacter (C. diversus, C. freundii,* and *C. intermedium).* Found in turtles, shellfish, chicken, fish, and pork.

d. *Klebsiella (K. ozaenae, K. pneumoniae* [Friedländer's bacillus)], and *K. rhinoscleromatis)*, *Enterobacter,* and *Serratia (S. liquefaciens, S. marcescens,* and *S. rubidaea).*

e. *Proteus* is found in the soil, water, and normal fecal flora *(P. mirabilis, P. morganii, P. rettgeri,* and *P. vulgaris). Providencia (P. alcalifaciens* and *P. stuartii)* is closely related to *Proteus* and *Morganella.*

f. *Hafnia (Enterobacter hafnia)*

g. *Erwinia (E. herbicola)* may be found on skin, in wounds, and in abscesses and can cause bacteremia traced to infusion pumps.

h. *Yersinia* (former *Pasteurella* sp.), exemplified by *Y. enterocolitica, Y. pseudotuberculosis,* and *Y. pestis* ("black death," "plague")

3. Other gram-negative bacilli require CO_2, in an enriched medium, to grow. These include *Campylobacter, Cardiobacterium, Actinobacillus, Bordetella, Brucella,* and *Francisella.* Newer genera include *Ewingella, Kluyvera, Cedecea, Rahnella, Tatumella,* and *Buttiauxella.*

4. *Pseudomonas* and other gram-negative rods. Among the nonfermentative, "water-loving" gram-negative rods, *Pseudomonas aeruginosa (Bacillus pyocyaneus)* is the most important organism; it is identified by a sweet fruity odor. Ultraviolet light may be used to demonstrate its yellow-blue-green presence in clinical infections. The fluorescent group includes *P. aeruginosa, P. putida,* and *P. fluorescens. Pseudomonas* may be either a normal constituent of pedal skin or a pathogen, given the appropriate conditions (burns). Miscellaneous groups that may produce opportunistic infections include *P. pseudomallei, P. acidovorans, P. achromobacter, P. xanthomonas, P. flavobacterium,* and *P. alcaligenes,* among others.

5. Anaerobic gram-negative bacilli. Anaerobic gram-negative rods are being increasingly recognized as pathogens in a variety of pedal infections. Often, the term bacteroides is applied to include all anaerobic nonsporulating gram negative rods (Fig. 4-4, *A* and *B*). These include species of the following genera:

a. *Bacteroides* species (kanamycin-vancomycin laced blood agar), such as *B. corrodens, B. fragilis, B. melaninogenicus, M. oralis, B. pneumosintes, P. ruminicola, P. serpens.*

b. *Fusobacterium* species such as: *F. meningosepticum* or *Flavobacterium* I, II, and III.

c. *Leptotrichia* is part of the normal flora of the mouth and urogenital tract *(L. buccalis).*

H. Actinomycetes have structural branches that resemble fungal elements *(Actinomyces bovis, A. israelii, A. naeslundii, A. odontolyticus).*

I. Mycoplasmas (pleuropneumonia-like organisms [PPLOs]) have been cultivated from the lungs, respiratory tract, gastrointestinal and genitourinary tracts, bones, and joints *(M. hominis, M. salivarium, M. orale,* and *M. pneumoniae).*

J. Rickettsiae are minute gram-negative, intracellular coccobacilli that are transmitted by arthropods and produce fever and rash *(R. akari, R. canada, R. mooseri, R. rickettsii,* and *R. typhi).*

BONE BIOPSY

A definitive diagnosis of contaminated bone (osteomyelitis) is made only through the invasive process of bone tissue biopsy, performed under sterile conditions. Biopsies are from clean and noninvolved areas, sinus tracts are generally not cultured, and, if possible, antibiotics are suspended for 48 hours prior to sampling. All other tests, although beneficial, are presumptive. Samples are taken for aerobes, anaerobes, mycobacteria, and fungi. This may be done through open surgery in the operatory under general anesthesia or percutaneously using local anesthesia. C-arm fluoroscopic control aids in the retrieval of a specimen from the exact area of interest.

In the presence of closed wounds or where open biopsy is not feasible, needle aspiration may be performed in an attempt to identify organism(s) responsible for osteomyelitis or deep abscess formation. The risk of inadvertent bacterial seeding from infected soft tissue must be considered, and the surgical approach to questionable areas of bone should be through noninflamed and noninfected soft tissues. Results may still be suspect.

If the biopsy is performed percutaneously, a Jamshidi (Perfectum Corp., Hyde Park, N.Y.) sternal bone marrow, 11-gauge, 6-inch, self-contained bone needle biopsy kit is ideal for the task in smaller pedal bones. It consists of an outer stainless steel cannula with trochar and plastic handle, with inner stylet for tissue clearance. The blunt inner stylet is used to disengage aberrant soft tissue structures without trauma. The sharp needle itself is directed accurately toward the suspicious area under fluoroscopic guidance (C-arm). In the absence of fluoroscopic equipment, needle position may be confirmed by standard radiographic techniques, with flat-plate x-rays in two or three cardinal body planes (translocation). Utilization of imaging techniques decreases the likelihood of aspiration or biopsy from uninvolved areas, as well as aiding in the prevention of damage to implanted polymers, prosthetic devices, or fixation hardware. If aspirated material cannot be obtained for Gram stain or cultural evaluation, and radiographs confirm the appropriate needle placement, the wound may be flushed with nonbacteriostatic saline and the wash aspirated for microbial analysis.[6]

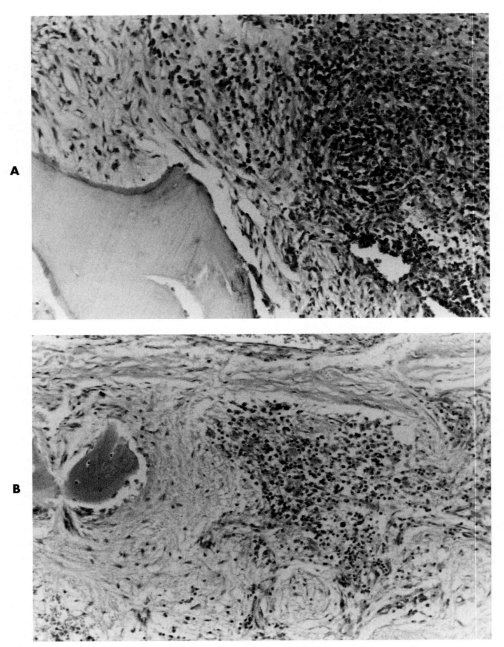

Fig. 4-4 A, *E. coli*–induced osteomyelitis (Brodie's abscess), right tibia, in a 64-year-old female patient with polycythemia rubra vera (PRV). Hematoxylin and eosin–stained section shows multiple fragments of bone with focal area of intramedullary chronic inflammation, with many plasma cells, some lymphocytes, histiocytes, and surrounding fibrosis. (×100.) *(Courtesy Dr. J. Otis, Atlanta, Ga.)* **B,** A 19-year-old female who sustained an open fracture of the right ankle and subsequent chronic · osteomyelitis, due to coagulase-positive *S. aureus, Aerobacter* sp., *Citrobacter* sp., and *Pseudomonas* sp. Hematoxylin and eosin stain shows foreign body lymphocytic inflammatory reaction, granulocytes, and plasma cells. Invasion extends into the periosteum, through cortical bone, and into cancellous bone. (×100.)

The larger pedal bones of the midfoot, rearfoot, and ankle may require use of a Michelle hand trephine for bone biopsy. Available in ⅛-inch and ³⁄₁₆-inch sizes, the trephine is used in a manner similar to that for the Jamshidi biopsy kit. An additional feature is the self-graduated core, which records the depth of osseous penetration in more substantial bones (Fig. 4-4, *C* to *F*).

Finally, an open surgical bone biopsy allows soft tissue and osseous structures to be visualized, manipulated, palpated, and debrided, if needed. It can be performed with a

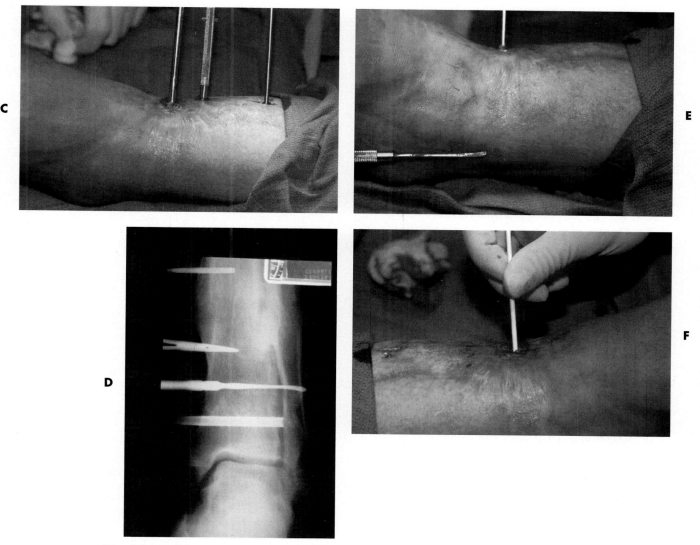

Fig. 4-4, cont'd **C,** Leg bone biopsy site identified through clinical translocation using four sterile probes. **D,** Radiographic view of probes. The second most distal probe was the suspicious site. **E,** Marker indicating depth of trephine penetration needed to secure valid bone biopsy specimen. **F,** Gram stain with culture and sensitivity testing performed through same surgical site.

multiple-drill-hole "perforation" technique or with power instrumentation to "window" a portion of cortico-cancellous bone for examination. The risks and benefits must be evaluated relative to contamination of uninvolved adjacent structures and infrastructural weakening of supporting skeletal stroma.

HOSPITALIZATION OF THE INFECTED PATIENT

Ultimately, there may come a time when the patient with an infected or potentially infected foot must be considered for hospitalization. The following criteria for hospitalization are suggested[20,21]:

1. Systemic manifestations and constitutional signs
   a. Fever (greater than 101° F—oral)
   b. Lymphangitis, ascending cellulitis, lymphadenopathy
   c. Malaise, chills, shakes
   d. Tachycardia (>100 beats/min)
2. Debilitated patient
   a. Diabetes mellitus
   b. Peripheral vascular disease
   c. Alcoholic
   d. Nutritionally deficient (failure to thrive)
   e. Immunodeficient (HIV)
   f. Elderly patient
   g. Miscellaneous systemic conditions
3. Infections requiring parenteral antibiotics
   a. Resistant organisms
   b. Gram-negative or anaerobic infections
   c. Deep space infections

d. Suspected bone involvement (osteomyelitis)
(1) Acute and symptomatic
(2) Chronic and symptomatic
5. Failure of outpatient therapy
6. Surgical debridement of bone and soft tissue

CONCLUSION

The clinical signs of the infectious process have been examined in this chapter. Emphasis has been placed on the clinical difference between inflammation and infection, since the first is a benign process and the second is pathologic. Finally, various cultural and radiographic diagnostic modalities have been briefly reviewed.

REFERENCES

1. Weiner JP, Steinwachs DM, Frank RG, Schwartz KJ: Elective foot surgery: relative roles of doctors of podiatric medicine and orthopedic surgeons, *Am J Public Health* 8: 987, 1987.
2. Bouchard JL: A 3½-year study of nosocomial infections in a community hospital and the effects on podiatric patients, *J Am Podiatry Assoc* 67:497, 1977.
3. Martin WJ, Mandracchia VJ, Beckett DE: The incidence of post-operative infection in outpatient podiatric surgery, *J Am Podiatry Assoc* 74:89, 1984.
4. Oloff LM, Thornton C: Clinical scenario of the fetid foot. In Marcinko DE, ed: *Medical and surgical therapeutics of the foot and ankle,* Baltimore, 1992, Williams & Wilkins.
5. Miller SJ: Temperature regulation and post-operative fever: a preliminary study, *J Am Podiatry Assoc* 74: 373, 1984.
6. Marcinko DE: *Advanced protocol for the diagnosis and treatment of pedal infections,* revised edition, Brentwood, Tenn, 1990, Podiatry Insurance Company of America.
7. Agoada D: Angiology of the lower extremity. In Marcinko DE, ed: *Medical and surgical therapeutics of the foot and ankle,* Baltimore, 1992, Williams & Wilkins.
8. Kidawa A: Angiology of the lower extremity. In Marcinko DE, ed: *Medical and surgical therapeutics of the foot and ankle,* Baltimore, 1992, Williams & Wilkins.
9. Heden RI, Lemont H: Early diagnosis of osteomyelitis with technetium bone scan, *J Am Podiatry Assoc.* 67:733, 1977.
10. Karl RD, Hammes CS: Nuclear medicine imaging in podiatric disorders, *Clin Podiatr Med Surg* 5:909, 1988.
11. Schlefman BS: Radiology. In McGlamry ED, ed: *Fundamentals of foot surgery,* ed 2, Baltimore, 1992, Williams & Wilkins.
12. Hirsch BE, Udupa JK, Roberts D: Three dimensional reconstruction of the foot from computed tomography scans, *J Am Podiatr Med Assoc* 79:384, 1989.
13. Huff HR, Kravette MA: Computed tomography of the foot and ankle, *J Am Podiatr Med Assoc* 76:375, 1986.
14. Downey M: Magnetic resonance imaging (MRI) vs. computed tomography (CT): clinical applications in the foot and ankle. In McGlamry ED, ed: *Reconstructive surgery of the foot and leg—* update 1989, Tucker, Georgia, 1989, Podiatry Institute Publishing Co.
15. Sartoris DJ, Resnick D: Magnetic resonance imaging of podiatric disorders: a pictorial essay, *J Foot Surg* 26:336, 1987.
16. Clark WD, Fann TR, McCrea JD, Venson JN: Use of bone scanning in podiatric medicine, *J Am Podiatry Assoc* 68:621, 1978.
17. Hetherington VJ: Technetium and combined gallium and technetium scans in the neurotrophic foot, *J Am Podiatr Assoc* 72:458, 1982.
18. Schlefman BS: Radiographic modalities and interpretation. In Marcinko DE, ed: *Medical and surgical therapeutics of the foot and ankle,* Baltimore, 1992, Williams & Wilkins.
19. Goldman F, Manzi J, Carver A, Torre RJ, Richter R: Sinography in diagnosis of foot infections, *J Am Podiatry Assoc* 71:497, 1981.
20. Marcinko DE: The anatomy of hospital charting (a simplified approach to infected admissions), *Curr Podiatr Med* 9:23, 1985.
21. Dennis KJ: The historical inquisition. In Marcinko DE, ed: *Medical and surgical therapeutics of the foot and ankle,* Baltimore, 1992, Williams & Wilkins.

ADDITIONAL READINGS

An approach to the evaluation of quality indicators of the outcome of care in hospitalized patients, with a focus on nosocomial infection indicators: The Quality Indicator Study Group, *Am J Infect Control* 23: 215, 1995.

Kelta-Perse O, Gaynes RP: Severity of illness scoring systems to adjust nosocomial infection rates: a review and commentary, *Am J Infect Control* 24(6):429, 1996.

Medina-Cuadros M, Sillero-Arenas M, Martinez-Gallego G, Delgado-Rodriguez M: Surgical wound infections diagnosed after discharge from hospital: epidemiologic differences with in-hospital infections, *Am J Infect Control* 24(6):421, 1996.

Salemi C, Morgan J, Padilla S: Association between severity of illness and mortality from nosocomial infections, *Am J Infect Control* 23:188, 1995.

5

Bacteriology and the Role of Glycocalyx in Diabetic Foot Infections

Dwight W. Lambe, Jr.
Kaethe P. Ferguson

I desire no other epitaph—no hurry about it, I may say—than the statement that I taught medical students in the wards, as I regard this as by far the most useful and important work I have been called upon to do. Sir William Osler

The role of bacteria in diabetic foot infections, and the number and species of aerobic and anaerobic microorganisms, will be reviewed in this chapter. The role of glycocalyx and several models of animal and human osteomyelitis will also be presented. In addition, the treatment of staphylococcal osteomyelitis with the antibiotic clindamycin will be discussed.

BACTERIOLOGY OF FOOT INFECTIONS IN DIABETIC PATIENTS

Foot infections are the most common septic problem requiring hospitalization of the diabetic patient, with about 25% of diabetics developing them.[1,2] These infections tend to be polymicrobic, with greater than four species isolated per specimen from deep tissue infections.[3-5] Aerobic organisms such as *Staphylococcus aureus,* coagulase-negative staphylococci, aerobic streptococci, and gram-negative aerobic bacilli have been reported from foot lesions.[2,6] Lambe and Ferguson[7] cultured multiple types of lower extremity infections from 434 diabetic patients. They found that the most common aerobic species included *S. aureus, Staphylococcus epidermidis, Enterococcus, Pseudomonas aeruginosa, Proteus mirabilis,* group B *Streptococcus,* alpha *Streptococcus, Escherichia coli, Klebsiella pneumoniae,* and *Acinetobacter calcoaceticus.*

The association of a putrid odor and soft tissue gas with foot lesions has long been observed, suggesting that anaerobic bacteria play a role in the etiology of diabetic foot lesions.[8] With improvement in methods of specimen collection, transport, and culture in recent years, numerous investigators have shown that anaerobes indeed play a major role in these infections.[3-5,7,9,10]

In reports of bacteria in specimens from foot infections in diabetic patients, the numbers and species of aerobes and anaerobes have varied greatly because each study has sampled a slightly different patient population and used different specimen sources.[3-12] For example, specimens obtained by scraping the base of the foot ulcer or the deep portion of a wound edge were cultured at the bedside in one study of 20 patients.[5]

Another retrospective study reviewed 30 diabetic patients who had undergone surgery for lower limb infections. Specimens were taken during surgery, or deep wound aspirates, taken within the first 48 hours of hospitalization, were analyzed.[9] This study yielded a low incidence of *Clostridium,*[9] also observed by Wheat et al[3] and Lambe and Ferguson.[7] However, specimens from 13 diabetic patients scheduled for lower limb amputations yielded a high percentage of *Clostridium* species.[4] Wheat et al[3] evaluated 131 foot infections in 103 diabetic patients over a 2-year period, culturing specimens from ulcers, abscesses, cutaneous bullae, and bone and soft tissue infections. This group divided specimens into two categories: "unreliable," if the specimen had come into contact with the ulcer or other open draining lesion, and "reliable" if the specimen was not so contaminated. Differences in the incidence of various species of bacteria isolated from unreliable versus reliable sources were noted. Deep surgical specimens from 250 patients with diabetic foot ulcers and bone biopsies from 250 patients with osteomyelitis of one of the bones of the foot were cultured by Klainer and Bisaccia.[7,10] Many species of aerobes and anaerobes have been isolated, and the importance of these species should not be underestimated.

The variation in species identification procedures from different laboratories and changes in taxonomic classification contribute to confusion in comparing different studies. Some authors grouped organisms belonging to *Peptostreptococcus, Peptococcus, Porphyromonas* (formerly *Bacteroides*), *Prevotella* (formerly *Bacteroides*), or *Clostridium* genera without speciating. *Peptostreptococcus magnus, Peptostreptococcus prevotii, Peptostreptococcus asaccharolyticus,* and *Peptostreptococcus anaerobius* represented 58% of anaerobes isolated by Lambe and Ferguson.[7] *Porphyromonas asaccharolytica* (formerly *Bacteroides asaccharolyticus*) and *Prevotella intermedia* (formerly *Bacteroides intermedius*) were reported only by Lambe and Ferguson; these two species plus *Prevotella melaninogenica* (formerly *Bacteroides melaninogenicus*) constituted 12% of anaerobes isolated.

Recent studies that speciated anaerobes reported a high incidence of anaerobes, including *P. asaccharolytica, P. intermedia, P. melaninogenica, Bacteroides fragilis,* other *Bacteroides* species, members of the genus *Peptostreptococcus,* including *P. magnus, P. prevotii, P. asaccharolyticus,* and *P. anaerobius,* other *Peptostreptococcus* species, anaerobic *Streptococcus* species, *Peptococcus* species, *Veillonella parvula, Propionibacterium* species, and various species of *Clostridium,* including *C. perfringens.*[3-5,7,9-11] The ten most common anaerobic species isolated by Lambe and Ferguson included *P. magnus, P. prevotii, P. asaccharolyticus, P. asaccharolytica, Propionibacterium acnes, B. fragilis, P. anaerobius, P. melaninogenica, V. parvula,* and *Eubacterium lentum.*[7] Two important points are noteworthy. First, black-pigmented anaerobes, including *P. asaccharolytica, P. melaninogenica,* and *P. intermedia,* the twelfth most common anaerobe isolated by Lambe and Ferguson, were isolated with very high frequency from these infections. These extremely fastidious anaerobes were notably absent in reports of many studies. These, and other fastidious, organisms require freshly prepared, reduced or prereduced, anaerobically sterilized (PRAS) agar media and an incubation period of up to 10 days for growth. Many strains of the genera *Prevotella* and *Porphyromonas* may take 7 to 10 days of incubation to grow and produce black pigment. Second, *E. lentum,* another slow-growing anaerobe, may take 7 or more days to produce visible colonies. The identification of the black-pigmenting anaerobic bacilli (*P. asaccharolytica, P. melaninogenica,* and *P. intermedia*) is important because this group of bacilli produce important toxins, such as endotoxin, collagenase, fibrinolysin, deoxyribonuclease, and ribonuclease.[13] This group of bacilli are important pathogens in head and neck infections[14] as well as in diabetic foot infections.

Anaerobic bacteria are particularly prevalent in more serious infections, such as necrotizing infections and those involving osteomyelitis.[3] Sapico et al[4] reported that anaerobes outnumbered aerobes 10 to 1 in a study in which deep tissue samples were cultured.

MODE OF BACTERIAL GROWTH IN DIABETIC INFECTIONS AND OSTEOMYELITIS

The microbiology of osteomyelitis

In about one third of diabetic patients hospitalized with foot infections, the soft tissue infection spreads to the medullary cavity of the bone, causing osteomyelitis.[3,15] Osteomyelitis generally requires longer-term antibiotic therapy than soft tissue infections,[15] and surgical intervention is frequently necessary.[15,16]

Numerous reports have reviewed the microbiology of osteomyelitis.[17-23] Generally, there are two types of osteomyelitis, with different organisms involved. Acute osteomyelitis is frequently found in children with associated skin or soft tissue infections, or in adults associated with intravenous drug abuse. These infections usually involve one organism, frequently *S. aureus,* and respond well to antimicrobial therapy.[23] Chronic osteomyelitis is usually associated with an older age group, and may follow trauma or skeletal surgery, frequently with the implantation of a prosthetic device. Lower extremities are usually involved. The microbiology of this type of osteomyelitis is quite different from that of acute osteomyelitis, and the disease is much more difficult to treat. There is usually a polymicrobic infection, involving anaerobes and aerobes.

Until recently, the incidence of anaerobes in bone infection was underestimated. An early report by Taylor and Davies[24] demonstrated that anaerobes were common in long bones of patients who had had war injuries. Their techniques of anaerobic isolation and identification were primitive compared with those of today, and clostridia were primarily isolated. Although sporadic reports of anaerobic involvement in osteomyelitis appeared throughout the century, the importance of anaerobes was not emphasized until Ziment and colleagues' 1968 report in which they described features of osteomyelitis involving anaerobes, including foul odor, failure to isolate aerobic pathogens, soft tissue gas, and the presence of black discharge and necrotic tissue.[17] Specimens from 17 patients with foot infections (8 cases), skull infections (5 cases), and long bone infections (4 cases) all yielded anaerobes, including *B. fragilis, Peptostreptococcus, Peptococcus, Sphaerophorus, Fusobacterium,* and *Bifidobacterium.* With the improvement of transport and culture techniques for anaerobes, the importance of these organisms in osteomyelitis became apparent. Lewis and associates' review of anaerobes in bone infections, through 1975, cites over 700 cases of anaerobic osteomyelitis reported in the literature.[19] The anaerobes most frequently isolated have been *B. fragilis,* black-pigmented anaerobic gram-negative rods, and anaerobic cocci, although numerous species of anaerobes have been reported. The longer the duration of chronic disease, the greater the number of anaerobic species that have been isolated.[20]

Generally, surgery is required, with removal of necrotic tissue and any implanted foreign body, along with long-term antibiotic therapy. Gristina et al[25] have emphasized the importance of adherent bacteria in the persistence of osteomyelitis.

Bacterial glycocalyx

Bacterial growth on a bone surface contributes to the development and persistence of chronic diseases such as osteomyelitis.[26-29] The mode of growth involves the glycocalyx, which is a network of exopolysaccharide polymers elaborated by bacteria.[30] The term glycocalyx includes the capsule surrounding the bacterial cell, as well as the "slime" that detaches from the cell, floats away, and adheres to surrounding tissue.

The glycocalyx mediates attachment of the bacterial cells to each other, forming microcolonies, and to a wide variety of surfaces, including substrates in the natural environment, bone, and artificial prostheses.[30] The microcolonies form thick biofilms composed of bacteria and glycocalyx, which render the bacteria resistant to surfactants[31] and antibiotics[32] and to destruction by host defense mechanisms such as antibodies[33] and phagocytosis.[34-36]

Bacterial glycocalyces are present in chronic diseases such as cystic fibrosis,[37] and in foreign body–related infections.[38-40] The glycocalyx therefore plays a role in the persistence of many chronic diseases, including osteomyelitis.[25] Ultrastructural studies in animal models of experimentally induced osteomyelitis have shown that glycocalyces are formed by *S. aureus, Prevotella bivia* (formerly *Bacteroides bivius*), *Prevotella disiens* (formerly *Bacteroides disiens*), *Bacteroides thetaiotaomicron, B. fragilis,* and *P. intermedia.*[28,41,42] The same mode of growth observed in animal models is seen in human osteomyelitis.[26,27,29,42] Foreign bodies such as surgically implanted biomaterials and prosthetic devices are reported to increase infection rates,[43,44] presumably by serving as substrates for sessile, glycocalyx-enclosed microorganisms.

Osteomyelitis is a disease that is recalcitrant to medical and surgical forms of treatment, although reasons for this were unknown until the role of the glycocalyx was elucidated. We established several rabbit models of osteomyelitis, which demonstrated that the mode of bacterial growth and the production of glycocalyx were important factors in treating osteomyelitis. A description of these animal models and the mode of bacterial growth follows.

Staphylococcus aureus rabbit model of osteomyelitis

Osteomyelitis was induced in rabbits by using *S. aureus.*[27] A piece of silicone-coated rubber catheter (foreign body) was surgically implanted in the marrow cavity of a rabbit tibia, with the introduction of a sclerosing agent and bacterial cells. Osteomyelitis developed in 60% of animals infected with *S. aureus,* as determined by radiologic and histologic examination. Organisms were recovered from infected samples of animals with osteomyelitis. Samples of bone marrow, bone chips, and foreign bodies were examined by transmission electron microscopy (TEM) and scanning electron microscopy (SEM). Infection with the accompanying production of glycocalyx advanced from the injection site into nearby bone and the foreign body.

The model of osteomyelitis in the rabbit shares many similarities with the human disease. Animals that developed osteomyelitis showed weight loss and radiologic evidence of progressive disease. Histologic samples of rabbit tibia showed striking morphologic changes in infected animals

consistent with a diagnosis of osteomyelitis. This model showed a high rate of induction of osteomyelitis, with recovery of *S. aureus* in pure culture from infected tibia, and gram-positive cocci were seen histologically.

Ultrastructural studies performed using this model showed that large quantities of *S. aureus* glycocalyx were present in the infection. TEM of samples from bone scrapings and bone marrow showed microcolonies of gram-positive cocci surrounded by glycocalyx either condensed on the bacterial cell surface or in a fibrous intracellular network. Material from the interior of the foreign body showed masses of gram-positive cocci embedded in glycocalyx. It appears that this mode of growth—that is, large amounts of glycocalyx surrounding masses of bacterial microcolonies—is typical of osteomyelitis. Thus, it is not surprising that this disease is so difficult to treat with antibiotics, which fail to penetrate the glycocalyx.[45]

A view of the surface of the infected bone and foreign body was provided by SEM.[27] Normal topographic features of the bone were altered dramatically by copious material adhering to the bone. Further magnification of this material revealed coccoid forms embedded in a matrix of accreted material. The accretions were observed on the interior and exterior surfaces of the foreign body. The accreted material observed for the rabbit model of osteomyelitis was far more extensive than has been previously described for the adhesion of uropathogens to polypropylene surfaces.

S. aureus cells in this rabbit model grew in thick, adherent, glycocalyx-enclosed biofilms. This aggregated mode of growth of the pathogen presented a fibrous exopolysaccharide bacterial cell surface to the host defense mechanisms and a thick anionic barrier to the penetration of antibiotics. This mode of growth helps to explain the persistence of these pathogens in osteomyelitis.

Additional rabbit models of osteomyelitis with gram-negative anaerobes and *Staphylococcus*

Following the development of the *S. aureus* osteomyelitis rabbit model, other bacteria were studied in this animal model to determine if a similar mode of growth was occurring with certain gram-negative anaerobes and staphylococci. The organisms examined included *B. fragilis, B. thetaiotaomicron, P. bivia, P. disiens, S. aureus,* and *S. epidermidis,* alone or in combination.[28,42,46] The mode of growth and the formation of glycocalyx found with these bacteria in osteomyelitis were similar to those observed with *S. aureus* alone. A description of the bacterial growth on the foreign body, in bone marrow, and on the bone surface follows.

Figs. 5-1 to 5-4 are electron micrographs of material from foreign bodies removed from rabbits infected with various combinations of gram-negative anaerobes and *Staphylococcus.* A low-magnification overview of the biofilm (bacteria plus glycocalyx in the form of innumerable microcolonies covered with slime) covering the foreign body is seen in Fig. 5-1. This foreign body from a rabbit infected with *B. thetaiotaomicron* and *S. aureus* is heavily encrusted with

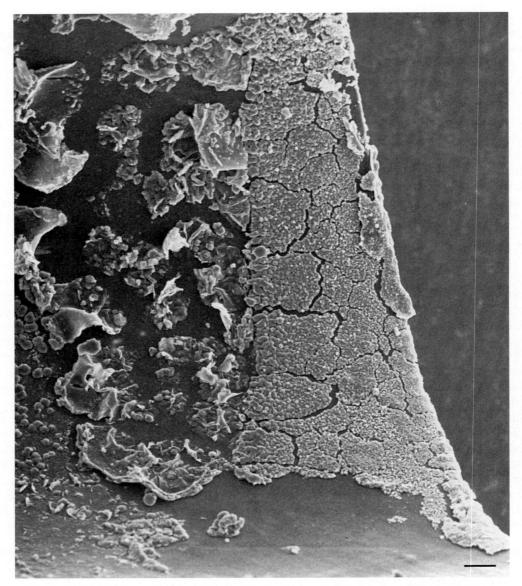

Fig. 5-1 SEM of an overview of the catheter (foreign body) from a rabbit infected with *B. thetaiotaomicron* and *S. aureus.* Extensive biofilm covers the foreign body surface. (Bar = 50 µm.)

a biofilm of bacteria and glycocalyx. Fig. 5-2, the SEM view of a foreign body sample from the same rabbit, shows a preponderance of cocci, heavily encased in a sticky glycocalyx. We have observed that in a mixed infection involving *Bacteroides* and *Staphylococcus* species, the *Bacteroides* appear to heavily colonize the bone, while more cocci are observed on the foreign body implant.[28,46,47] However, a TEM view of a foreign body scraping from a rabbit infected with *B. fragilis* alone shows that the *Bacteroides* do adhere to the foreign body.[28] Individual cells are surrounded by large amounts of glycocalyx (Fig. 5-3). In rabbits infected with *Bacteroides* and *Staphylococcus*, small numbers of gram-negative rods are observed sticking to the foreign body, as in 5-4. Note the large amount of glycocalyx

surrounding this cell of *B. thetaiotaomicron,* which contributes to its ability to adhere to the foreign body.[47] Samples taken from bone marrow show rods and cocci enmeshed in glycocalyx.[28] Fig. 5-5 shows the marrow from a rabbit monoinfected with *B. fragilis.* Numerous rod-shaped bacteria were present on exposed surfaces of the marrow. The cells appeared to penetrate the marrow and lie partially buried within it. The marrow from a rabbit infected with *B. thetaiotaomicron* and *S. aureus* reveals a particularly sticky glycocalyx covering bacteria profile (Fig. 5-6). Fig. 5-7 shows the marrow from a rabbit infected with *B. thetaiotaomicron* and *S. epidermidis* with a foreign body implant and with *B. thetaiotaomicron* and *S. aureus* without a foreign body implant. Numerous rods and cocci were observed in the

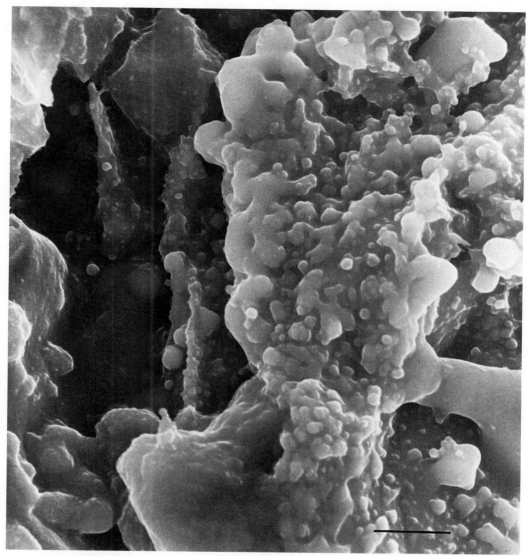

Fig. 5-2 SEM of the surface of the foreign body from a rabbit infected with *B. thetaiotaomicron* and *S. aureus*. Bacterial accretions extend from an extremely viscous matrix of glycocalyx. The foreign body surface is completely obscured. (Bar = 5 μm.)

marrow.[47] When rabbits were infected with *B. fragilis* alone or in combination with *S. epidermidis,* 100% of rabbits developed osteomyelitis.[7] Fig. 5-8, an SEM view of a bone chip, shows heavy colonization by adherent microcolonies of rod-shaped bacteria that tend to form chains. Fig. 5-9, a bone chip from a rabbit infected with *B. thetaiotaomicron* and *S. epidermidis,* also shows bone largely colonized by rods. Masses of bacteria, partially or almost entirely encased in glycocalyx, are present. Again, in a mixed infection, the rods predominated on the bone surface, while cocci predominated on the foreign body.[28,46,47]

The pathogenicity of the organisms tested in the rabbit model varied. *B. fragilis* induced osteomyelitis at high rates, alone or in combination with *S. epidermidis.* The *B. fragilis*

isolates, when the rabbit model came from a patient with osteomyelitis, are more virulent than strains isolated from other types of clinical infection.[48] *B. thetaiotaomicron* and *S. epidermidis* can induce osteomyelitis alone or in combination. However, the incidence of osteomyelitis is higher in polymicrobic infection (95%) than in animals infected with either species alone. In addition, the presence of a foreign body enhanced the incidence of osteomyelitis in monoinfected rabbits.[42] However, when a foreign body was present in combination with *S. epidermidis* and *B. thetaiotaomicron,* 73% of rabbits developed osteomyelitis, compared with 25% infected with *S. epidermidis* alone.[42] Thus, there is an important synergistic relationship between *S. epidermidis* and certain anaerobic gram-negative bacilli.

Text continued on p. 61

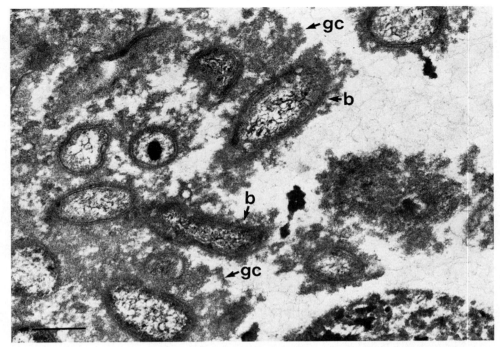

Fig. 5-3 TEM of a section of ruthenium red–stained biofilm scraped from the surface of the foreign body from a rabbit infected with *B. fragilis.* Gram-negative rod-shaped bacterial cells *(arrows, b)* enclosed in extensive fibrous anionic glycocalyces *(arrows, gc)* were found throughout this accreted material. (Bar = 0.5 μm.) *(From Lambe DW Jr et al.[28])*

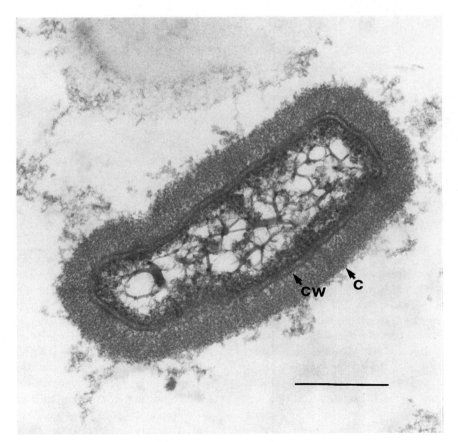

Fig. 5-4 TEM of a thin section of a sample of material scraped from the surface of a foreign body from a rabbit infected with *B. thetaiotaomicron* and *S. epidermidis.* A thick, ruthenium red–stained capsule *(arrow, c)* extends beyond the gram-negative bacterial cell wall *(arrow, cw).* (Bar = 0.5 μm.) *(From Mayberry-Carson KJ et al.[47])*

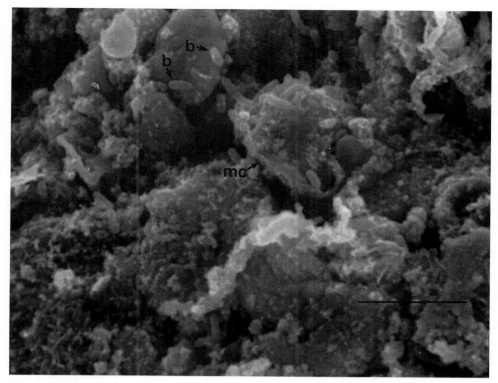

Fig. 5-5 SEM of bone marrow from the tibia of a rabbit infected with *B. fragilis.* Rod-shaped bacterial cells *(arrows, b)* were present on exposed surfaces of the marrow. Many cells appeared to penetrate this material and to lie partially buried within it. Some apparent bacterial microcolonies *(arrow, mc)* were present in the marrow where aggregates of bacteria appeared to coalesce to form large masses. (Bar = 5 μm.) *(From Lambe DW Jr et al.[28])*

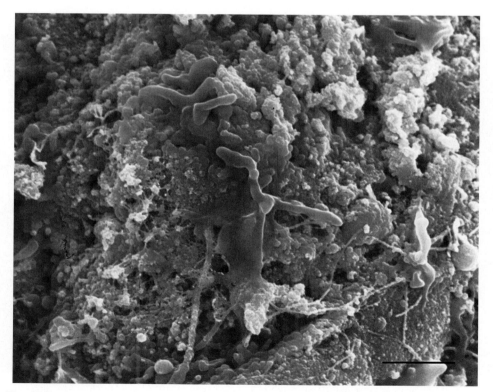

Fig. 5-6 SEM of bone marrow from the tibia of a rabbit infected with *B. thetaiotaomicron* and *S. aureus.* A very extensive biofilm can be seen, with bacterial accretions in the shape of rods and cocci extending from the surface. The glycocalyx surrounding the masses of cells appears quite viscous in some areas. (Bar = 5 μm.)

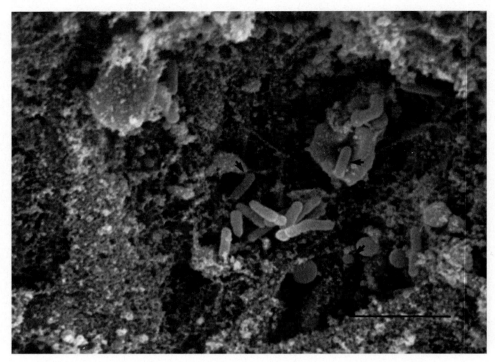

Fig. 5-7 SEM of bone marrow from the tibia of a rabbit infected with *B. thetaiotaomicron* and *S. epidermidis*. Cocci and rods *(arrows)* were observed in the marrow. (Bar = 5 μm.) *(From Mayberry-Carson KJ et al.[46])*

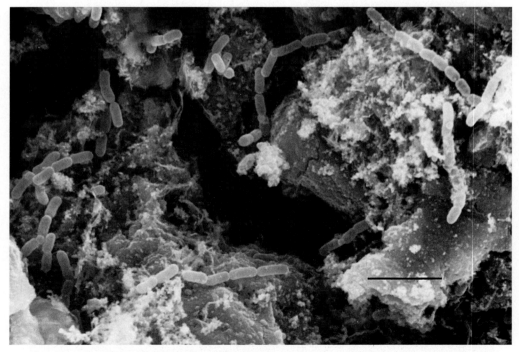

Fig. 5-8 SEM of a bone chip from a rabbit infected with *B. fragilis*. The surface of the bone chip was heavily colonized by adherent microcolonies of rod-shaped bacteria that formed chains. (Bar = 5 μm.)

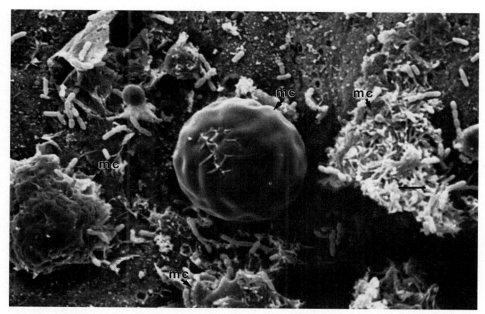

Fig. 5-9 SEM of a bone chip from the tibia of a rabbit infected with both *B. thetaiotaomicron* and *S. epidermidis,* with a foreign body implant. The bone surface was covered with predominantly microcolonies *(arrows, mc)* of rod-shaped bacteria. (Bar = 5 µm.) *(From Mayberry-Carson KJ et al.[46])*

TREATMENT OF STAPHYLOCOCCAL OSTEOMYELITIS WITH CLINDAMYCIN

After induction of experimental osteomyelitis with *S. aureus,* animals were treated with clindamycin phosphate for 1-, 2-, or 3-week periods.[49] SEM of infected bone samples showed masses of coccoid profiles embedded in a matrix of condensed glycocalyx. This material was present in untreated animals and those treated with clindamycin for 1 week. Fig. 5-10, an SEM view of biofilm covering a bone chip from an untreated, infected animal, shows coccoid bacterial profiles in an amorphous glycocalyx matrix. After 2 to 3 weeks of clindamycin treatment, SEM revealed few coccoid profiles adhering to the bone and marrow. Fig. 5-11, an SEM image of material from the tibia of a *S. aureus*–infected rabbit after 3 weeks of treatment with clindamycin phosphate, shows clearance of the biofilm. Cultures of bone marrow and bone were negative.

Many aspects of the rabbit model of osteomyelitis are quite similar to human osteomyelitis. Roentgenographic evidence of progressive disease was seen in animals with osteomyelitis, and histologic observations showed changes in the tissues consistent with human osteomyelitis. Infecting microorganisms can also be recovered from sites of infection in the animal model, as with human osteomyelitis.[49]

HUMAN OSTEOMYELITIS

Ultrastructural studies of specimens from patients with osteomyelitis show that the mode of bacterial growth is the same in human and experimentally induced osteomyelitis.[29] A 69-year-old diabetic man developed osteomyelitis in the right hallux, which was amputated. A presurgical specimen cultured by the hospital clinical laboratory yielded beta-hemolytic *Streptococcus* and *Staphylococcus*. A portion of bone from the amputated toe cultured in the hospital laboratory was negative for anaerobes and aerobes. Another portion of the bone was placed in a sterile Petri plate in an anaerobe jar, and transported to an anaerobe chamber within 20 minutes of removal from the patient. Culture of this bone yielded no aerobes, but the anaerobes *B. fragilis, P. asaccharolytica, P. anaerobius, P. magnus,* and *P. acnes* were found.[29] SEM of the bone surface showed bacilli connected by strands of glycocalyx (Fig. 5-12). Another bone surface, at a greater magnification, showed a bacillus surrounded by a profusion of glycocalyx strands (Fig. 5-13). Figs. 5-14 and 5-15 demonstrate cocci of various sizes, ranging from 0.8 µm, the size range of *P. anaerobius,* to 5.0 µm, the size range of *P. magnus*.[29] The organisms observed in Figs. 5-12 to 5-15, embedded in varying amounts of glycocalyx on the bone surface, were quite similar in appearance to the previous figures showing bone surfaces of rabbits with bacterial osteomyelitis (Figs. 5-1 to 5-9).

Fig. 5-16 is an SEM view of the bone surface from another diabetic patient with osteomyelitis. *P. aeruginosa* was cultured from this amputated toe.[7] Copious amounts of glycocalyx surround and connect bacilli. The similarity between this photograph and Fig. 5-8, showing bacilli on the bone surface of a rabbit with osteomyelitis, is marked.

Text continued on p. 65

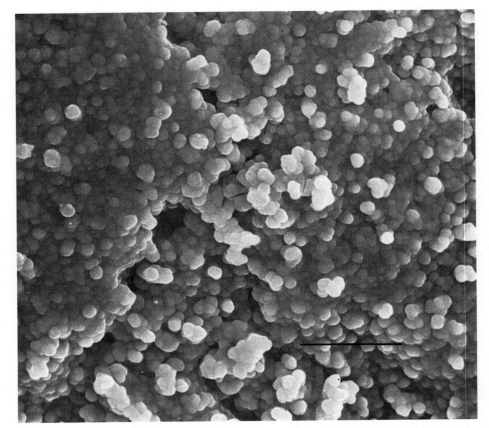

Fig. 5-10 SEM of a bone sample from the tibia of a rabbit infected with *S. aureus*. The surface of the bone is completely obscured by a biofilm showing coccoid profiles in an amorphous glycocalyx matrix. (Bar = 5 μm.) *(From Mayberry-Carson KJ et al.[49])*

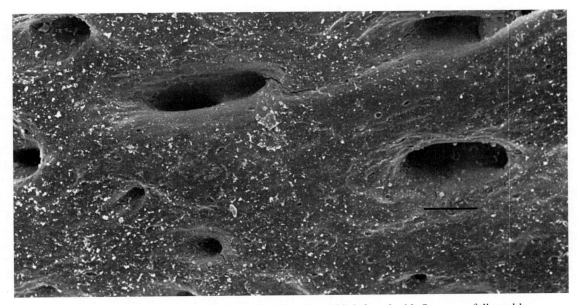

Fig. 5-11 SEM of a bone sample from the tibia of a rabbit infected with *S. aureus*, followed by three weeks of treatment with clindamycin phosphate. The biofilm has been cleared from the bone surface. (Bar = 100 μm.) *(From Mayberry-Carson et al.[49])*

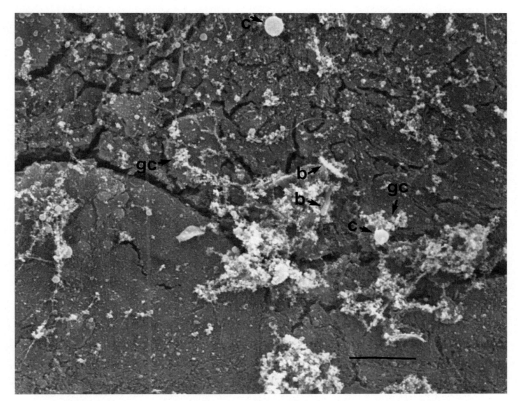

Fig. 5-12 SEM of bone chip from a patient with osteomyelitis. Bacilli *(arrows, b),* cocci *(arrows, c),* and glycocalyx *(arrows, gc)* were visible. (Bar = 5 μm.) *(From Lambe DW Jr et al.[29])*

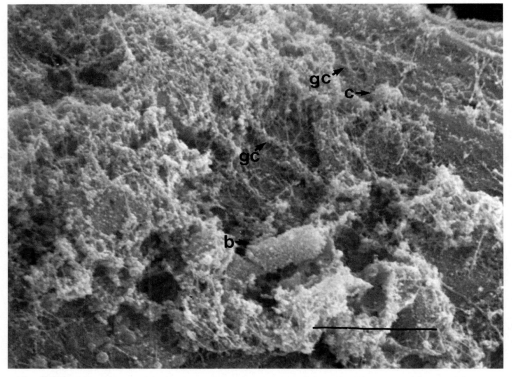

Fig. 5-13 SEM of bone chip from a patient with osteomyelitis. A bacillus *(arrow, b),* cocci *(arrow, c)* and tangled masses of glycocalyx *(arrows, gc)* attached to the bone surface. (Bar = 5 μm.) *(From Lambe DW Jr et al.[29])*

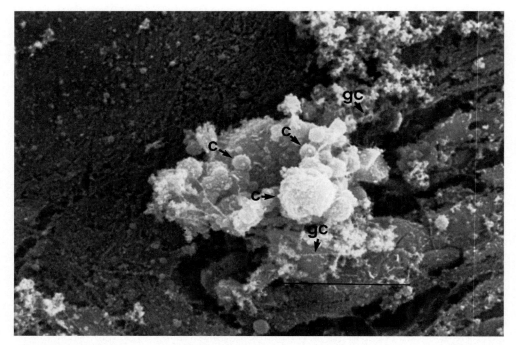

Fig. 5-14 SEM of bone surface from a patient with osteomyelitis. A clump of cocci of varying sizes *(arrows, c)* was present. Glycocalyx strands *(arrows, gc)* attached cocci to the bone surface. (Bar = 5 μm.) *(From Lambe DW Jr et al.[29])*

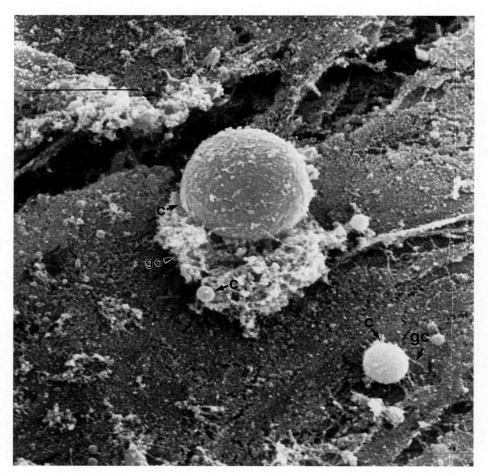

Fig. 5-15 SEM of bone surface from a patient with osteomyelitis. This enlargement showed cocci 1.8 to 5 μm in diameter, the size of *P. magnus,* and cocci 0.8 to 1.0 μm in diameter, the size of *P. anaerobius.* Glycocalyx strands *(arrows, gc)* connected cocci *(arrows, c)* to bone surface. (Bar = 5 μm.) *(From Lambe DW Jr et al. [29])*

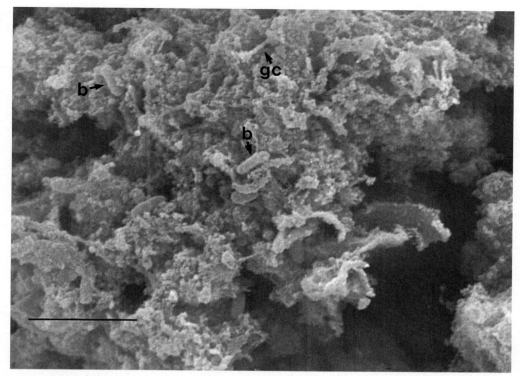

Fig. 5-16 SEM of the bone surface from a diabetic patient with osteomyelitis, from which *Pseudomonas aeruginosa* was cultured. A massive biofilm occludes the bone surface. Bacillary profiles *(arrows, b)* protrude from the biofilm, surrounded by glycocalyx *(arrow, gc)*. (Bar = 5 μm.) *(From Lambe DW and Ferguson KP.[7])*

INFLUENCE OF GLYCOCALYX ON INFECTION

Bacterial adherence to bone inhibited by clindamycin

In an in vitro study to examine the effect of subinhibitory concentrations of clindamycin on the adherence of bacteria to bone, *S. aureus* and *P. intermedia* were grown in broth media containing discs of rabbit tibia in the absence or presence of varying concentrations of clindamycin.[50] In the absence of clindamycin, *S. aureus* colonized the bone surface extensively, and formed large microcolonies surrounded by glycocalyx (Fig. 5-17). When grown in 0.1 minimal inhibitory concentration (MIC) of clindamycin, *S. aureus* adherence to bone surfaces decreased 80%, with fewer and smaller microcolonies present (Fig. 5-18). At a concentration of 0.25 MIC clindamycin, only a rare microcolony was seen, with most of the bone surface uncolonized (Fig. 5-19). No colonization occurred at 0.5 MIC clindamycin.[50]

Fig. 5-20 shows heavy colonization of the bone surface by *P. intermedia* in the absence of antibiotic.[7,29] Unlike *S. aureus*, 0.1 MIC clindamycin had little effect upon adherence of *P. intermedia*. A concentration of 0.25 MIC clindamycin was required to dislodge 80% of *P. intermedia* from the bone.[7,29] At a concentration of 0.5 MIC clin-

damycin, single cells and small microcolonies were still observed, with much bone surface visible (Fig. 5-21). In the presence of 1.0 MIC clindamycin, no colonization was observed.[7,29]

Inhibition of phagocytosis by glycocalyx

Veringa et al[51] showed that subinhibitory concentrations of clindamycin and trospectomycin significantly enhanced the phagocytosis of glycocalyx-enclosed *Bacteroides*. Without antibiotic treatment, few bacterial cells were phagocytized. The bacterial cells that were phagocytized contained little or no glycocalyx. Fig. 5-22 shows a polymorphonuclear leukocyte containing a large number of cells of *B. thetaiotaomicron* that had been cultured in 0.5 MIC clindamycin. *B. fragilis* grown in 0.5 MIC clindamycin was also more susceptible to phagocytosis (Fig. 5-23). A moderate amount of glycocalyx was observed surrounding *B. thetaiotaomicron*, but a thick layer surrounded clindamycin-treated *B. fragilis* cells. Homologous or heterologous glycocalyx added to preopsonized, preadhered *B. fragilis*, *B. thetaiotaomicron*, or *S. epidermidis* prior to incubation with polymorphonuclear leukocytes had no effect upon phagocytosis of untreated bacteria, because the untreated bacterial cells already had glycocalyx that was antiphagocytic. However, when isolated glycocalyx from *B. thetaiotaomicron* or *B. fragilis* was added to clindamycin- or trospectomycin-treated bacteria, phagocytosis was significantly reduced.

This effect of glycocalyx on phagocytosis was quantitative[35,36]; the more glycocalyx added, the less phagocytosis. The antibiotic altered the glycocalyx in some unknown way so that the glycocalyx was no longer antiphagocytic. The decrease in phagocytosis caused by the addition of glycocalyx to antibiotic-treated cells demonstrates that glycocalyx *per se* is antiphagocytic. Glycocalyx preparations from *Bacteroides* and *Staphylococcus* significantly inhibited the chemiluminescence and chemotactic responses of viable polymorphonuclear leukocytes, without toxicity to the polymorphonuclear leukocytes.[52]

These studies showed that the glycocalyx specifically inhibits phagocytosis, chemiluminescence, and chemotactic responses of viable PMNLs. Certain other antibiotics, such as amdinocillin, ceftriaxone, and ciprofloxacin, did not alter the glycocalyx; thus they did not enhance phagocytosis.

Inhibition of lymphocyte proliferation by glycocalyx

Ten to 100 µg/ml of glycocalyx isolated from *Staphylococcus lugdunensis* or *S. epidermidis* and partially purified under endotoxin-free conditions inhibited the phytohemagglutinin-stimulated proliferation of peripheral-blood mononuclear cells.[53] When peripheral-blood mononuclear cells were depleted of adherent monocytes, the phytohemagglutinin-stimulated proliferation of nonadherent cells (PBML) occurred in the presence or absence of glycocalyx. Therefore, the mechanism of glycocalyx-mediated inhibition required the presence of adherent

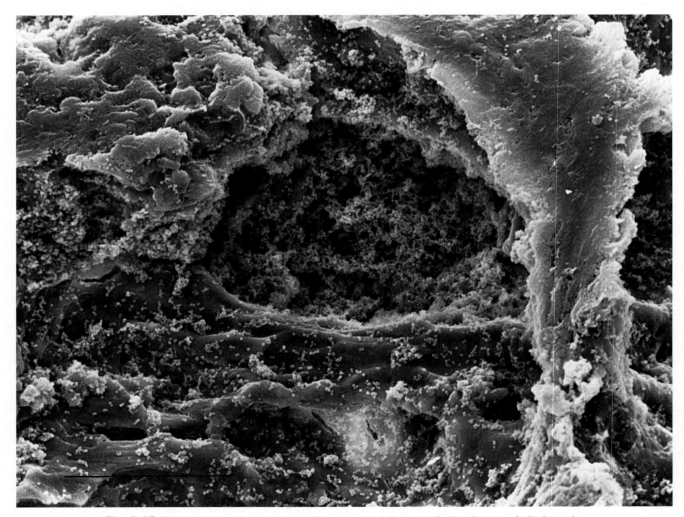

Fig. 5-17 SEM of the surface of a bone disc exposed to *S. aureus* in the absence of clindamycin, for 48 hours. There is extensive colonization of the bone. (Bar = 50 µm.) *(From Mayberry-Carson KJ et al.[50])*

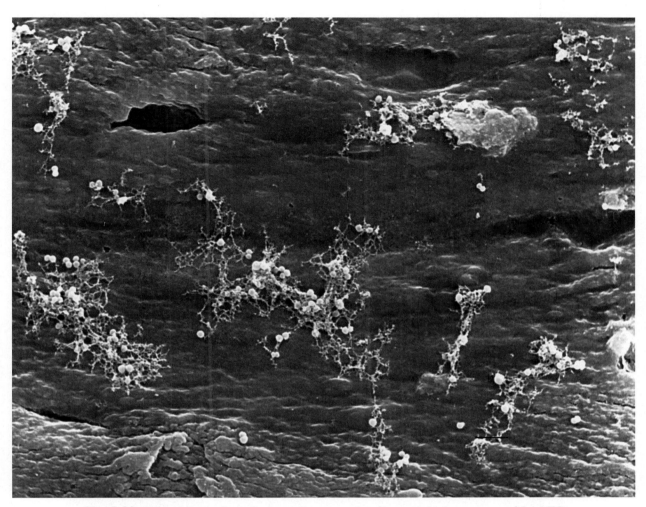

Fig. 5-18 SEM of the surface of a bone disc exposed to *S. aureus* in the presence of 0.1 MIC clindamycin, for 48 hours. Clindamycin decreased colonization of the bone by 80%. Discrete-matrix-enclosed microcolonies can be seen on the bone surface. (Bar = 5 μm.) *(From Mayberry-Carson KJ et al.[50])*

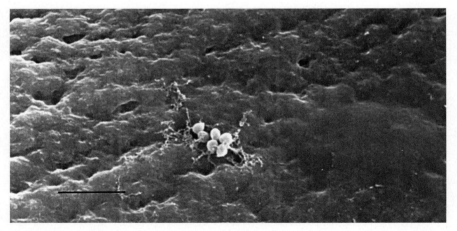

Fig. 5-19 SEM of the surface of a bone disc exposed to *S. aureus* in the presence of 0.25 MIC clindamycin, for 48 hours. The bone surface is sparsely colonized by bacteria in microcolonies surrounded by relatively small amounts of condensed extracellular material. (Bar = 5 μm.) *(From Mayberry-Carson KJ et al.[50])*

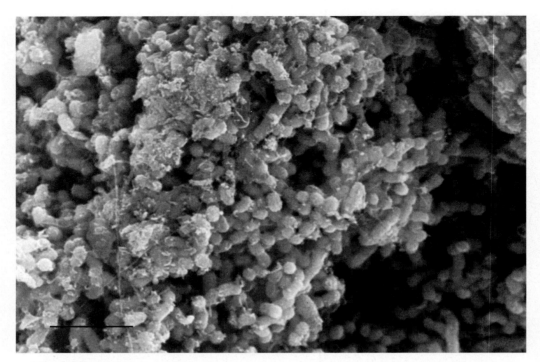

Fig. 5-20 SEM of the surface of a bone disc exposed to *P. intermedius* in the absence of clindamycin, for 48 hours. There is extensive colonization of the bone. Massive numbers of bacilli colonized the bone surface. (Bar = 5 μm.) *(From Lambe DW Jr et al.[29])*

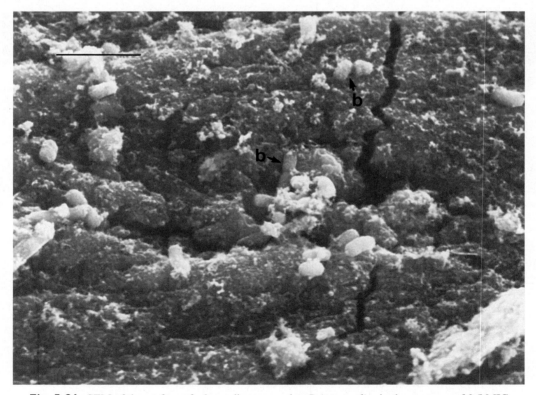

Fig. 5-21 SEM of the surface of a bone disc exposed to *P. intermedius* in the presence of 0.5 MIC clindamycin, for 48 hours. Few bacilli *(arrows, b)* with little glycocalyx remained adhered to the bone, with much of the bone surface exposed. (Bar = 5 μm.) *(From Lambe DW and Ferguson KP.[7])*

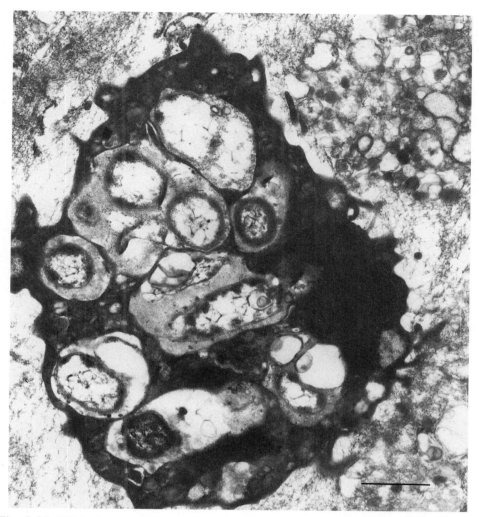

Fig. 5-22 TEM of *B. thetaiotaomicron* treated overnight with 0.5 MIC clindamycin. Bacteria were opsonized in 40% heated specific antiserum for 15 minutes and incubated with PMNs for 15 minutes. A PMN contains such a large number of bacteria that the nucleus is pushed to the side of the cell. A moderate amount of glycocalyx is present around some cells. (Bar = 1 μm.) *(From Veringa EM et al.[51])*

monocytes. Culture supernatants of monocytes stimulated by glycocalyx contained a soluble factor that inhibited proliferation of monocyte-depleted peripheral blood mononuclear cells. The soluble factor was not produced in the absence of glycocalyx. Nor was it produced when glycocalyx was added to peripheral-blood mononuclear cells along with indomethacin, which inhibits the synthesis of prostaglandin E_2, a product of adherent blood monocytes. Therefore, the glycocalyx does not have a direct effect upon T lymphocytes, but rather inhibits proliferation indirectly by stimulating monocyte production of prostaglandin E_2, which in turn inhibits lymphocyte proliferation.[53]

CONCLUSION

The role of bacteria in diabetic foot infections, and the number and species of aerobic and anaerobic microorganisms, were reviewed in this chapter. The role of glycocalyx and several models of animal and human osteomyelitis were also presented. Finally, the treatment of staphylococcal osteomyelitis with the antibiotic clindamycin was elucidated.

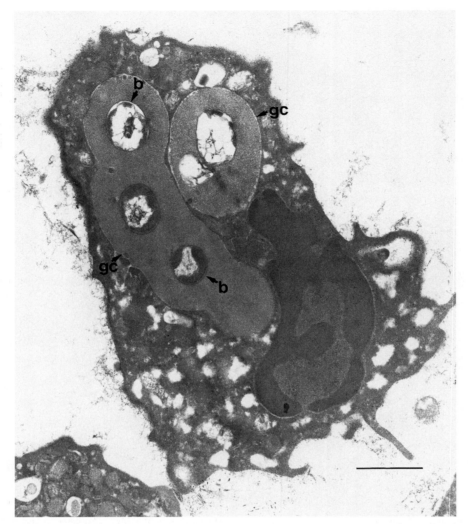

Fig. 5-23 TEM of *B. fragilis* treated overnight with 0.5 MIC clindamycin. Bacteria were opsonized in 40% heated specific antiserum for 15 minutes and incubated with PMNs for 15 minutes. A PMN contains bacterial cells *(arrows, b)* surrounded by glycocalyx *(arrows, gc)*. (Bar = 1 μm.)

REFERENCES

1. Drury T, Danchik K, Harris M: Sociodemographic characteristics of adult diabetics. In Harris M, Hamman R, eds: Diabetes in America, Washington, D.C., 1988, U.S. Government Printing Office, VII.1-VII.37.
2. Pratt TC: Gangrene and infection in the diabetic, *Med Clin North Am* 49:987-1004, 1965.
3. Fineberg N, Norton J: Diabetic foot infections: bacteriologic analysis, *Arch Intern Med* 146:1935-1940, 1986.
4. Sapico FL, Canawati NH, Witte JL, Montgomerie JZ, Wagner FW, Bessman AN: Quantitative aerobic and anaerobic bacteriology of infected diabetic feet, *J Clin Microbiol* 12:413-420, 1980.
5. Louie TJ, Bartlett JG, Tally FP, Gorbach SL: Aerobic and anaerobic bacteria in diabetic foot ulcers, *Ann Intern Med* 85:461-463, 1976.
6. Sharp CS, Bessman AN, Wagner FW Jr, Garland D: Microbiology of deep tissue in diabetic gangrene, *Diabetes Care* 1:289-292, 1978.
7. Lambe DW, Ferguson KP: Microbial nature of diabetic foot infections. In Bakker K, Nieuwenhuijzen Kruseman AC, eds: *Proceedings of the 1st International Symposium on the Diabetic Foot,* Noordwijkerhout, The Netherlands, 1991, Excerpta Medica, pp 83-97.
8. Meleney FL: Gangrene of the extremity in the diabetic, *Ann Surg* 110:723, 1939.

9. Fierer J, Daniel D, Davis C: The fetid foot: lower-extremity infections in patients with diabetes mellitus, *Rev Infect Dis* 1:210-217, 1979.
10. Klainer AS, Bisaccia E: Antibiotic therapy in the treatment of diabetic foot infections. In Bakker K, Nieuwenhuijzen Kruseman AC, eds: *Proceedings of the 1st International Symposium on the Diabetic Foot,* Noordwijkerhout, The Netherlands; 1991, pp 98-105.
11. Klainer AS: Clindamycin in the treatment of diabetic foot infections. In Zambrano D, ed: *Clindamycin in the treatment of human infections,* Kalamazoo, Mich, 1992, The Upjohn Co, pp 9.1-9.16.
12. Gibbons GE, Eliopoulas GM: Infection of the diabetic foot. In Kozak GP, Hoar CS Jr, Rowbotham JL, eds: *Management of diabetic foot problems,* Philadelphia, 1984, WB Saunders, pp 97-102.
13. Lambe DW Jr: Serology of *Bacteroidaceae.* In Lambe DW Jr, Genco RJ, Mayberry-Carson KJ, eds: *Anaerobic bacteria, selected topics.* New York, 1980, Plenum Press, pp 141-153.
14. Finegold SM: Ear, nose, throat, and head and neck infections. In Finegold SM, ed: *Anaerobic bacteria in human disease,* New York, 1977, Academic Press, pp 115-154.
15. Lipsky BA, Pecoraro RE, Wheat LJ: The diabetic foot: soft tissue and bone infection, *Infect Dis North Am* 4:483-492, 1990.

16. Bamberger DM, Daus GP, Gerding DN: Osteomyelitis in the feet of diabetic patients: long term results, prognostic factors and the role of antimicrobial and surgical therapy, *Am J Med* 83:653-660, 1987.

17. Ziment I, Miller LG, Finegold SM: Nonsporulating anaerobic bacteria in osteomyelitis, *Antimicrob Agents Chemother* 7:77-85, 1968.

18. Finegold SM: Bone and joint infections. In Finegold SM, ed: *Anaerobic bacteria in human disease,* New York, 1977, Academic Press, pp 433-454.

19. Lewis RP, Sutter VL, Finegold SM: Bone infections involving anaerobic bacteria, *Medicine* 57:279-305, 1978.

20. Raff MJ, Melo JC: Anaerobic osteomyelitis, *Medicine* 57:83-103, 1978.

21. Nakata MM, Lewis RP: Anaerobic bacteria in bone and joint infections, *Rev Infect Dis* 6:s165-s170, 1984.

22. Templeton WC III, Wawrukiewicz A, Melo JC, Schiller MG, Raff MJ: Anaerobic osteomyelitis of long bones, *Rev Infect Dis* 5:692-712, 1983.

23. Gentry LO. Osteomyelitis: options for diagnosis and management, *J Antimicrob Chemother* 21 (suppl C):115-128.

24. Taylor K, Davies M: Persistence of bacteria within sequestra, *Ann Surg* 66:522-528, 1917.

25. Gristina AG, Oga M, Webb LX, Hobgood CD: Adherent bacterial colonization in the pathogenesis of osteomyelitis, *Science* 228:990-993, 1985.

26. Marrie JW, Costerton JW: Mode of growth of bacterial pathogens in chronic polymicrobial human osteomyelitis, *J Clin Microbiol* 22:924-933, 1985.

27. Mayberry-Carson KJ, Tober-Meyer B, Smith JK, Lambe DW Jr, Costerton JW: Bacterial adherence and glycocalyx formation in osteomyelitis experimentally induced with *Staphylococcus aureus,* *Infect Immun* 43:825-833, 1984.

28. Lambe DW Jr, Ferguson KP, Mayberry-Carson KJ, Tober-Meyer B, Costerton JW: Foreign-body-associated experimental osteomyelitis induced with *Bacteroides fragilis* and *Staphylococcus epidermidis* in rabbits, *Clin Orthop* 266:285-294, 1991.

29. Lambe DW Jr, Mayberry-Carson KJ, Mayberry WR, Tober-Meyer BK, Costerton JW: The effect of subinhibitory concentrations of clindamycin on the adherence and role of glycocalyx in *Staphylococcus aureus* and *Bacteroides* species in vitro and in vivo. In Szentivanyi A, Friedman H, Gillissen, eds: *Antibiosis and host immunity,* New York, 1987, Plenum, pp 35-49.

30. Costerton JW, Irvin RT, Cheng K-J: The bacterial glycocalyx in nature and disease, *Annu Rev Microbiol* 35:299-324, 1981.

31. Govan JRW: Mucoid strains of *Pseudomonas aeruginosa:* the influence of culture medium on the stability of mucus production, *J Med Microbiol* 8:513-522, 1975.

32. Costerton JW: Cell envelope as a barrier to antibiotics. In Schlessinger D, ed: *Microbiology—1977,* Washington, D.C, 1977, American Society for Microbiology, pp 151-157.

33. Baltimore RS, Mitchell M: Immunologic investigation of mucoid strains of *Pseudomonas aeruginosa:* comparison of susceptibility to opsonic antibody in mucoid and non-mucoid strains, *J Infect Dis* 141:238-247, 1980.

34. Schwarzmann S, Boring JR III: Antiphagocytic effect of slime from a mucoid strain of *Pseudomonas aeruginosa,* *Infect Immun* 3:762-767, 1971.

35. Veringa EM, Ferguson DA Jr, Lambe DW Jr, Verhoef J: The role of glycocalyx in surface phagocytosis of *Bacteroides* spp., in the presence and absence of clindamycin, *J Antimicrob Chemother* 23:711-720, 1989.

36. Veringa EM, Ferguson DA Jr, Lambe DW Jr, Verhoef J: Trospectomycin enhances surface phagocytosis of *Bacteroides* and *Staphylococcus* by altering the bacterial glycocalyx, *Zbl Bakt* 271:311-320, 1989.

37. Marrie TJ, Harding GKM, Ronald AR, et al: Influence of antibody coating of *Pseudomonas aeruginosa, J Infect Dis* 19:357-361, 1979.

38. Marrie TJ, Nelligan J, Costerton JW: A scanning and transmission electron microscopic study of an infected endocardial pacemaker lead, *Circulation* 66:1339-1341, 1982.

39. Marrie TJ, Costerton JW: Scanning electron microscopic study of uropathogen adherence to a plastic surface, *Appl Environ Microbiol* 45:1018-1024, 1983.

40. Marrie TJ, Noble MA, Costerton JW: Examination of the morphology of bacteria adhering to peritoneal dialysis catheters by scanning and transmission electron microscopy, *J Clin Microbiol* 18:1388-1398, 1983.

41. Lambe DW Jr, Mayberry-Carson KJ, Tober-Meyer B, Costerton JW: The role of glycocalyx in osteomyelitis, *Hyg Med* 12:55-57, 1987.

42. Lambe DW Jr, Mayberry-Carson KJ, Tober-Meyer B, Costerton JW, Ferguson KP: The role of anaerobes in foreign body–associated osteomyelitis. In Peterson PK, Fleer A, eds: *3rd European Congress of Clinical Microbiology Symposium on Foreign Body–Related Infections,* Amsterdam, 1987, Excerpta Medica, pp 36-47.

43. Dougherty SH: Pathobiology of infection in prosthetic devices, *Rev Infect Dis* 10:1102-1117, 1988.

44. Mayberry-Carson KJ, Tober-Meyer B, Gill LR, Lambe DW Jr, Mayberry WR: Effect of ciprofloxacin on subcutaneous abscesses induced with *Staphylococcus epidermidis* and a foreign body implant in the mouse, *Microbios* 54:45-59, 1988.

45. Dudman WF: The role of surface polysaccharides in natural environments. In Sutherland I, ed: *Surface carbohydrates of the prokaryotic cell,* New York, 1977, Academic Press, pp 357-414.

46. Mayberry-Carson KJ, Tober-Meyer B, Lambe DW Jr, Costerton JW: Osteomyelitis induced in rabbit tibia by *S. aureus* and other experimental models, *Microbios* 69:53-65, 1995.

47. Mayberry-Carson KJ, Tober-Meyer B, Gill LR, Lambe DW Jr, Hossler FE: Effect of ciprofloxacin on experimental osteomyelitis in the rabbit tibia, induced with a mixed infection of *S. epidermidis* and *B. thetaiotaomicron, Microbios* 64:49-66, 1990.

48. Norden CW: Experimental osteomyelitis: I. A description of the model, *J Infect Disease* 122,410-418, 1970.

49. Mayberry-Carson KJ, Tober-Meyer B, Lambe DW Jr, Costerton JW: An electron microscopic study of the effect of clindamycin therapy in experimental *S. aureus* osteomyelitis, *Microbios* 48:189-206, 1986.

50. Mayberry-Carson KJ, Mayberry WR, Tober-Meyer BK, Costerton JW, Lambe DW Jr: An electron microscopic study of the effect of clindamycin on adherence of *S. aureus* to bone surfaces, *Microbios* 45:21-32, 1986.

51. Veringa EM, Lambe DW Jr, Ferguson DA Jr, Verhoef J: Enhancement of opsonophagocytosis of *Bacteroides* spp. by clindamycin in subinhibitory concentrations, *J Antimicrob Chemother* 23:577-587, 1989.

52. Ferguson DA, Veringa EM, Mayberry WR, Overbeek BP, Lambe DW Jr, Verhoef J: *Bacteroides* and *Staphylococcus* glycocalyx: chemical analysis, and the effects on chemiluminescence and chemotaxis on human polymorphonuclear leukocytes, *Microbios* 69:53-65, 1992.

53. Stout RD, Ferguson KP, Li Y-N, Lambe DW Jr: Staphylococcal exopolysaccharides inhibit lymphocyte proliferative responses by activation of monocyte prostaglandin production, *Infect Immun* 60:922-927, 1992.

Section Two

Laboratory and Radiographic Diagnostic Modalities

6

Diagnostic Laboratory Analysis of Foot Infections

Kenrick J. Dennis

Medical theory is truly useful, only when its practical results are beneficial. To judge correctly of these results, we must have recourse to the phenomena presented to clinical observers. Andrew M'Call

Perhaps there is no place in medical practice where the clinical examination is more important than in the diagnosis of the infectious process. However, to support the clinical diagnosis, and then to implement definitive treatment, requires the assistance of laboratory analysis. By thoroughly understanding how laboratory parameters change in the infectious process, the practitioner will be able to more effectively order appropriate diagnostic tests and interpret the ensuing results. Since the accurate collection of culture material is as important as the appropriate interpretation of laboratory results, a sequential approach to obtaining laboratory information is critical in order to avoid obfuscating the clinical situation as the treatment regimen unfolds. Moreover, it must be recalled that each individual clinical laboratory possesses its own techniques and will also have its own specific parameter of normal values. Most have a normal range that has a 95% confidence level (plus or minus two standard deviations from the mean).

In this chapter, each test will be focused on the topic of foot infections. The reader is directed to recent medical literature, such as the treatise by Dennis, for more common blood collection techniques, laboratory parameters, and normal values in other situations.[1]

SPECIMEN COLLECTION

The accuracy of a laboratory evaluation is only as good as the quality and quantity of the specimen obtained. In general, the specimen sent for laboratory analysis should be representative of the entire disease process. Contamination of any type, whether it be bacterial during blood cultures, air during an anaerobic culture, or viral during a spinal fluid tap, will ruin the culture.

The *site* from which the specimen is obtained must be meticulously clean. For example, in a superficial ulcera-

tion the surface of the wound is quite likely to be contaminated with normal skin flora. The depth of the sinus tract or ulceration should be curetted to obtain a good specimen.

Scraping is a useful technique when the sample is scaling. Either a sterile wooden tongue depressor or a sterile scalpel blade may be used to scrape off a representative sample. The sample may then be evaluated by direct visualization or culture. If the area is very sensitive, the area may be hydrated first with sterile water and then swabbed for a culture.

When a practitioner is *swabbing* a wound for culture, special attention is needed because specimens are easily contaminated by wound-colonizing microbes. Organisms proliferate at different rates, and a contaminant picked up by careless collection may overgrow the true pathogen. Whenever possible, the culture should be taken from the depth of the wound.

Aspiration is the classic sampling technique for an abscess. It is important to remember that organisms may not be evenly distributed throughout an abscess. For this reason, cultures should be obtained from the central portion of the abscess as well as from the interface between viable tissue and the abscess. For example, an ascending cellulitis presents a challenge for accurate specimen collection. Historically, aspiration or biopsy of the leading edge has been utilized; however, this technique has been criticized for allowing false-positive as well as false-negative readings.

Osteomyelitis is difficult to evaluate and treat, both clinically and with laboratory examination. Open bone biopsy remains the single most useful diagnostic tool. It is both definitive and invasive.[2]

Tables 6-1 and 6-2 list some common soft tissue infections and infestations of the foot and their respective diagnostic tests.

TABLE 6-1   Common soft tissue foot infections and diagnostic tests

Diagnosis	Organism	Test
Erysipelas	*Streptococcus pyogenes*	Aspirate
Erythema chronicum (Lyme disease)	*Borrelia burgdorferi*	Serology, biopsy
Erythrasma	*Corynebacterium minutissimum*	Wood's light, scales
Eumycetoma	*Madurella* sp.	Biopsy (sulfur grains)
Hepatitis B	Hepatitis B virus	Clinical, serology
Herpes simplex	Herpes virus hominis	Tzanck smear (FA)
Impetigo (bullous)	*Staphylococcus aureus/pyogenes*	Gram stain, culture
Infectious mononucleosis	Epstein-Barr virus	Clinical, serology
Leprosy	*Mycobacterium leprae*	Biopsy
Puncture wound culture	Polymicrobial	Gram stain
Ringworm	Dermatophytes	KOH, culture
Scabies	*Sarcoptes scabiei*	Scraping (KOH), biopsy
Scalded skin	*S. aureus*	Culture
Shingles	Varicella-zoster virus	History, serology
Swimming granuloma	*M. marinum*	Mycobacteria culture
Syphilis (secondary)	*Treponema pallidum*	Serology, dark-field exam
Tinea	*Trichophyton* sp.	KOH, culture
Ulcers	Polymicrobial	Gram stain, culture
Warts	Papillomavirus (human type)	Clinical, biopsy

Modified from Howanitz JH, Howanitz PJ: *Laboratory medicine: test selection and interpretation,* New York, 1991, Churchill Livingstone.

TABLE 6-2   Common soft tissue foot infestations and diagnostic tests

Diagnosis	Organism	Test
Body lice	*Pediculus humanus*	Clinical
Chigger bites	*Trombicula irritans*	Clinical

Modified from Howanitz JH, Howanitz PJ: *Laboratory medicine: test selection and interpretation,* New York, 1991, Churchill Livingstone.

TABLE 6-3   Sample preparation for direct visual examination

Diagnosis	Specimen	Test
Dermatophytes, *Candida*	Hair, skin, nails	KOH, culture
Tinea	Skin	Scraping, KOH
Scabies	Burrow	Scraping, KOH
Herpes	Vesicle, scraping	Tzanck test
Infection (cellulitis, abscess)	Pus, aspirate	Gram stain

Modified from Howanitz JH, Howanitz PJ: *Laboratory medicine: test selection and interpretation,* New York, 1991, Churchill Livingstone.

DIRECT VISUAL EXAMINATION

After successful collection of the specimen, empiric treatment may begin after direct visual examination. It is always critically important to remember the clinical examination. Normal skin flora may be isolated from a wound culture and can be identified simply as a contaminant; however, with the right clinical setting this skin flora may be the true pathogen. Under direct microscopy, polymorphonuclear leukocytes (PMNLs) should be readily visualized in the infectious process. Table 6-3 shows the appropriate sample preparation for direct visualization with several common diagnoses.

GRAM STAIN

The Gram stain is the most common direct microscopic examination method available for evaluating a purulent exudate. It was originally developed by Hans Christian Gram over 100 years ago.[2] The Gram stain technique is described in Table 6-4.

Different species of bacteria have different chemical constituents to their cell walls, which give them the ability to retain gentian violet even after a treatment with a mixture of a decolorizer, such as alcohol, and acetone. Gentian violet serves as the primary stain in the Gram stain technique. Bacteria that retain the gentian violet dye appear blue/black when observed under the microscope (gram-positive bacteria). Certain other bacteria have a high lipid content in their cell walls, which causes them to lose the gentian violet when the combination of alcohol and acetone is applied. These bacteria will then pick up safranin counterstain, as the last step in the technique, and will appear red when observed under the microscope (gram-negative bacteria).[2] The more common appearances of bacteria are shown in Table 6-5.

TABLE 6-4   Gram stain technique

1. Make a thin specimen smear on a slide and allow to air dry.
2. Pass the slide through a flame to fix the sample to the glass.
3. Cover the specimen with gentian (crystal) violet solution.
4. After 1 minute, wash the slide with distilled water.
5. Cover the specimen with Gram's iodine (mordant) solution.
6. After 1 minute wash the slide with distilled water.
7. Apply a few drops of acetone-alcohol decolorizer until no more violet washes out, in about 10 seconds.
8. Rinse with running water.
9. Cover the specimen with safranin counterstain.
10. After 1 minute rinse under running water.
11. Drain off excess water and let dry before examining under 10- to 30-power oil immersion microscopy.

Reagent	Time	Gram Positive	Gram Negative
Primary stain: gentian violet	20 seconds	Purple	Purple
Mordant: Gram's iodine	1 minute	Purple	Purple
Decolorizing agent: 95% alcohol	10-20 seconds	Purple	Colorless
Counterstain: safranin	20 seconds	Purple	Pink

Modified from Dennis KJ: Clinical laboratory evaluation. In Marcinko DE, ed: *Medical and surgical therapeutics of the foot and ankle,* Baltimore, 1992, Williams & Wilkins.

TABLE 6-5   Common bacteria appearances on gram stain

Appearance	Bacteria
Gram-positive cocci in clusters	Staphylococci
Gram-positive cocci in chains	Streptococci
Gram-positive lancet-shaped diplococci	*Streptococcus pneumoniae*
Gram-negative biscuit-shaped diplococci	*Neisseria* sp.
Large gram-positive bacilli	*Bacillus* or *Clostridium* sp.
Small gram-positive bacilli	*Listeria* or *Corynebacterium* sp.
Gram-negative bacilli	Enterobacteriaceae or *Campylobacter* sp.

Modified from Horowitz JH, Horowitz PJ: *Laboratory medicine: test selection and interpretation,* New York, 1991, Churchill Livingstone.

ACID-FAST STAINS

Mycobacteria have a thick waxy material that coats the cell wall and is extremely resistant to staining. The primary stain, carbolfuchsin, is used to penetrate the waxy material of the acid-fast bacilli. After the stain is applied, the sample is heated to near boiling in order to help penetration. Once the stain has been absorbed, the bacterial cells resist decolorization by almost all solvents. The acid-fastness of an organism may vary with age and drugs. Also, although *M.*

tuberculosis is consistently acid-fast, *M. leprae, Nocardia,* and *Actinomyces* are not.

Cold acid-fast stains, such as the Kinyoun and Putt stains, may also be used to identify nonbacterial organisms. Under oil-immersion microscopic examination, acid-fast rods appear slightly curved and beaded. Artifacts are not recorded, and only definitive organisms are considered acid-fast rods.

METHYLENE BLUE STAIN

Loeffler's methylene blue stain is used to identify the metachromatic granules of *Corynebacterium diphtheriae* and diarrheal stool for leukocytes.

FUNGAL STAINS

The microscopic examination for fungal elements requires direct mounts of unfixed specimens. Several of the more common stain types are listed below.

Potassium hydroxide stain

The potassium hydroxide (KOH) examination is one of the easiest and most efficient laboratory tests that can be performed in the office, and it can be utilized for any suspected mycotic infection. The sample may consist of a scraping of the skin, a piece of the nail, or hair. A negative KOH preparation does not completely rule out a fungal infection and should be followed up with a fungal culture. The test may require overnight incubation for complete disintegration of nail or skin debris. The presence of hyphae after gentle heating with 10% KOH is indicative of a positive result.

Periodic acid–Shiff stain (PAS)

In the face of a negative KOH mount, the PAS technique (same procedure as for KOH) should be used for increased sensitivity.

Nigrosin stain

The cellular capsules of *Candida, Cryptococcus, Torulopsis, Rhodotorula,* and *Trichosporon* may be detectable with nigrosin, by providing a homogenous background without precipitates. Capsular identification is diagnostic. The quellung ("swelling") reaction is an immunologic reaction wherein cellular capsules are rendered refractile and visible by exposure to antibodies directed against specific antigens. Newer immunologic tests are now more often used.

Giemsa and Wright stains

The Giemsa and Wright stains are used to detect rickettsiae, chlamydiae, the parasitic organisms of malaria, and the parasitic yeast cell forms of *Histoplasma capsulatum.* The latter intracellular organism typically stains light to dark blue and is surrounded by a transparent halo that represents artifacts, not capsules. Further immediate information from these stains includes the differentiation of inflammatory cells, eosinophils, and inclusion bodies.

LABORATORY SKIN TESTS

The *Tzanck test* seeks to identify the presence of multinucleated giant cells, which suggest a herpes zoster infection. It is done by scraping the base of a vesicle onto a glass slide and fixing it with methanol stain. The test is also used for the diagnosis of viral diseases such as herpes simplex and molluscum contagiosum.

A *skin biopsy* requires a prepped and anesthetized area. A 2- to 8-mm disposable sterile punch is rotated through to the subcutaneous layer. The biopsy should be deep, contain both suspicious and normal skin, or come from the apex of the lesion.

Immunofluorescent microscopy may be either direct or indirect. In direct immunofluorescence, the skin biopsy is stained with fluoresceinated antihuman immunoglobulin and anticomplement reagents and examined under a fluorescent microscope. In indirect immunofluorescent microscopy, the patient's serum is tested with the same reagents. Both are useful in diagnosing vesiculobullous disorders.

A *Wood's light examination* is used for erythrasma, a toe web infection caused by *Corynebacterium minutissimum.* It fluoresces coral-red or pink-orange under the special light. *Pseudomonas aeruginosa,* on the other hand, produces a yellowish green fluorescence. Patients who are taking tetracycline will fluorescence pink at the toenail bed lunule.

Special dermatologic tests include (1) *diascopy,* which uses a clear glass slide pressed against the skin lesion to observe either small blood vessel integrity or intravascular blood (apple jelly sign) without vessel integrity, as seen in granulomatous or purpuretic lesions; (2) the *Auspitz sign,* or pinpoint bleeding when a psoriatic scale is removed; (3) the *Koebner (isomorphic) phenomenon,* the appearance, on uninvolved skin, of an eruption, such as psoriasis or lichen planus, that is of the same type as that present at a site of trauma; and (4) the *Nikolsky sign,* epidermal detachment from a lack of skin cohesion.

FEVER OF UNKNOWN ORIGIN

Three criteria are needed to define a fever of unknown origin (FUO): (1) fever on multiple occasions greater than 100° F (37.8° C) orally or greater than 101° F (38.3° C) rectally; (2) fever for at least 3 weeks and; (3) inability to diagnose the fever, for at least 1 week, after a complete physical examination and routine diagnostic tests such as urine and blood studies, chest x-rays, and cultural examination. Causes include infection (tuberculosis, spirochetes, leptospirosis, rickettsiae, chlamydiae, viruses, fungi, and parasites), neoplastic disorders, hypersensitivity and autoimmune reac-

TABLE 6-6 Normal values for the complete blood count

Red blood cells (RBC)	Male: $4.3\text{-}5.9 \times 10^6/mm^3$ Female: $3.5\text{-}5.5 \times 10^6/mm^3$
Hemoglobin (Hgb)	Male: 13.9-18 g/dl Female: 12.0-16 g/dl
Hematocrit (Hct)	Male: 39% to 55% Female: 36% to 48%
White blood cells (WBC)	$4.0\text{-}10.5 \times 10^3/mm^3$
Platelets	$140\text{-}440 \times 10^3/mm^3$
Differential	
PMNLs	45% to 75%
Band cells (bands)	0% to 5%
Metaphylls (meta)	0%
Lymphocytes	20% to 45%
Monocytes	0% to 10%
Eosinophils	0% to 6%
Basophils	0% to 2%

The following is a simple notation method for recording CBC results:

Hgb   Segs/Bands/Lymphs/Monos/Eosinos

WBC> _____ MCV _____ MCH _____ MCHC

                      Hct _____

Example: 10.1   41S, 20B, 30L, 5M, 3B, 5E

    11,100> _____ 80/29/30

      30.5   283,100

tions, inherited disorders, CNS disorders, osteomyelitis, and urinary tract infections (UTIs). Finally, drug reactions may alter results.

One of the most important functions of the complete blood count (CBC), relative to the chronic infectious disease process, is the identification of anemia. Anemia is a condition in which there is a low red cell count, a low hemoglobin, or a combination of the two. Anemias may be classified by the morphology of the red blood cells. The mean corpuscular hemoglobin concentration (MCHC) indicates the hemoglobin concentration of the erythrocytes. The mean corpuscular volume (MCV) indicates the size of the erythrocytes. Normal values for a complete blood count are listed in Table 6-6.

WHITE BLOOD CELL COUNT AND DIFFERENTIAL

The white blood cell (WBC) count identifies the number of cells found in a cubic millimeter of whole blood. The normal range is 4,000 to 10,000. White blood cells, which are also known as leukocytes, may be increased (leukocytosis) with any type of stress (such as exercise), by as much as 2,000. The white count may also be sensitive to medications, such as metronidazole, griseofulvin, lincomycin, amoxicillin, ampicillin, carbenicillin, nafcillin, oxacillin, penicillin, ticarcillin, diazepam, indomethacin, mefenamic acid, phenylbutazone, allopurinol, and colchicine.

When tissues are inflamed, such as in an infection, a substance is released that is known as leukocytosis-promoting factor (LPF). As this factor diffuses into blood and is finally delivered to bone marrow, it has two actions. First, within hours it will cause the release of many neutrophils into the blood; these neutrophils have been stored in the bone marrow. As a result of their release, the neutrophil count may become as high as 20,000 to 30,000 per cubic millimeter of blood. Second, the rate of production of neutrophils is increased. It is unknown whether this is a direct result of the LPF or results from the depletion of neutrophils because of the large number that have just been released. As long as the leukocyte-promoting factor is being produced by inflamed tissue, the bone marrow will continue to produce large numbers of neutrophils. However, at this increased production rate, many immature neutrophils will be released, which leads to what is known as a "left shift" because of the abundance of precursor cells.

Within 6 to 12 hours after initiation of the inflammatory response, neutrophils reach their maximum effectiveness. Macrophages and monocytes are also present. As the neutrophils and macrophages engulf large amounts of bacteria and necrotic tissue, they too eventually die. Within the inflamed tissue, an area of necrotic tissue and dead macrophages and neutrophils develops, and this mixture is commonly termed pus (purulence).

The white blood cell differential count provides more specific information about the immune system than the white blood count. This test divides white blood cells, on a stained film of peripheral blood, into the numerous granulocytes (basophils, eosinophils, and neutrophils) and nongranulocytes, and determines the percentage of each component. The following conditions may occur.

Neutrophilia ("left shift")

The daily production of PMNLs is about 10 to 11 cells, with an average extravascular survival range of 7 hours to 4 days. Intravascular pool (circulating and marginating) half-life is 6 to 8 hours. Neutrophilia is characterized by an increase in the number of neutrophils mobilized from mature granulocytes in bone marrow and found on the differential examination. A left shift may be indicative of acute, local, or general bacterial infections, spirochetes, rickettettsiae, viruses, protozoa, helminths, acute necrotic inflammation, pain, exercise, stress, sunlight, allergies, lithium carbonate, convulsions, or burns.

Neutropenia ("right shift")

Neutropenia is characterized by a decrease in the number of neutrophils seen on the differential smear. The lower limit of normal is 1500 to 2000/mm^3. Below about 500/mm^3, there is a dramatic increase in the incidence of infection.

A right shift may be indicative of bone marrow depression, bone marrow replacement, autoantibodies, pyogenic organisms, salmonellosis, brucellosis, phenothiazines, sulfonamides, penicillins, chephalosporins, vancomycin, chloramphenicol, or viral or fungal infections. Cyclic neutropenia is a rare autosomal dominant defect of myelopoiesis characterized by episodic decreases in neutrophils from the circulation. Prednisolone therapy is supportive.

Lymphocytic evaluation

Lymphocytic evaluation may be abnormal even in the face of a normal white blood count. Lymphocytes are also produced within the bone marrow and appear to be a multipotential cell. Under the right conditions, they may become erythroblastic, myeloblastic, fibroblastic, etc. Lymphocytes appear to play a special role in the process of immunity. Lymphocytosis may be indicative of many viral infections as well as mumps, measles, and hepatitis.

Monocytosis

Monocytosis on the differential analysis may indicate monocytic leukemia, tuberculosis, brucellosis, syphilis, Hodgkin's disease, collagen vascular disease, sarcoidosis, certain protozoal infections, or subacute bacterial endocarditis (SBE).

Eosinophils

The eosinophils normally range between 1% and 3% of the white blood count. Although they are phagocytic, they are not as effective as the neutrophils. They are found in especially high numbers in the mucosa of the intestines as well as lung tissues, where foreign proteins may enter the body. It appears that their job is to wall off and detoxify these foreign substances before damage can occur. Eosinophils also migrate to blood clots, where they apparently release profibrinolysin. They play an important role in the dissolution of old clots and are most commonly seen as the result of an allergic reaction. They may also indicate a parasitic infection, pemphigus, scarlet fever, or pernicious anemia. Drugs implicated in eosinophilia commonly include cephalosporins, penicillins, tetracyclines, streptomycin, and rifampin.

A decrease in the eosinophils (eosinopenia) may indicate Cushing's disease, or an overproduction of adrenocorticotropic hormone (ACTH), or an oversupply of adrenal hormones or steroids. Eosinopenia is also commonly found during labor, with shock, or as a result of surgical trauma. Drugs implicated in eosinopenia include indomethacin and procaine.

Basophils

Basophils are found in very small numbers in the white blood cell differential. They function very similarly to mast cells in the body in that they liberate heparin into the blood. In a prolonged inflammatory process, there is an increased tendency for red blood cells to coagulate. Basophils are increased in this process and appear to help block this coagulation by release of heparin.

TABLE 6-7 Erythrocyte sedimentation rates

Male	Under 50 years old: <15 mm/hr
	Over 50 years old: <20 mm/hr
Female	Under 50 years old: <20 mm/hr
	Over 50 years old: <30 mm/hr

ERYTHROCYTE SEDIMENTATION RATE

Standard ESR values are listed in Table 6-7.

C-REACTIVE PROTEIN

The C-reactive protein (CRP) is a constituent of plasma, with concentration ranges from 70 ng/ml (neonates) to 580 ng/ml (adults). It is similar to the ESR in that it is a nonspecific indicator of inflammation and tissue trauma. An end result of inflammation is a change in the plasma concentrations of acute-phase reactants (APRs), which include fibrinogen and alpha$_1$-antitrypsin. APRs can be grouped into "negative" APRs and "positive" APRs. The concentrations of negative APRs decrease with inflammation, while the concentration of positive APRs increase. Three groups of positive APRs are present in the blood. The first two groups rarely increase by more than 50% in the face of inflammation. The third group of positive APRs increases very quickly and dramatically in the face of inflammation. These are the C-reactive proteins. The C-reactive proteins rise very early in acute inflammation (4 to 6 hours) to levels several hundred to a thousand times the normal concentration of less than 0.9 µg/dl. They will return to normal levels after the acute phase of inflammation is over, which is usually in 3 to 6 days.

CRP was discovered in the 1930s in the serum of patients with pneumonia, because it precipitated the C-polysaccharide present in the cell walls of *Streptococcus pneumoniae*. For many years the assays were only qualitative, but now quantitative analysis is available. CRP is an excellent indicator of bacterial infections in patients with chronic inflammatory diseases or with neoplastic conditions, postsurgical patients, neonates, and neutropenic patients. CRP is a better monitor than the ESR in rheumatic diseases, as well as postoperatively and in post-transplantation rejection and inflammatory valve disease.

TEICHOIC ACID TITERS

Teichoic acids (teichos = wall) are polyolphosphate polymers found in the cell walls of certain gram-positive bacteria (i.e., staphylococci, streptococci, lactobacilli, and *Bacillus* sp.). The serum titer may be obtained to give an indication of a staphylococcal infection. In 60% of patients with staphylococcal endocarditis, the teichoic acid titer is greater than 1:4. Ten percent of patients with staphylococcal

infections that are not secondary to endocarditis will have a titer greater than 1:2. Therefore, most laboratories consider a finding greater than 1:4 to be positive for staphylococcal endocarditis and less than 1:4 a negative finding. The titer closely follows the infection and decreases as the infection resolves.

ANTI-STREPTOLYSIN O TITERS

ASO titers may be used to confirm ongoing or recent infections with beta-hemolytic streptococci. They also may facilitate distinguishing between rheumatic fever, rheumatoid arthritis, and infection when there is prolonged and unexplained joint pain. Normal values are anything less than 85 Todd units.

BLOOD CULTURES

A positive blood culture remains one of the most effective and accurate diagnostic tools in serious infections. Normal flora may gain access to the circulatory system through wounds, the gastrointestinal tract, the urinary tract, or the pulmonary system or by direct inoculation by insect or animal vectors, trauma, or blood transfusion. Once in the circulatory system, the infectious agent may fluorish and enjoy widespread dissemination, resulting in serious infection. Arterial blood cultures are of little added value, while bone marrow cultures may be helpful in unusual cases.

Fever and chills are the hallmark of clinical symptoms associated with bacteremia. Other clinical signs include tachycardia, hypotension, leukocytosis, and possible changes in mental status. In patients with a difficult wound, blood cultures may be useful in establishing the etiologic factor of the wound infection.

Blood cultures must be done with strictly aseptic technique. Do not draw cultures through an indwelling line or palpate the venipuncture site after antiseptic preparation. Bacteremia occurs most commonly prior to an acute episode of fever and chills. Since it is difficult to anticipate the onset of fever, cultures should be done at the onset of fever. Three cultures spaced over a 60-minute period should be sufficient to detect almost all bacteremia episodes. To ensure optimum samples for interpretation, at least 10 to 20 ml of blood per culture is needed.

There are three methods of culturing blood for bacteria. These include broth, biphasic, and lysis centrifugation. Each method is different in its sensitivity, specificity, the time required to detect and identify various bacteria, and the ability to provide a quantitative result. Interpretation of blood cultures requires a complete knowledge of the clinical examination. Negative cultures do not necessarily exclude bacteremia. Pathogens may be extremely fragile or may be collected in such small amounts as to limit growth. Conversely, a positive culture does not necessarily indicate bacteremia. Contaminants are a common cause of positive cultures. As a result, the most difficult results to interpret are those which show the pathogen to be a member of the normal skin flora. Whenever a culture identifies a gram-negative bacillus, anaerobes, or fungal elements, these should all be considered pathogens until proven otherwise.

VENEREAL DISEASE RESEARCH LABORATORY (VDRL) TEST

The VDRL test is used to screen for primary or secondary syphilis or to confirm primary or secondary syphilis in the presence of skin lesions. Biologic false positives may result from viral infections, bacterial infections, chronic systemic disease, or nonsyphilitic treponemal infections. Positive results should be further evaluated with the fluorescent treponemal antibody absorption test (FTA-ABS). Similar serologic tests are available for Lyme disease and AIDS.

SERODIAGNOSIS

The thought of deciphering all the choices in a large battery of serologic tests can be both intimidating and frustrating, even to the most experienced clinician. There are five reasons why serologic testing may be performed: (1) It can be done to detect the presence of antibodies, since the presence of IgG establishes exposure to infection, and to indicate immunity to further infection. (2) Change in the quantity of antibody may indicate acute infection. (3) The long incubation periods needed to grow some microorganisms, and the presence of antibodies, may provide a more efficacious means of detection. (4) The presence of antibodies serves to differentiate a systemic infection from normal colonization of superficial flora. (5) The presence of antibodies may help direct further invasive procedures (e.g., the presence of antibodies to hepatitis B would reduce the need for a liver biopsy).

The presence of specific antibodies is a useful and important detection tool for various conditions. However, in samples more than 1 month old, IgM antibodies may no longer be detectable. Specific methods of serodiagnosis are shown in Tables 6-8 and 6-9.

Serologic tests are the diagnostic tool of choice for most viral, chlamydial, and mycoplasmal infections because they are more readily available and less costly than cultures. In fact, cultures are not available for some viruses. For most viral infections, serologic diagnosis can help direct treatment course. Serologic studies also are useful in determining the immune status against a particular virus (such as a screening test for immunity of women of childbearing age to rubella virus). Since serum can be frozen and stored, it may be collected early in the disease process and stored for potential follow-up testing.

Agglutination

"Agglutinins" was the term given to the substances that caused clumping of bacteria in the serum of infected patients

TABLE 6-8 Specific methods of serodiagnosis

Immunodiffusion (ID)
Agglutination reactions (AR)
Complement fixation test (CF)
Radioimmunoassay (RIA)
Enzyme-linked immunoassay (ELISA)
Enzyme immunoassay (EIA)
Indirect immunofluorescence (IFA)

TABLE 6-9 Serologic tests for specific organisms

Organism	Test	Accuracy
Salmonella	Agglutination	Inaccurate, culture preferred
Brucella	Agglutination	Excellent, faster than culture
T. pallidum	Agglutination/IFA	Good results
Rickettsiae	Agglutination	Inaccurate
Chlamydiae	IFA/EIA	Inaccurate
Fungi	Immunodiffusion	Good results
T. gondii	IFA/EIA	Good results
Cytomegalovirus	EIA	Excellent
Epstein-Barr virus	Agglutination	Excellent
Herpes simplex virus	IFA/EIA	Inaccurate
Influenza virus	CF/EIA	Excellent
Rubella virus	Agglutination	Excellent
Varicella zoster virus	IFA/EIA	Excellent

in the late nineteenth century. Agglutination remains one of the simplest and fastest laboratory tests available today. This test detects the presence of antibodies to a specific pathogen. Serum (not plasma) is the most accurate test medium. In the presence of antibody, the commercially available agglutination methods cause a grossly visible clumping after being thoroughly mixed. An estimate of the amount of antibody present may be made after serial dilutions are obtained. This test is easy to perform and may yield results in 10 to 15 minutes.

Agglutination findings may be nonspecific, however, leaving interpretation potentially difficult. With high concentrations of antibodies, a false-negative result (prozone phenomenon) may be obtained.

Complement fixation

Complement fixation (CF), although cumbersome and tedious, is a very sensitive test. One weakness of CF is that it is not able to identify the class of antibody present. As a result, complement fixation is not useful in the diagnosis of acute infections. The test itself measures the competition between the antigen-antibody complex being measured and an indicator system for complement. If complement is bound to the antibody being evaluated, none remains available to be bound to the indicator system. If there is little antibody present, the indicator cells will bind the complement, resulting in lysis of the indicator cells. The results are reported as a dilution titer.

IMMUNOFLUORESCENCE

Radioimmunoassay (RIA), enzyme-linked immunoassay (ELISA), enzyme immunoassay (EIA), and indirect immunofluorescence (IFA) are similar tests that are commonly used today. In all these tests, the antigen of the test system is attached chemically to the surface of a tube or polystyrene beads. A sample of serum is added and allowed to interact with the antigen. Excess immunoglobulin is washed free after a specified incubation period, which is critical to the accuracy and reproducibility of the test. Radioactive antisera to human immunoglobulin are then used to detect antibody. The excess marker is again washed, and at this point the test system consists of a solid support, with antigens, specific antigens, specific antibodies, and the detecting antibody with marker left in place. These tests are generally referred to as "sandwich assays" because of this layering of reagents.

These tests are the most sensitive of all serodiagnostic methods. Any of the methods described are able to provide qualitative, semiquantitative, or quantitative results. RIA tests are the most sensitive of all those described, being able to detect quantities of protein in the picogram range. RIA is also more easily reproducible than the rest. For most infections, however, this degree of sensitivity and reproducibility is not necessary. EIA methods are useful in that no radioactive material is utilized and there is a greater storage potential for the reagents. The IFA methods are the most specific of all the analyses; however, interpretation and analysis are significantly more subjective than with either EIA or RIA.

If a fungal infection is suspected, cultures and histologic studies are more effective than serologic assays in determining the pathologic agent. Radioimmunoassay and enzyme-linked immunoassay are extremely sensitive tests but lack specificity. Conversely, another technique, known as immunodiffusion, is a very specific test but lacks sensitivity. The use of a serologic diagnosis is much less reliable in identifying an opportunistic fungal infection, such as aspergillosis or candidiasis. It is much more reliable in diagnosing nonopportunistic fungal infections, such as coccidioidomycosis, histoplasmosis, and blastomycosis.

ANTIMICROBIAL TESTING

As clinicians become more sophisticated in the treatment of infections, so do the bacteria and other infectious agents in their resistance to conventional care. The number of organisms with 100% susceptibility to specific drugs is quickly shrinking. Still, not every culture requires the determination of extensive susceptibilities.

TABLE 6-10 Factors affecting clinical antibiotic efficacy

Protein binding of the antibiotic
Dosage and route of administration
Fluctuations in the concentration of antibiotics
Ability of antibiotic to penetrate systems
Renal and hepatic function
In vivo environment (i.e., pH, oxygen level, etc.)
Immune status
Virulence of bacteria
Bacterial resistance
Other miscellaneous drugs
Minimal bactericidal concentration

Antimicrobial susceptibility tests are indicated in patients who are not responding as expected to the initial therapy. In such a case, the identification of a more effective drug would be the goal. Patients taking broad-spectrum drugs could be converted to more narrow-spectrum drugs as the results of antimicrobial susceptibility tests became available. Long-term therapy with costly medications might also be a good indication for reevaluating antimicrobial susceptibility. If an infection were not acute, a patient would not begin initial therapy until antimicrobial susceptibility had been identified. Finally, in a patient who had an allergy or contraindication to the drug of choice, antimicrobial susceptibility tests would help identify a second-line medication.

The three antimicrobial susceptibility tests commonly used today are disc diffusion, disc dilution, and disc elution methods. In general, the results of antimicrobial susceptibility tests are reported in similar fashion. Each laboratory will be slightly different in reporting, but listings of "susceptible," "intermediate," or "resistant" categories will be utilized.

When dilution susceptibility testing is used, minimal inhibitory concentrations (MIC) may be provided. This information is useful in cases of serious infection, in which peak and trough levels of antibiotic must be monitored closely.

To effectively use MIC results, one must try to obtain a drug concentration at the site of infection that is four times the MIC of the infecting organism. A common mistake is to blindly choose the lowest MIC value reported, since the pharmacokinetics of the potential drug treatments must be considered. For example, with an infection in which ampicillin and gentamicin are considered for treatment, although the gentamicin may have a lower MIC, it has significantly higher toxicity. If the MIC of the less toxic ampicillin could be obtained, it would be considered the drug of choice. It is important to remember that the MIC and all susceptibility testing are laboratory tests and do not take into account many clinical factors. Factors affecting the in vivo effectiveness of antibiotics are included in Table 6-10.

TABLE 6-11 Common susceptibility panels

Gram-positive panel:
Ampicillin ⎫
Cefazolin ⎬ One of these three
Cephalothin ⎭
Chloramphenicol
Clindamycin
Erythromycin
Gentamicin
Methicillin
Nafcillin ⎫
Oxacillin ⎬ One of these two
Penicillin
Sulfisoxazole-trimethoprim
Tetracycline
Vancomycin
Gram-negative panel:
Amikacin
Ampicillin
Carbenicillin
Cefamandole
Cefoxitin
Cephalothin
Gentamicin
Sulfisoxazole-trimethoprim
Tetracycline
Tobramycin

Modified from Howanitz JH, Howanitz PJ: *Laboratory medicine: test selection and interpretation,* New York, 1991, Churchill Livingstone.

The tests discussed to this point have described the ability of antimicrobial agents to inhibit growth of microorganisms. In order to eradicate the infecting organism, information on the bactericidal activity is needed. The minimal bactericidal concentration (MBC) is easily determined by taking a broth dilution MIC test one step further. Each of the dilutions tested in the MIC can be further subcultured on an agar medium, and any future growth would be indicative of inhibition versus bactericidal effect.

In patients with severe infections or osteomyelitis, serum bactericidal tests (SBTs), which were previously known as the Schlichter test, are useful to give an indication of the overall ability to fight the infection. These tests measure the ability of the antimicrobial agent, and any additional antibacterial factors in the serum that may be working to control the infecting organism.

Obviously, the clinical laboratory cannot test the susceptibility of every antibiotic available; therefore a panel of antibiotic medications is normally established for each type of infection. Table 6-11 shows the most common panels utilized.

RAPID BACTERIAL IDENTIFICATION

Once the diagnosis of infection has been established, there is inherent down time regarding the etiologic factor that is being identified. Although there is some inaccuracy in all laboratory testing, several "quick tests" are available

to focus the suspicion on the appropriate pathogen. The following rapid screening tests allow for good initial empiric treatment, and are available to further identify isolated colonies that have been grown from the initial culture.

Bile solubility

Bile solubility has proven to show the difference between *Streptococcus pneumoniae* and all other streptococcal species. *S. pneumoniae* is different because it has cells that are soluble in bile. A blue-green color (depending on the reagent used) within 20 seconds is a positive result.

Methyl red test

The methyl red test is utilized to identify Enterobacteriaceae. This test takes 18 to 24 hours to perform, yet it still cuts down on the conventional 5 days of incubation with previous testing. A well-isolated colony is inoculated into a broth and incubated for 18 to 24 hours. After 1 drop of methyl red is applied, a color change is noted. A yellow color is a negative result, a red color is a positive result, and an orange color is an equivocal result.

Fifty-degree urease test

The fifty-degree urease test is used to distinguish between *Klebsiella* sp. and *Enterobacter* sp. Although bacteria produce urease, only *Klebsiella* is able to continue urease activity at a temperature level of 50° C. This test is performed by inoculating a well-isolated colony into a culture medium and incubating that culture for 4 to 6 hours at 50° C. A pink to purple color is a positive indication. Negative results are indicated by yellow to white colors.

Germ tube formation test

The germ tube formation test is utilized to isolate *Candida albicans*. This test is performed by transferring an isolated colony to 0.5 ml of serum and incubating it for 3 hours at 35° C. *C. albicans* will produce filamentous outgrowth (germ tube) under these ideal conditions. If no germ tubes are identified under direct light microscopy, then follow-up tests are indicated.

Coagulase test

Staphylococcus aureus has historically been identified with a positive coagulase test. A single colony is transferred to 0.5 ml of brain-heart infusion (BHI) broth, and the sample is incubated for 4 to 6 hours at 35° C. Part of the broth is then transferred to a tube containing EDTA coagulase plasma. A positive coagulase test is indicated by clot formation. It can be seen when the tube is gently tilted. A thermonuclease test is performed with the rest of the medium after the BHI broth is heated to 100° C for 15 minutes. The broth is then inoculated into wells cut into a special DTM agar medium. After 4 hours the development of a pink halo around each well indicates a positive result.

Special bacterial studies

The following laboratory studies are not routinely done but may be useful to identify related bacterial isolates:

1. Phage typing, according to various phage type sensitivities, is particularly useful in *S. aureus* contamination (type 80/81). Typing of other organisms, such as *Clostridium difficile* and some enteric gram-negative species, is now possible, but many organisms cannot be differentiated by this technique.
2. Serotyping is useful to identify some gram-negative rods, such as *Klebsiella* sp., *Pseudomonas* sp., and *Legionella* sp.
3. Plasmid typing of self-replicating, transferable, and extrachromosomal bacterial DNA portions has been performed in eurokaryote organisms, through electrophoresis. Organisms identified in this manner include *Enterococcus faecalis*, *Staphylococcus epidermidis*, and *Bacillus catarrhalis*.
4. Identification may also be based on the particular physical characteristics of some microorganisms, such as specific proteins, pili, and chemical reactions found in *C. difficile* and *Haemophilus influenzae*.

Fungal serology

Fungal serology is used to isolate antifungal antibodies, aiding in the diagnosis of systemic mycotic infections. Table 6-12 lists several serum test titers for fungal infections possible in the foot.

BLOOD CHEMISTRY PROFILE

Blood chemistry analysis is not directly related to the diagnosis of foot infections. However, it does provide general evidence of clinical health status in many organ systems. Normal parameters for more common tests are listed in Table 6-13.

CONCLUSION

The laboratory tests discussed in this chapter will aid the clinician in the timely and accurate diagnosis of foot infections. No laboratory test or modality, however, will

TABLE 6-12 Serum titers of antifungal antibodies

Disease	Titer
Coccidioidomycosis (CF) (precipitin test)	<1:2 <1:16
Blastomycosis	<1:8
Histoplasmosis (histoplasmin fixation) (yeast fixation)	<1:8 <1:18
Aspergillosis	<1:8
Sporotrichosis	<1:40
Cryptococcosis	Negative antigen

Modified from Dennis KJ: Clinical laboratory evaluation. In Marcinko DE, ed: *Medical and surgical therapeutics of the foot and ankle*, Baltimore, 1992, Williams & Wilkins.

TABLE 6-13 Blood chemistry

Test Name	Units	Normal Value	Specimen Requirement	Clinical Significance
Creatine phosphokinase (CPK)	mU/ml	Male: 50 to 325 Female: 50 to 250	Red top 2 ml serum	Myocardial infarction
Globulin	g/dl	1.5 to 4.5	Red top 3 ml serum	
Glucose	mg/dl	Under 50 yr: 60 to 115	Red top 2 ml serum, fasting	Diabetes
Hematocrit (Hct)	%	Male: 39 to 55 Female: 36 to 48	Lavender top 7 ml blood	Decreased with excessive blood loss
Hemoglobin (Hgb), plasma	g/dl	Male: 13.9 to 18.0 Female: 12.0 to 16.0	Lavender top 7 ml blood	
Hemoglobin A1C			Lavender top 7 ml blood	Evaluate long-term control in diabetes
High-density lipoprotein (HDL)	mg/dl	Male: 30 to 70 Female: 35 to 75	Red top 2 ml serum	
Iron (Fe)	mg/dl	40 to 180	Red top 3 ml serum	Hepatitis (increased) Affected by anemias
Lactic acid	mg/dl	Venous: 5 to 20 Arterial: 3 to 7	Gray top 2 ml plasma	Increased in congestive heart failure, hemorrhage, shock
Lactate dehydrogenase (LDH)	IU/L	100 to 250	Red top 3 ml serum	
Magnesium (Mg)	mEq/L	1.3 to 2.4	Red top	
Phosphorus (P)	mg/dl	2.5 to 4.5 3 ml serum	Red top	
Potassium (K)	mEq/L	3.5 to 5.5 3 ml serum	Red top	

Modified from Roche Biomedical Laboratories, Inc., Burlington, NC. From Marcinko DE, ed: *Medical and surgical therapeutics of the foot and ankle*, Baltimore, 1992, Williams & Wilkins.

▌ **TABLE 6-13 Blood chemistry—cont'd**

Test Name	Units	Normal Value	Specimen Requirement	Clinical Significance
Protein (total)	g/dl	6.0 to 8.5 3 ml serum	Red top	
SGOT	IU/L	0 to 50	Red top	
PMNL (%)	<25	<25	>50775 usually	
Culture	(−)	(−)	(−)(+)	
Acid phosphatase	Sigma U/ml	Male: 0.13 to 0.63 Female: 0.01 to 0.56	Red top 1 ml serum: analyze immediately or freeze serum	Elevated in prostatic carcinoma
Albumin	g/dl	3.5 to 5.8	Red top 2 ml serum	May be increased in shock and decreased with hemorrhage
Alkaline phosphatase	IU/L	20 to 125	Red top 2 ml serum	Elevated in pregnancy
Amylase	Somogyi U/dl	60 to 160	Red top 3 ml serum	Elevated in pancreatitis and cirrhosis
Bilirubin	mg/dl	Total: 0.1 to 1.2 Direct: 0.1 to 1.2 Indirect: 0.1 to 1.0	Red top 3 ml serum: protect from light	Liver disease
Blood urea nitrogen (BUN)	mg/dl	7 to 26	Red top 2 ml serum	Renal disease
Calcium	mg/dl	8.5 to 10.6	Red top 2 ml serum	Bone
carbon dioxide (CO_2)	mEq/L mEq/L	Adult: 24 to 32 Infant: 18 to 24	Red top Centrifuge and refrigerate	Vomiting, diarrhea Respiratory distress
Chloride	mEq/L	94 to 109	Red top 3 ml serum	Renal disease (increased) Diabetes, diarrhea, vomiting, pneumonia, burns (decreased)
Cholesterol	mg/dl	<200	Red top 3 ml serum, fasting	
Creatinine	mg/dl	0.5 to 1.5	Red top 3 ml serum	Renal function
SGPT	IU/L	0 to 50 3 ml serum	Red top	
Sodium (Na)	mEq/L	135 to 148 3 ml serum	Red top	
Triglyceride	mg/dl	10 to 250 2 ml serum	Red top	
Uric acid	mg/dl	Male: 3.9 to 9.0 2 ml serum	Red top	
VDRL (RPR)		Female: 2.2 to 7.7 2 ml serum	Red top	

supplant an accurate physical examination. Tests are adjunctive verification and only serve to confirm clinical impressions. Thus, physical findings will remain the most efficient diagnostic modality for the experienced practitioner.

REFERENCES

1. Dennis KJ: Clinical laboratory evaluation. In Marcinko DE, ed: *Medical and Surgical Therapeutics of the Foot and Ankle,* Baltimore, 1992, Williams & Wilkins.
2. Howanitz JH, Howanitz PJ: *Laboratory medicine: test selection and interpretation,* New York, 1991, Churchill Livingstone, pp 619-625, 675-719, 789-795, 803-833.

ADDITIONAL READINGS

Abramson C, McCarthy DJ, Rupp MJ: *Infectious diseases of the lower extremity,* Baltimore, 1991, Williams & Wilkins, pp. 73-78.
Barry AL: Simple and rapid methods for bacterial identifications, *Clin Lab Med* 5(1):3-16, 1985.
Barry AL: Standardization of antimicrobial susceptibility testing, *Clin Lab Med* 9(2):203-207, 1989.
Calabrese LH: Autoimmune manifestations of human immunodeficiency virus (HIV) infection, *Clin Lab Med* 8(2):269-274, 1988.
Evans AS, Brachman PS: *Bacterial infections of humans: epidemiology and control,* New York, 1991, Plenum Medical Book Publishing.
Joseph WS: Clinical and laboratory diagnosis of lower extremity infections, *J Am Podiatr Med Assoc* 79:505-510, 1989.
Gilmour IJ, Boyle MJ, Streifel A: The effects of circuit and humidifier type on contamination potential during mechanical ventilation: a laboratory study, *Am J Infect Control* 23:65, 1995.
Koneman EW, Janda WM, Allen SD, Sommers HM, Dowell VR, Larsson S, Thelander U, Friberg S: C-reactive protein (CRP) levels after elective orthopedic surgery, *Clin Orthop Related Res* 275:237-242, 1992.
Mandell GL, Douglas RG, Bennett JE: *Principles and practice of infectious diseases,* ed 3, New York, 1990, Churchill Livingstone, pp 160-175.
Rupp M, Fravenhoffer S: Preoperative laboratory testing and podiatric surgery, *J Foot Surg* 26:493, 1987.
Schmidt NJ: Rapid viral diagnosis, *Clin Lab Med* 5(1):137-140, 1985.
Tilton RC, Balows A, Hohnadel DC, Reiss RF: *Clinical laboratory medicine,* St Louis, 1992, Mosby, pp. 402-405, 467-475, 545-559, 565-570.

7

Radiographic Impressions of the Infected Foot: A Photographic Review

David J. Sartoris
David Edward Marcinko

The three basic elements of the musculoskeletal system—bone, muscle and connective tissue—normally perform with perfect teamwork. Their mission is to support the body, shield its delicate internal organs and make it mobile. No task force was ever more meticulously equipped and organized. Alan E. Nourse

The traditional radiographic signs of soft tissue foot infections include abscess formation, gas, and an increase in soft tissue density and volume. Signs of bone contamination include periosteal elevation, bone destruction, sequestration (necrotic old bone formation), involucrum (new reparative bone formation), and cloaca formation. In most clinical settings, infection does not normally cross epiphyseal lines but may involve joint structures by contiguous contamination through sinuses, capsular tears, or other portal-of-entry sites. Since radiographic signs of contamination are not seen until the infection destroys enough bone (50%) to be visible on flat-plate x-rays, usually in 10 to 14 days, the diagnosis and subsequent treatment of osteomyelitis may be delayed. Serial or comparative radiographs are therefore helpful.[1-3]

Other radiographic modalities are used in foot infections to attempt earlier diagnosis. All are presumptive for osteomyelitis, and none are definitive. This chapter will consider these methodologies by using richly illustrated documentation to emphasize cognitive and interpretive skills, rather than technologic minutiae.

XERORADIOGRAPHY

Xeroradiography may be useful to delineate soft tissue masses such as neuromata or foreign bodies such as wood, rubber, glass, or cloth products. It may also be used for infection identification because it allows visualization of cortical margins, breaks, swelling, soft tissue tears, and joint integrity. Xerographic plates contain an aluminum base with a layer of selenium. Both positive and negative images can be produced. The plate is given an electrostatic charge and exposed to x-ray beams as in conventional techniques. After development, heat and pressure are used to produce the final plate. Unfortunately, the amount of

radiation exposure is greater than with conventional x-rays, and costs are increased. The technique is infrequently used today.[4]

COMPUTERIZED TOMOGRAPHY (CT) SCANS

CT scans reconstruct cross-sectional body planes with little superimposition of body structures. However, they cannot differentiate a homogeneous object of nonuniform thickness from a uniformly thick object of different composition. In cases of osteomyelitis, elevation of attenuated values in the marrow space may be an early but indirect sign of bone infection. The nonspecific destruction of cortical bone and new bone formation can be seen in this way, and the progression and/or recession of disease may be monitored. CAD/CAM (computer-aided design/computer-aided manufacturing) software programs can be used to reconstruct a three-dimensional image for better visualization.[5-7]

MAGNETIC RESONANCE IMAGING (MRI)

Magnetic resonance imaging distinguishes soft tissue structures more readily than any other imaging modality. It can differentiate osteonecrosis from aseptic necrosis, since most infarcts of bone occur in fatty tissue, which is easily imaged by MRI. This is because water has a high proton content and MRI measures water content of various body tissues (CT measures specific gravity). The more water (more protons), the higher the signal intensity. For example, fat, muscle, tendon and ligament, nerves, and blood vessels all have different imaging characteristics. Bone is white on a CT scan because of calcium (increased density); bone is white on an MRI scan because of high marrow content (increased intensity). These tissues are ranked on the relative Spin-Echo Grayscale, in the following order: fat, marrow, cancellous bone, brain, spinal cord, viscera, muscle, fluid-filled cavities, ligaments, tendons, blood vessels, compact bone, and air (brightest: short T1 and/or long T2; darkest: long T1 and/or short T2 and/or very low protein density). In foot and ankle injuries, a short trauma inversion recovery (STIR) sequence may be done in the sagittal plane. STIR represents a highly T1-weighted sequence in which the fat signal is suppressed and traumatic pathology appears with a brighter signal intensity.

The advantages of MRI include its noninvasive and harmless nature to the patient, who is exposed to no ionizing radiation or radioactive isotopes. It is similar to CT except uses magnetic equipment instead of moving x-ray tubes and detectors. Unfortunately, the relatively slow scan acquisition time results in artifacts caused by motion. Also, some patients experience claustrophobia because of the small bore of the magnet, and the strong magnetic field interferes with life support equipment. Calcium is a signal void and hinders evaluation of cortical bone. MRI is contraindicated in patients with aneurysm clips or cardiac pacemakers, as there is an attractive force between any ferromagnetic material and the static magnetic field.[8-10]

Major advantages of MRI over nuclear imaging for the diagnosis of osteomyelitis are its greater specificity and its ability to define drainable abscess collections. High-resolution studies using newer dual 3-inch surface magnetic coils, along with intravenous gadolinium injection therapy, are meaningful. On T1-weighted images, bone marrow will exhibit a decreased signal intensity. On T2 and fat-suppressed post-gadolinium T1 images, there will be increased signal intensity in the bone. Cellulitis will enhance post-gadolinium scans, whereas edema will not. In addition, abscesses and pus pockets will not be enhanced; they remain as relatively low signal areas expected in the fluid cavity. The signal characteristics of infection are not specific, although the clinical setting directs the suspicious clinician to the proper diagnosis.

MAGNETIC RESONANCE ANGIOGRAPHY

Magnetic resonance angiography (MRA) is a noninvasive technique used for visualization of the arterial vasculature of the lower limb, such as the anterior tibial artery, the posterior tibial artery, and the dorsalis pedis artery of the foot. MRA is essentially a series of pulse sequences performed on a conventional MRI scanner wherein the peripheral vasculature is considered a "two-dimensional time of flight."

A gradient echo is then used to acquire close axial images, as low as 1.5 to 2.5 mm in separation. These images are compressed, and a maximum-intensity projection is made in which the brightest pixel in a cardinal plane is selected. Unfortunately, since MRA is susceptible to turbulent blood flow, occlusive images are often exaggerated in size. In MRA, the anatomy distal to the stenosis can often be evaluated better than in traditional angiography, and operating decisions regarding an infectious infarction may be more accurately assessed.

NUCLEAR MEDICINE (BONE SCANNING)

Recent medical advances, especially within the realm of nuclear medicine, have resulted in tests that are sometimes necessary for early or precise diagnosis of soft tissue or bone infections. Although relatively expensive and not currently available in all hospitals, they have dramatically reduced the morbidity of the infected pedal patient. These tests and procedures include the following and may be ordered by the attending physician, infectious disease specialist, or other consultant.[11]

Technetium-99m methylene diphosphate (MDP) scans

Radioisotopic technetium is an osseous intensification agent because it binds to the hydroxyapatite crystals of metabolizing bone. Uptake will occur in the infectious process or any other condition involving increased bone growth turnover, such as arthrosis, fracture, altered weight-bearing stress, tumor formation, inflammation, or reactive periostitis.

Technetium has a physical half-life of 6 hours and is excreted by the kidneys in the well-hydrated patient. Technetium, as well as other radionuclides, arrives at its destination by the vascular "hot spot" network. Consequently, since one of the main factors in osteomyelitis is vascular embarrassment, the radionuclide may not be able to reach the area of infection, and hence a "cold spot" may be seen. It has been reported that technetium bone scans can identify a likely diagnosis of osteomyelitis, made in conjunction with clinical data, as early as 48 hours after the onset of osseous contamination.

Technetium-99m bone scintigraphy consists of four phases, and is highly sensitive but not specific. The first (angiogram) bone scan phase determines vascularity within intravascular compartments. The second (immediate postinjection) phase represents a "blood-pool" image that quantifies the relative hyperemia or ischemia of the body part along with information about the relative arterial blood present in the capillary and venous system, representing extracellular fluid. The third (delayed) phase, 3 to 4 hours later, visualizes regional rates of bone metabolism, while a fourth (late) bone scan phase is studied 24 hours after injection. It will show greater bone activity and less soft tissue activity in patients with marginal extremity perfusion. The latest portion of the fourth phase is most sensitive for bone contamination,[12] particularly for osteomyelitis in the diabetic foot.

Text continued on p. 116

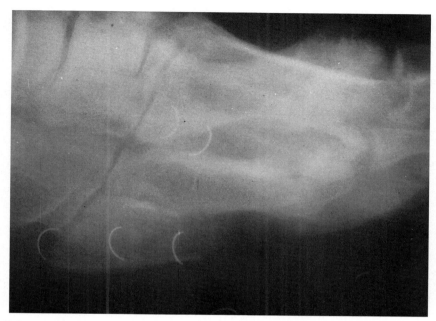

Fig. 7-1 Osteomyelitis following partial amputation of fifth metatarsal bone. Lateral radiograph demonstrates poorly defined osteolysis involving the remaining stump.

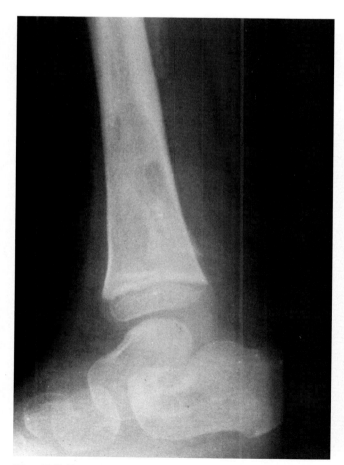

Fig. 7-2 Lateral radiograph of Brodie's abscess reveals a well-defined area of chronic osteomyelitis of the distal tibia.

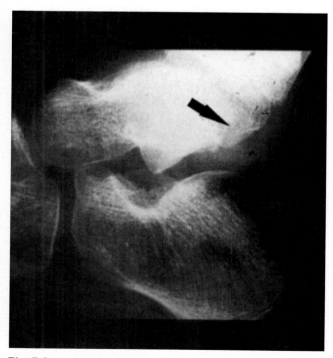

Fig. 7-3 Hematogenous parasitic *(Necator americanus)* osteomyelitis of the talus, demonstrating sclerosis and poorly defined osteolysis *(arrow)* involving the posterior aspect of the bone.

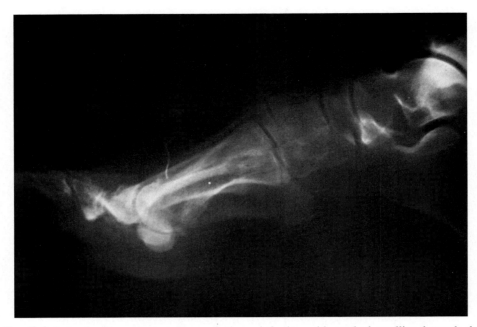

Fig. 7-4 Lateral radiograph reveals a soft tissue infection with marked swelling beneath the metatarsal heads.

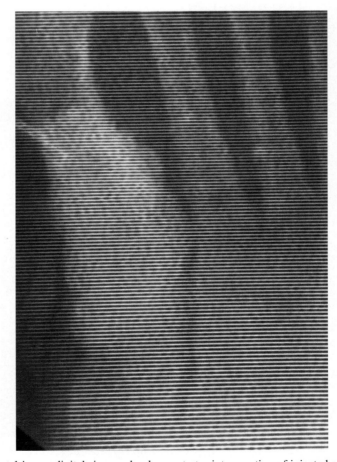

Fig. 7-5 Frontal-image digital sinography demonstrates intravasation of injected contrast material around the first metatarsal and medial (inner) cuneiform bone.

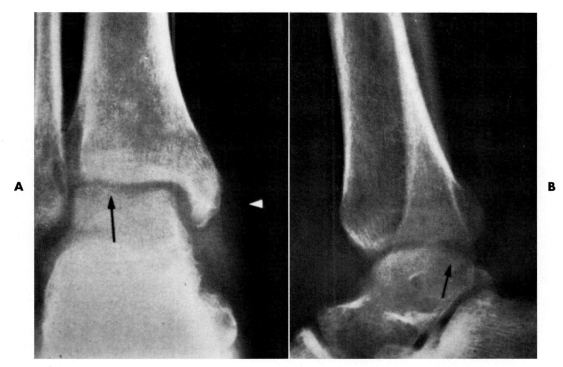

Fig. 7-6 Gonococcal arthritis: frontal **(A)** and lateral **(B)** radiographs reveal soft tissue swelling *(arrows)* and osseous erosions *(arrowhead)* with joint space narrowing involving the ankle (tibiotalar) joint.

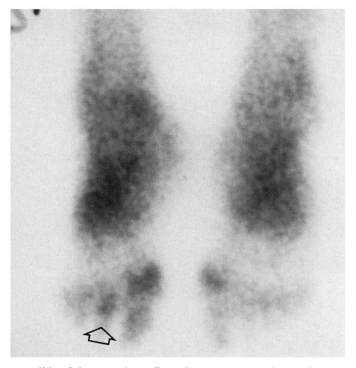

Fig. 7-7 Osteomyelitis of the second toe. Frontal gamma camera image demonstrates abnormal activity *(arrow)* at the site of infection (technetium-99m MDP bone scan).

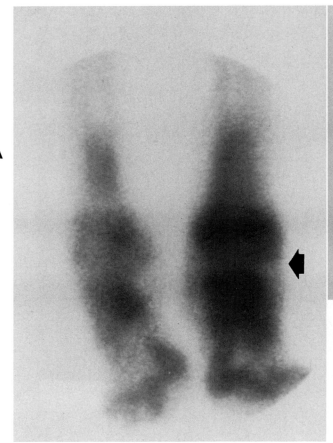

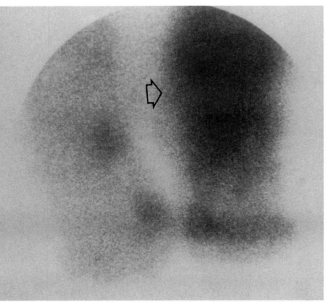

Fig. 7-8 Osteomyelitis and septic arthritis of the rearfoot. **A,** Frontal gamma camera image reveals intense radiopharmaceutical uptake *(arrow)* related to advanced infection (technetium-99m MDP bone scan). **B,** Corresponding gallium-67 citrate image *(arrow,* zone of infectious uptake).

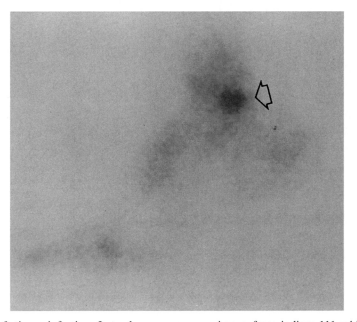

Fig. 7-9 Soft tissue infection. Lateral gamma camera image from indium-111 white cell scan demonstrates focus of abnormal uptake *(arrow)* adjacent to the ankle joint.

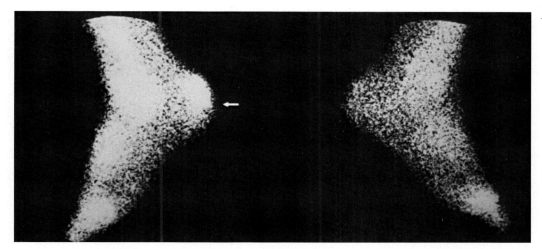

Fig. 7-10 Lateral blood-pool phase gamma camera images of cellulitis from a radionuclide bone scan, revealing hyperemia and increased activity overlying the left calcaneus *(arrow)*.

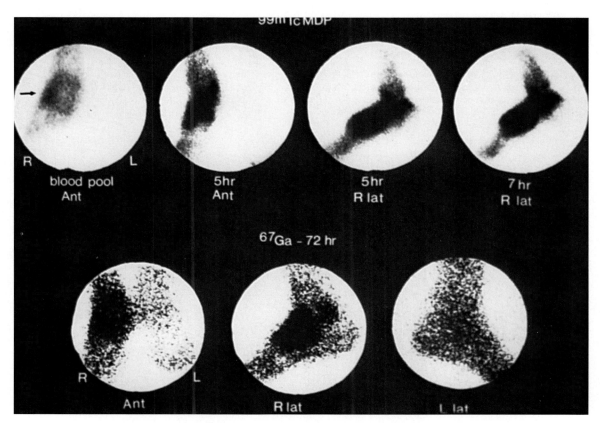

Fig. 7-11 Increased right midfoot activity *(arrow)* on both bone scan *(above)* and gallium scan images is characteristic of osteomyelitis. Left foot is normal.

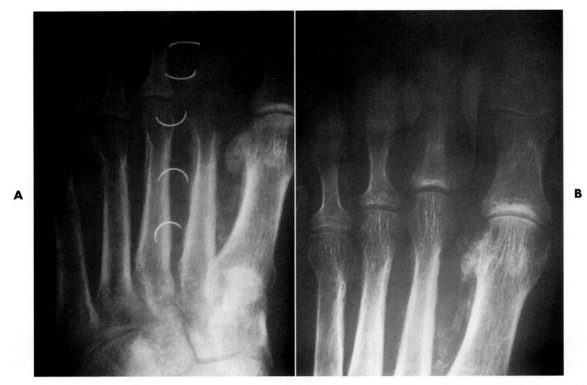

Fig. 7-12 Advanced osteomyelitis. **A,** Frontal radiograph demonstrates destruction of the distal second ray and immature periostitis, in a diabetic patient. **B,** An earlier T1-weighted MRI demonstrates decreased signal intensity in the marrow and subcutaneous fat.

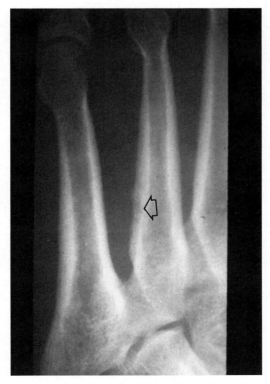

Fig. 7-13 Oblique radiograph reveals early osteomyelitis with subtle cortical erosion *(arrow)* secondary to adjacent soft tissue infection.

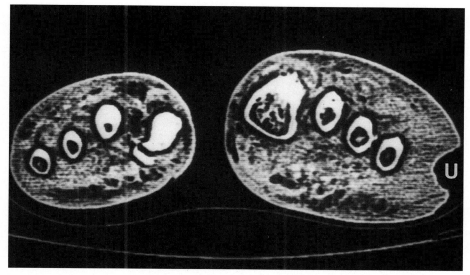

Fig. 7-14 Soft tissue ulceration (recurrent) following amputation. CT soft tissue window demonstrates large lateral defect *(U)* subjacent soft tissue infection.

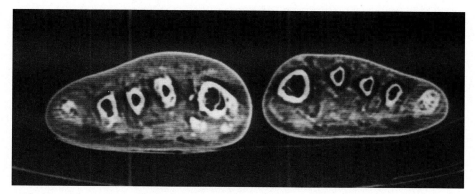

Fig. 7-15 Dorsal soft tissue infection, with CT window, reveals obliteration of fat planes on the dorsal aspect of left foot.

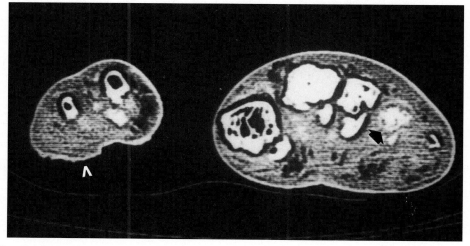

Fig. 7-16 Bilateral CT soft tissue infection window reveals large recurrent plantar ulcer on left *(arrow)* and secondary osteomyelitis on right *(arrow)*.

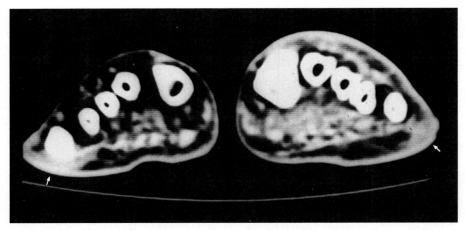

Fig. 7-17 Bilateral lateral-compartment soft tissue infection. CT soft tissue window demonstrates subcutaneous fluid accumulation *(arrow)*.

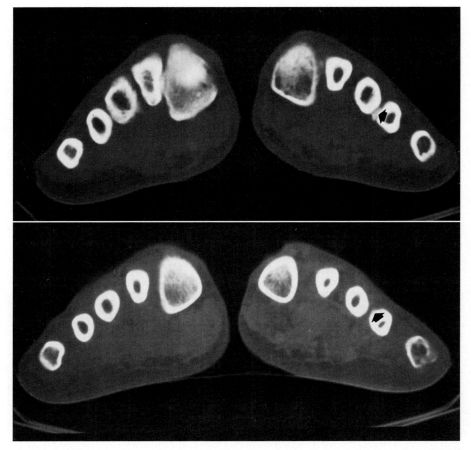

Fig. 7-18 Early osteomyelitis. Sequential CT bone window images reveal immature periostitis *(arrows)* affecting the fourth metatarsal.

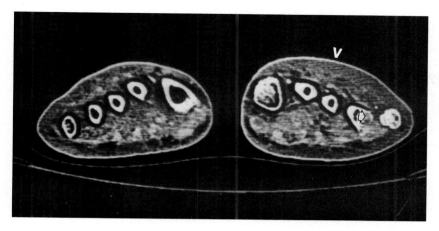

Fig. 7-19 Dorsal soft tissue infection *(arrow)* with early extension to the fourth metatarsal *(arrow)*. CT soft tissue window image.

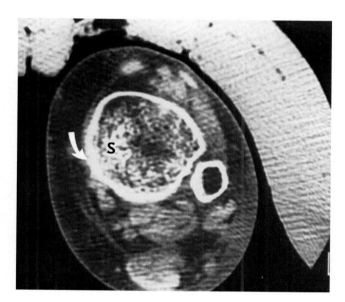

Fig. 7-20 Hematogenous osteomyelitis of the distal tibia. CT soft tissue window image reveals osteosclerosis *(S)* and periostitis *(arrow)*.

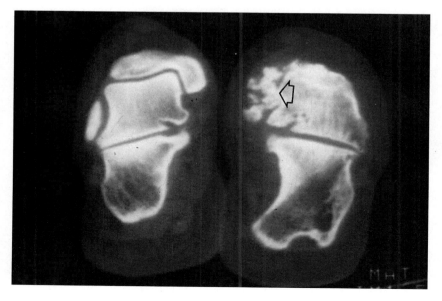

Fig. 7-21 CT bone window demonstrates dystrophic calcification *(arrow)* within an old tuberculous abscess adjacent to the talus.

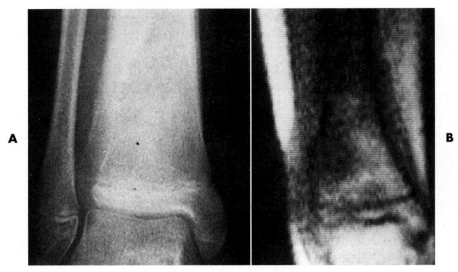

Fig. 7-22 Chronic osteomyelitis of the distal tibia. **A,** Frontal radiograph reveals diffuse osteosclerosis and periostitis. **B,** T1-weighted MRI demonstrates decreased signal intensity in the marrow and subcutaneous fat.

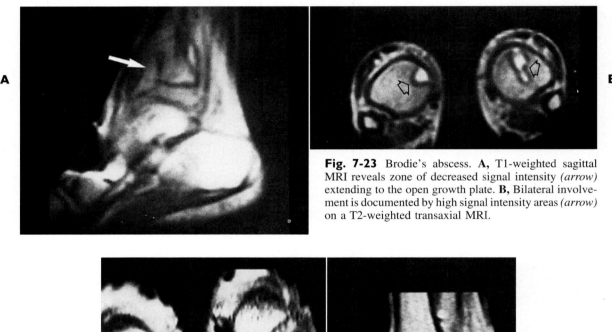

Fig. 7-23 Brodie's abscess. **A,** T1-weighted sagittal MRI reveals zone of decreased signal intensity *(arrow)* extending to the open growth plate. **B,** Bilateral involvement is documented by high signal intensity areas *(arrow)* on a T2-weighted transaxial MRI.

Fig. 7-24 Actinomycosis of the calcaneus. **A,** Transaxial T1-weighted MRI reveals diffuse decreased marrow signal intensity of the talus. **B,** Sagittal T2-weighted MRI demonstrates increased marrow signal intensity in the same distribution.

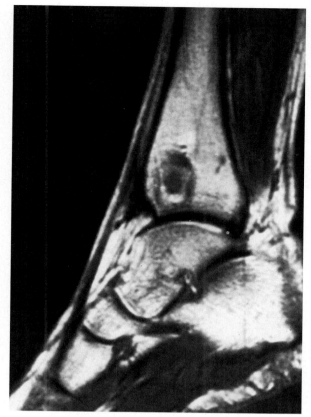

Fig. 7-25 Sagittal T1-weighted MRI of a Brodie's abscess reveals a well-defined lesion of low signal intensity in the distal tibia.

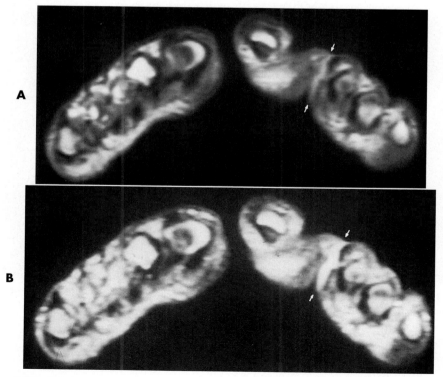

Fig. 7-26 Soft tissue sinus tract. Transaxial proton density weighted (**A**) and T2-weighted (**B**) MRIs demonstrate *(arrows)* linear zone of abnormal signal intensity at a site of prior amputation.

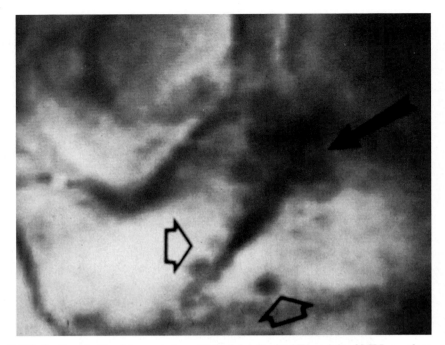

Fig. 7-27 Septic arthritis of the posterior subtalar joint. Sagittal T1-weighted MRI reveals synovial proliferation *(closed arrow)* and irregularity of the subchondral surfaces *(open arrows).*

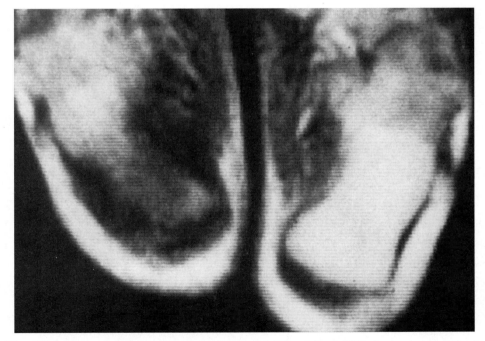

Fig. 7-28 Hematogenous osteomyelitis. Transaxial T1-weighted MRI demonstrates diffusely decreased marrow signal intensity within the left calcaneal tuberosity.

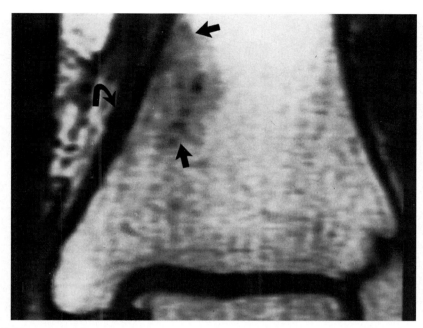

Fig. 7-29 Hematogenous osteomyelitis of the distal tibia. Coronal T1-weighted MRI reveals decreased marrow signal intensity *(straight arrows)* with associated periosteal reaction *(curved arrow).*

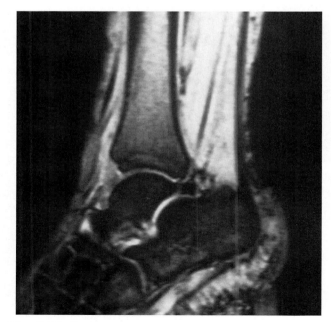

Fig. 7-30 Septic arthritis of the talo-calcaneo-navicular joint. Sagittal gradient echo MRI reveals high signal intensity fluid within the affected articulations.

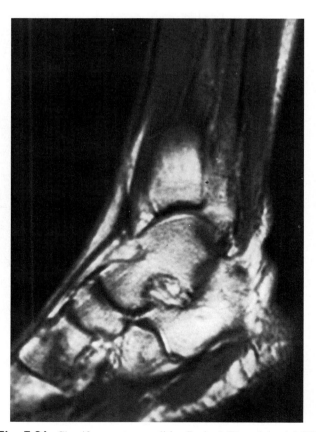

Fig. 7-31 Cuneiform osteomyelitis. Sagittal T1-weighted MRI demonstrates decreased marrow signal intensity within the affected bone.

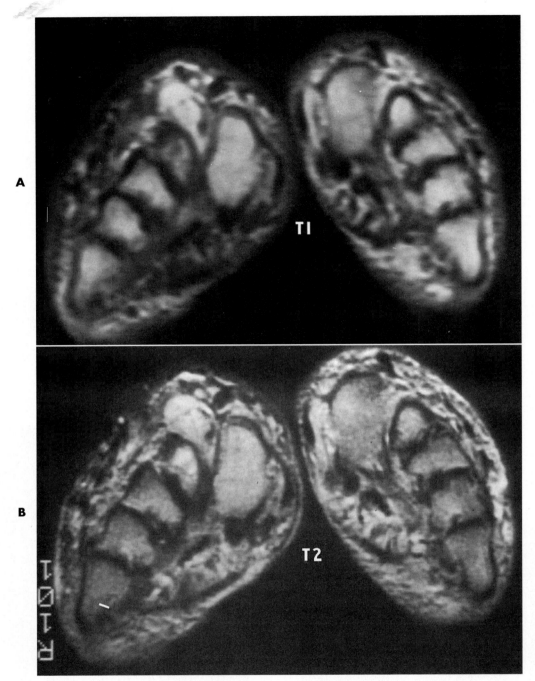

Fig. 7-32 Transaxial T1-weighted **(A)** and T2-weighted **(B)** MRIs reveal abnormal marrow signal in the second metatarsal base, compatible with osteomyelitis.

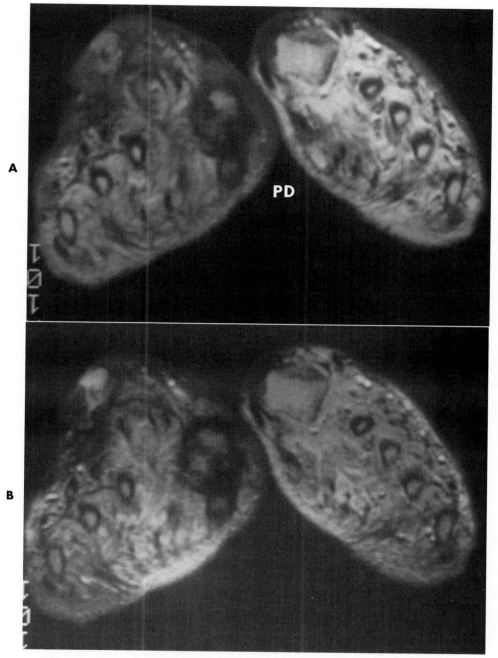

Fig. 7-33 Transaxial proton density (**A**) and T2-weighted (**B**) MRIs reveal dorsal soft tissue abscess in the postoperative patient.

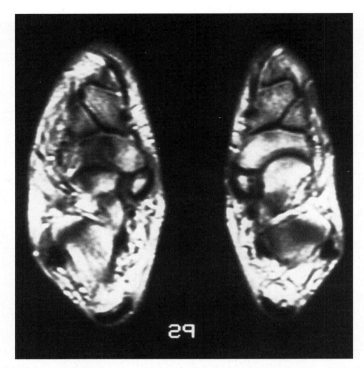

Fig. 7-34 T1-weighted MRI in plantar plane reveals low signal intensity in navicular bone marrow, compatible with osteomyelitis.

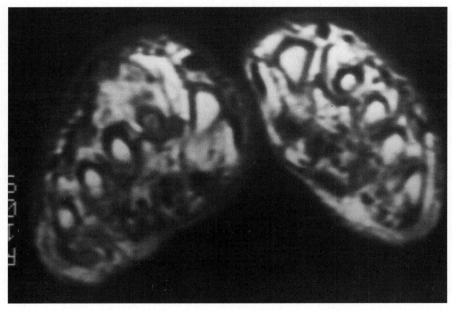

Fig. 7-35 Transaxial T1-weighted MRI reveals low signal intensity in second metatarsal shaft bone marrow, compatible with osteomyelitis.

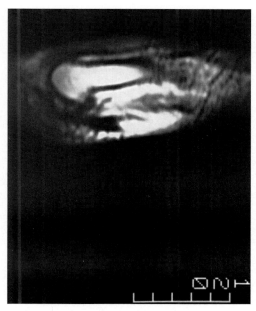

Fig. 7-36 Sagittal T1-weighted MRI of toe reveals soft tissue abscess dorsal to normal metatarsal.

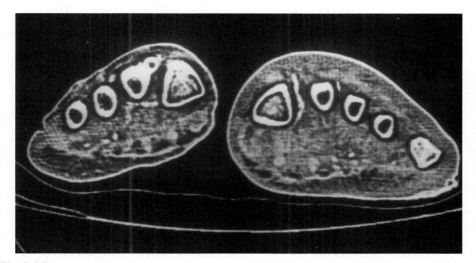

Fig. 7-37 CT soft tissue window reveals lateral compartment infection extending to dorsum of foot.

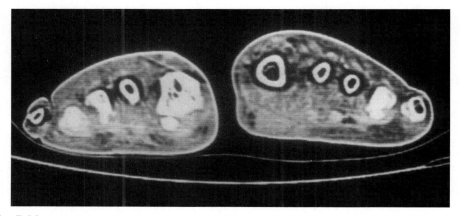

Fig. 7-38 CT soft tissue window reveals medial compartment infection *(right)* and cellulitis *(left)*.

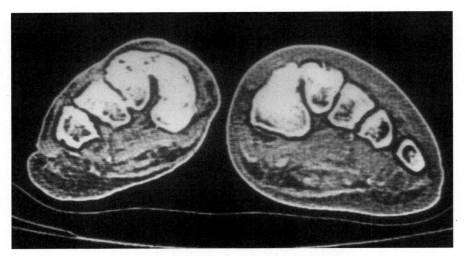

Fig. 7-39 CT soft tissue window reveals intermediate compartment infection extending into metatarsophalangeal joint.

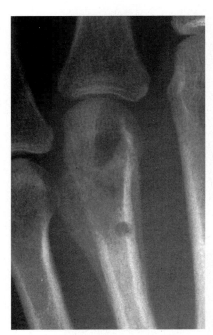

Fig. 7-40 Radiograph reveals osteomyelitis of the second metatarsal extending into the respective MPJ.

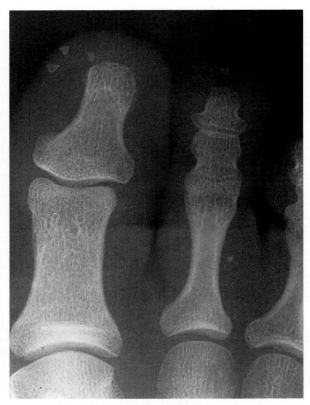

Fig. 7-41 Radiograph reveals soft tissue infection of great toe with evidence of secondary osteomyelitis.

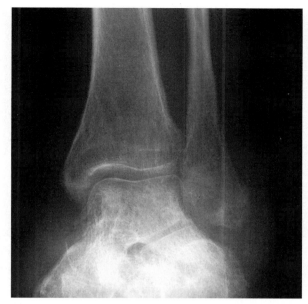

Fig. 7-42 Oblique radiograph reveals periarticular osteopenia in a case of early ankle septic arthritis.

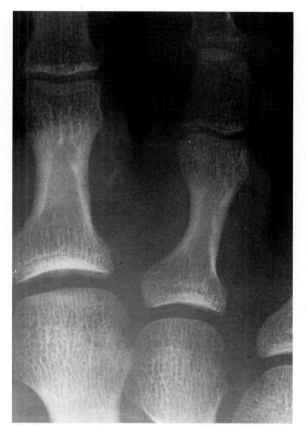

Fig. 7-43 Radiograph reveals periarticular osteopenia in a case of early septic fourth metatarsal arthritis.

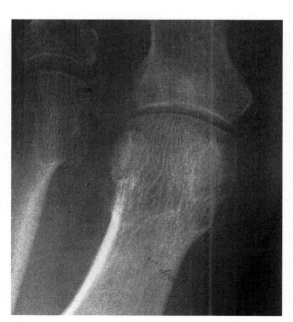

Fig. 7-44 Radiograph reveals narrowing of first MPJ and early medial erosion of metatarsal head in patient with septic arthritis and osteomyelitis.

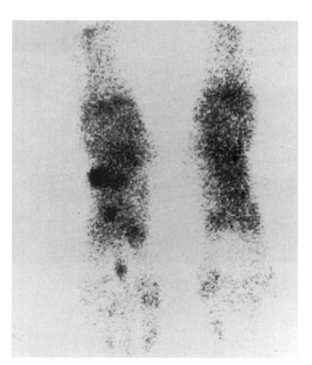

Fig. 7-45 Bone scan reveals increased uptake in anterolateral aspect of calcaneus, compatible with osteomyelitis.

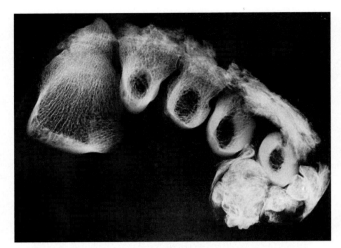

Fig. 7-46 Injected specimen radiograph showing spread of lateral compartment infection to dorsum of foot.

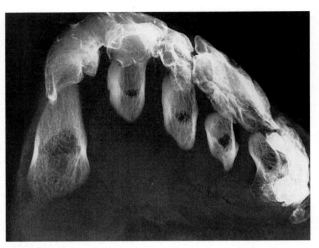

Fig. 7-47 Injected specimen radiograph showing dorsal compartment infection.

Fig. 7-48 **A,** Injected specimen radiograph showing intermediate compartment infection. **B,** Corresponding injected specimen.

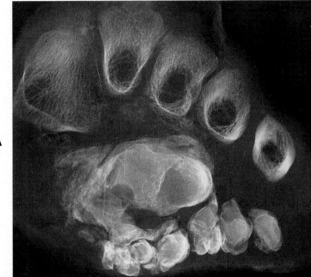

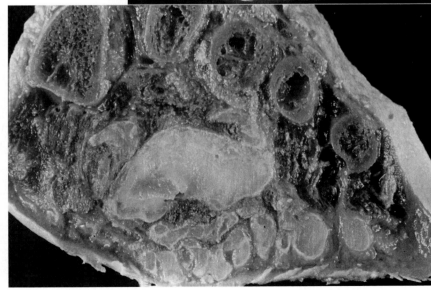

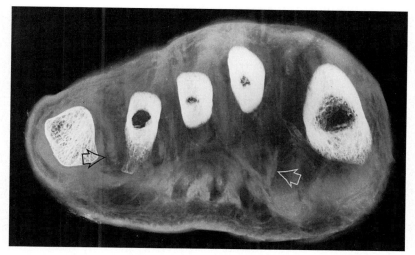

Fig. 7-49 Specimen radiograph demonstrating intermuscular fibrous septa *(black and white arrows)* separating three plantar compartments.

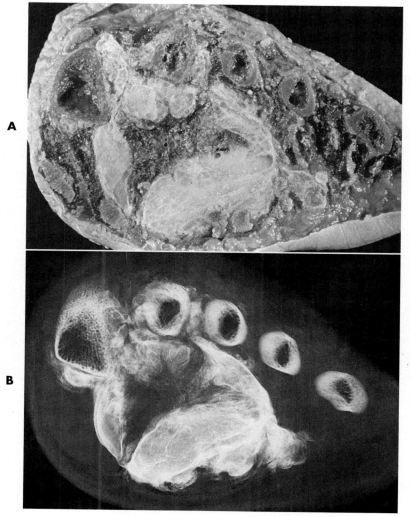

Fig. 7-50 Injected specimen **(A)** and injected specimen radiograph **(B)** showing spread of intermediate compartment infection to dorsum of foot.

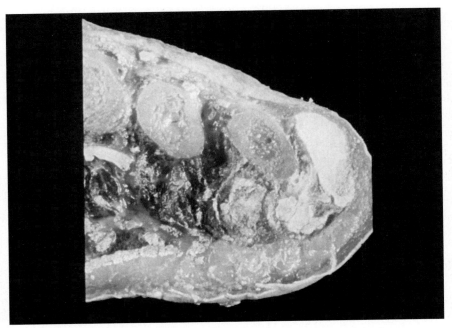

Fig. 7-51 Injected specimen showing lateral compartment infection.

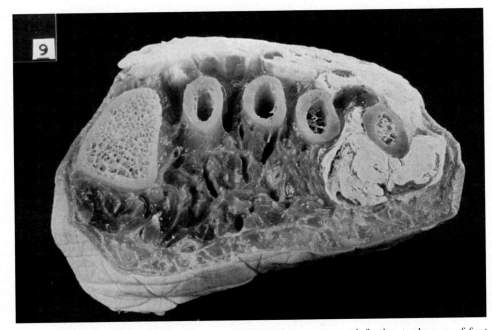

Fig. 7-52 Injected specimen showing spread of lateral compartment infection to dorsum of foot.

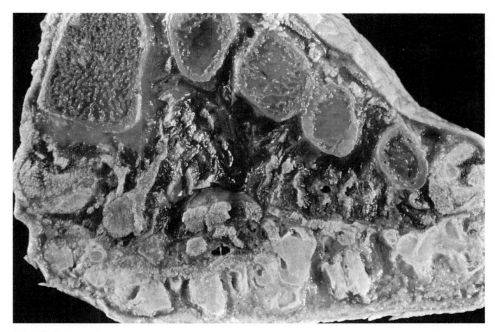

Fig. 7-53 Injected specimen showing spread of lateral compartment infection into plantar fat.

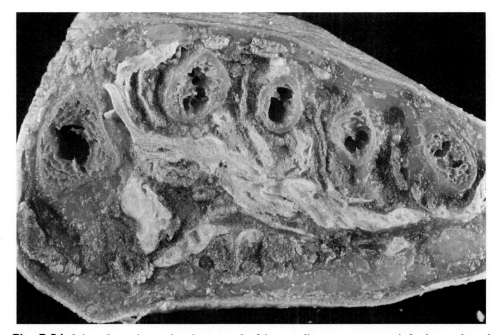

Fig. 7-54 Injected specimen showing spread of intermediate compartment infection to lateral compartment and dorsum of foot.

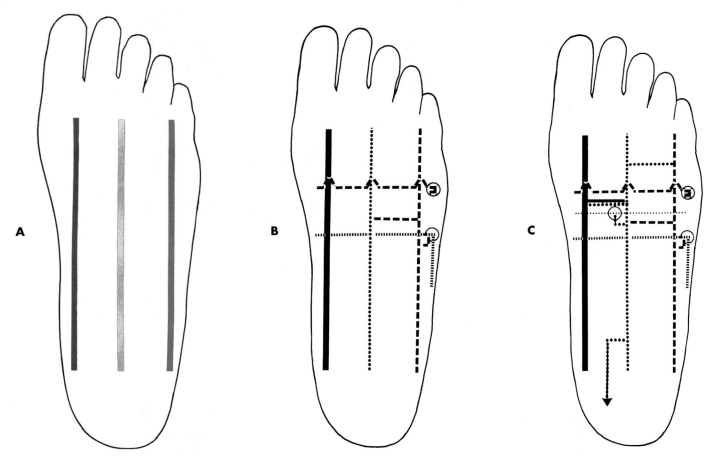

Fig. 7-55 Distribution of plantar compartments **(A),** with pathways of potential spread **(B** and **C).**

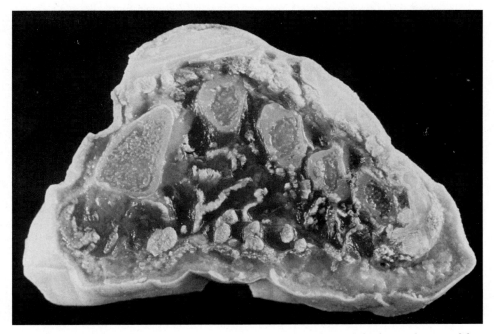

Fig. 7-56 Injected specimen showing spread of lateral compartment infection to dorsum of foot.

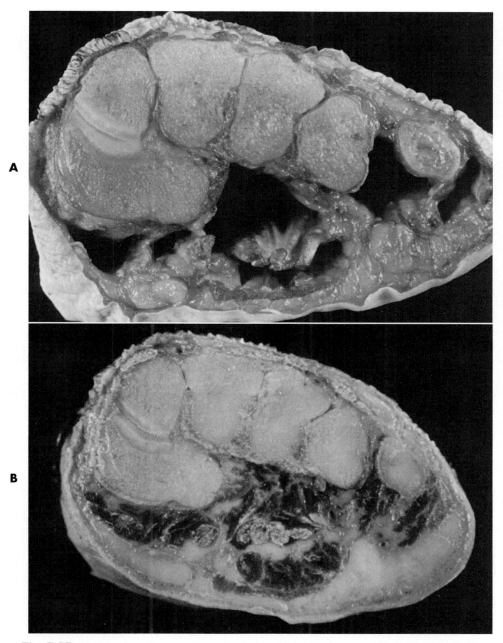

Fig. 7-57 A, Specimen showing three plantar compartments separated by intermuscular fibrotic septa. **B,** With muscles intact.

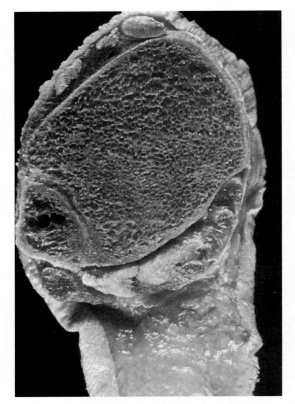

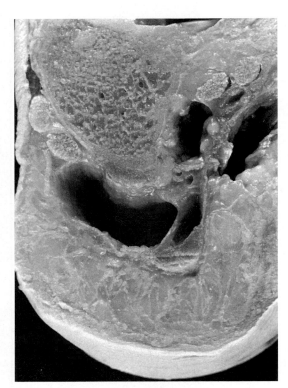

Fig. 7-58 Injected specimen showing spread of intermediate compartment infection into posterior compartment of calf.

Fig. 7-59 Specimen showing distribution of intermediate compartment in the rearfoot.

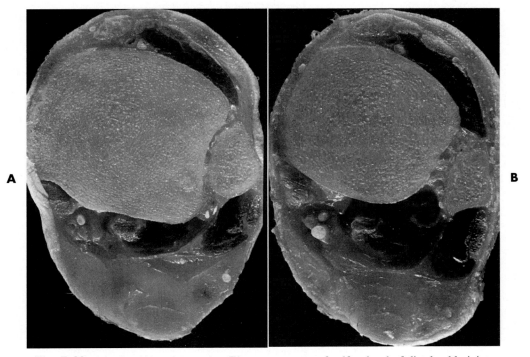

Fig. 7-60 Anterior (**A**) and posterior (**B**) compartments of calf at level of distal ankle joint.

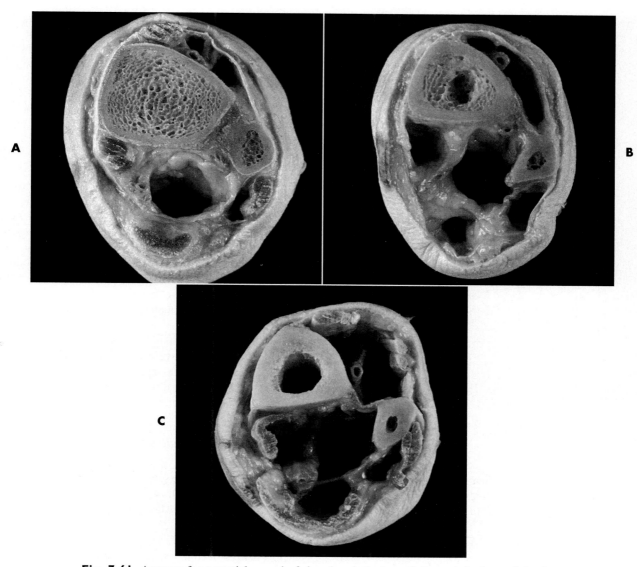

Fig. 7-61 Avenues for potential spread of dorsal and plantar soft tissue infections of the foot into the anterior and posterior compartments of the calf, respectively. **A** to **C,** Distal to proximal levels.

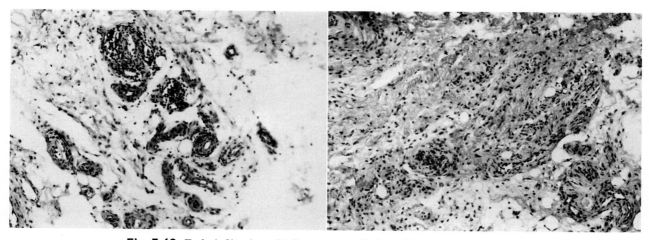

Fig. 7-62 Early infiltration of inflammatory cells in pedal soft tissue infections.

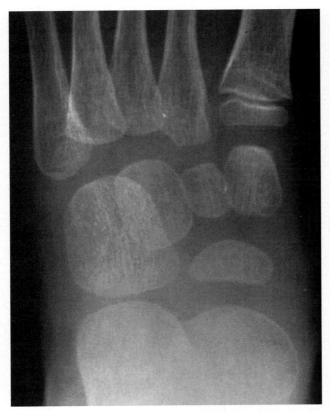

Fig. 7-63 Radiograph demonstrates soft tissue swelling without evidence of osteomyelitis, in a pediatric infection caused by a puncture wound.

A differential diagnostic scheme for a bone scan that is hot in all three phases, and becomes more focused with each subsequent phase, might look like the following:

Hot first phase
1. Acute fracture
2. Osteomyelitis
3. Recent surgery or debridement
4. Reflex sympathetic dystrophy (RSD)
5. Charcot joint(s)
6. Hypervascular tumor

Hot second phase
1. Subacute fracture
2. Surgery (months) in the recent past
3. Charcot joint(s)

Hot third phase
1. Degenerative bone and joint disease
2. Stress reaction and altered weight bearing
3. Surgery or fracture more than 1 year ago
4. Stable Charcot joint(s)
5. Tumor

Gallium-67 citrate scans

Gallium is considered an inflammatory imaging agent because it accumulates at the sites of plasma proteins, white blood cells, ferritin, transferrin, and siderophores. A gallium scan is performed 6 to 48 hours following a 3- to 5-mCi injection. Unlike technetium, gallium is not dependent on blood flow, possesses a 78-hour half-life, and is excreted by the kidneys. In serious cases of pedal infection, technetium is combined with gallium scans in order to obtain the most complete evaluation possible of the pathologic process. If both agents are used, technetium should be given first, followed in 24 to 48 hours by gallium.[13]

Indium-111 oxine (8-hydroxyquinoline) scans

Indium-111 is an inflammatory imaging radiopharmaceutical that binds to the cytoplasmic components of the white blood cell membrane. It may be more accurate in detecting acute infections, while gallium-67 may be more sensitive in assessing subacute and chronic infections. When this agent is used, autologous leukocytes are isolated from blood and labeled with the indium-111 oxine. The prepared cells are then introduced into the patient, and scanning is done 24 hours later.[14] Unfortunately, some patients may demonstrate multiple "hot spots" at a very early stage of *Staphylococcus aureus* septicemia that do not progress to bone infection. Moreover, a negative scan with a confirmed case of osteomyelitis may occur as a result of impaired blood supply. There may even be difficulty in differentiating normal bone repair from bone infection, producing a biologic false-positive reaction.

Combination nuclear scans

Combination scans, or multiple tracer studies, may be performed when necessary, but the bone scan should precede the gallium scan by 24 to 48 hours. The following scheme lists clinical scenarios when multiple tracer studies may be used:
A. Acute osteomyelitis
   1. Positive technetium-99m MDP scan in all three phases (weak, moderate, and strong)
   2. Positive gallium-67 scan focal uptake
   3. Positive indium-111 scan
B. Chronic inactive osteomyelitis
   1. Positive technetium-99m MDP scan in three phases (weak, moderate, and very strong)
   2. Negative gallium-67 scan
   3. Negative indium-111 scan
C. Acute cellulitis
   1. Positive technetium-99m MDP scan in three phases (strong, moderate, and weak)
   2. Positive gallium-67 scan with diffuse uptake
   3. Positive indium-111 scan
D. Infected implant(s)
   1. Positive technetium-99m MDP scan
   2. Strongly positive gallium-67 scan
E. Charcot joint(s)
   1. Positive technetium-99m MDP scan in four increasing phases
   2. Negative gallium-67 scan
   3. Negative indium-111 scan

HMPAO labeled leukocytes

Recently, technetium-99 hexamethylpropylamine oxine (HMPAO; Ceretic* labeled leukocytes have been developed as a cost effective alternative to indium-111 labeled cells, due to a similar biodistribution and function. The more favorable radiation dosimetry of the technetium label permits a larger dose of radiation to be administered. Images of the lower extremities can be rapidly acquired and are more readily interpreted because of the larger amount of localized activity. Although clinical experience with this technique is limited, preliminary studies suggest that HMPAO labeled WBC scintigraphy is a simple, accurate, sensitive (90%), and specific (86%) test for the detection of pedal osteomyelitis.[15-18]

MISCELLANEOUS TESTS

Sinograms, tenograms, arthrograms, and fistulograms are used in infection evaluation to help identify contaminated soft tissue planes, dead spaces, joints, or sinus tracts. Initially, a soft-tipped catheter is used to inject a radiocontrast medium into a suspected contaminated area to determine its extent. Care is taken to avoid the creation of new contaminated tissue planes, through the avoidance of too much back pressure. Upon removal of the catheter, the wound is sealed and radiographs are taken in three planes. When needed, sinography may be combined with fluoroscopy or CT scanning in order to derive information from the combination of tests which normally would not be ascertained by the use of either modality separately.[19]

CONCLUSION

Many radiographic techniques are used in the identification of foot infections. This chapter reviews these modalities in an illustrated format. It is hoped that diagnostic and clinical understanding is enhanced with this photographic case review style. Nonclinical material may be acquired from more traditional texts.

REFERENCES

1. Weissman S: Standard radiographic techniques for the foot and ankle, *Clin Podiatr Med Surg* 5:767, 1988.
2. Schlefman BSS: Radiographic modalities and interpretation. In Marcinko DE, ed: *Medical and Surgical Therapeutics of the Foot and Ankle,* Baltimore, 1992, Williams & Wilkins.
3. Kirby KA, Loendorf AJ, Gregorio R: Anterior axial projection of the foot, *J Am Podiatr Med Assoc* 78:159, 1988.
4. Schlefman BS: Radiology. In McGlamry ED, ed: *Fundamentals of Foot Surgery,* Baltimore, 1987, Williams & Wilkins.
5. Hirsch BE, Udupa JK, Roberts D: Three dimensional reconstruction of the foot from computed tomography scans, *J Am Podiatr Med Assoc* 79:384, 1989.
6. Huff HR, Kravette MA: Computed tomography of the foot and ankle, *J Am Podiatr Med Assoc* 76:375, 1986.
7. Oloff-Solomon J, Solomon MA: Computed tomographic scanning of the foot and ankle, *Clin Podiatr Med Surg* 5:931, 1988.
8. Sartoris DJ, Resnick D: Magnetic resonance imaging of podiatric disorders: a pictorial essay, *J Foot Surg* 26:336, 1987.
9. Downey M: Magnetic resonance imaging (MRI) vs. computed tomography (CT): clinical applications in the foot and ankle. In McGlamry ED, ed: *Reconstructive surgery of the foot and leg—update 1989,* Tucker, Ga, 1989, Podiatry Institute Publishing Co.
10. Sartoris D, Resnick D: Magnetic resonance imaging of the foot: technical aspects, *J Foot Surg* 26:351, 1987.
11. Karl RD, Hammes CS: Nuclear medicine imaging in podiatric disorders, *Clin Podiatr Med Surg* 5:909, 1988.
12. Visser HJ, Jacobs AM, Oloff L, Drago JJ: The use of differential scintigraphy in the clinical diagnosis of osseous and soft tissue changes affecting the diabetic foot, *J Foot Surg* 23:85, 1984.
13. Hetherington VJ: Technetium and combined gallium and technetium scans in the neurotrophic foot, *J Am Podiatry Assoc* 72:458, 1982.
14. Techner LM, Eiser CA: Pathology in the rearfoot, *J Foot Surg* 26:266, 1987.
15. Blume PA, Dey HM, Daley LJ: Diagnosis of pedal osteomyelitis with Tc-99m HMPAO labeled leukocytes, *JFAS* 36:120-126, 1997.
16. Loredo R, Metter D: Imaging of the diabetic foot: emphasis on nuclear medicine and magnetic resonance imaging, *Clin Podiatr Med Surg* 14(2)235-265, 1997.
17. Lau LS, Bin G, Suphaneewan J: Cost effectiveness of magnetic resonance imaging in diagnosis of *Pseudomonas aeruginosa* infection after puncture wound, *JFAS* 36:36-43, 1997.
18. DiMarcangenelo, Yu TC: Diagnostic imaging of heel pain and plantar fasciitis, *Clin Podiatr Med Surg* 14(2)281-303, 1997.
19. Ross JA, Lepow GM: The use of CT in the foot, *J Foot Surg* 21:11, 1982.

ADDITIONAL READINGS

Juhl JH, Crummy AB: *Essentials of radiographic images,* Philadelphia, 1993, JB Lippincott.
Mayer DP, Hirsch BE, Simon WH: *Foot and ankle: a sectional imaging atlas,* Philadelphia, 1993, WB Saunders.
Sartoris DJ, Resnick D: Pictorial analysis: computed tomography of trauma to the ankle and hindfoot, *J Foot Surg* 27:80, 1988.
Sartoris DJ, Resnick D: Podiatric imaging quiz, *J Foot Surg* 27:178, 1988.
Silverman FN, Kuhn JP: *Caffey's pediatric x-ray diagnosis,* St Louis, 1993, Mosby.
Singer JM: Hershey board certification review outline study guide, Camp Hill, Pa, 1997, Pennsylvania Podiatric Medical Association Press.
Solomon MA, Oloff-Solomon J: Magnetic resonance imaging in the foot and ankle, *Clin Podiatr Med Surg* 5:945, 1988.

---

* Amersham Healthcare, Arlington Heights, Ill.

Section Three

The Spectrum and
Clinical Variety of
Foot Infections

8

Skin, Subcutaneous, and Soft Tissue Foot Infections

Frederick J. Bartolomei

Everyone has a skin disease of one kind or another, sooner or later.
What they do about it is often amusing. R.L. Sutton, Jr.

The skin and subcutaneous tissues serve as a mechanical and physiological barrier between the environment and the underlying soft tissues and osseous stroma. In the foot, the skin is both anatomically and ecologically unique and easily susceptible to infectious contamination from all types of pathologic microorganisms. Therefore, the purpose of this chapter is to review some of the more common bacterial, viral, and fungal organisms that may colonize the pedal skin and produce disease. It is hoped that a high index of suspicion, coupled with the appropriate cultures, biopsies, and tests, will alert the clinician and encourage both prompt diagnosis and effective treatment of these infectious skin and soft tissue entities.

ANATOMY OF THE INTEGUMENTARY BARRIER

The human skin serves as a mechanical, physiological, and biochemical barrier between the internal milieu and the external environment. This cutaneous shield consists of superficial epidermal layers and deeper dermal strata. The structure varies at different sites, even on the human foot.

Embryologically, the skin evolves from three distinct founts. The epidermis arises from the ectoderm. The dermis arises from connective tissue, and vascular elements come from the mesoderm. Melanocytes and other specialized migratory cells develop from the neural ectoderm.

Human epidermis possesses four layers: the stratum basale, the stratum spinosum, the stratum granulosum, and the stratum corneum. The deepest layer, the stratum basale, is separated from the underlying dermal strata by the basement membrane.

The stratum basale, also referred to as the stratum germinativum, contains cells of a low columnar or high cuboidal morphology. The predominant feature of the cells in this layer is a strongly basophilic, ovoid nucleus. Free ribosomes and filaments are abundant. Cells of the stratum

basale maintain a steady state with the adjacent dermis, and the interface area is increased by projections known as rete pegs.

The stratum spinosum lies directly above the stratum basale. The cells of this layer assume an increasingly parallel orientation to the external or exposed layer of the skin, or they migrate outward. Intracellular features characteristic of the stratum spinosum include thinning of the nucleus, as well as increased quantities of rough endoplasmic reticulum and Gogli apparatus. At low powers of magnification under the light microscope, the stratum spinosum appears to have bridges across the tight intercellular spaces. This erroneous image of many sharp points (processes) led to the designation of the "prickle cell" or "prickle cell layer."

The stratum granulosum is the most superficial of the three layers (basale-spinosum-granulosum) that constitute the stratum malpighii, or living portion of the epidermis. The stratum granulosum is intensely basophilic and contrasts sharply with adjacent layers under light microscopy. Keratohyalin granules are a characteristic of the layer. The granules come together into an amorphous ground substance. The typical morphology of cells in this stratum is even more flattened than the previous layer and with swollen nuclei.

The so-called "lucidum" layer represents an artifact of fixation, as early microscopists observed a clear zone between the stratum granulosum and the outermost epidermal layers (stratum corneum). The void occurs during fixation, and no such layer actually exists. The stratum corneum comprises the visible skin. This layer represents the first line of protection against invasion of microorganisms in the intact host. The stratum corneum of the plantar foot is subject to the unique challenge of bipedal locomotion. Cells of the stratum corneum contain an amorphous intracellular composition typically lacking organelles. Under scanning electron microscopy (SEM) the free surface of healthy stratum corneum appears to be composed of more or less regularly arranged cubes with a crazed covering.

The epidermal-dermal junction (basement membrane) divides the two distinct sections of skin. Constitutional components of the basement membrane originate from both the deepest portion of the epidermis and the most superficial portion of the dermis. The basement membrane is PAS-positive.

The dermis, like the epidermis, can be broken into superficial and deep sections. The papillary dermis is superficial, while the reticular dermis rests deeper. The papillary dermis meshes with the epidermis via papillae, which consist of columns of dermis that jut out into cavitations between the rete pegs of the epidermis. The papillary dermis is significantly richer in neurovascular and lymphatic structures than the deeper reticular dermis. Likewise, the papillary portion contains an abundance of cellular constituents (lymphocytes, fibrocytes, and histiocytes) relative to the reticular portion. The reticular dermis possesses an amorphous stroma or matrix interspersed with aggregate of collagen.

The subcutaneous layer (hypodermis) is considered by some to belong to the skin. If viewed in that perspective, the subcutaneous layer becomes the deepest and thickest stratum. The predominant cell of the hypodermis is the lipocyte. The cytoplasm of a lipocyte demonstrates a nucleus smashed against the periphery as a result of the enormous quantity of intracellular fat. Triglycerides are the principal component of fat. Lipocytes become subdivided into fat lobules by intervening sheets of collagen. Subcutaneous fatty deposits are distributed in different thicknesses throughout the body. Even the human foot demonstrates marked variations in depth of the layer; especially when one considers the difference between the weight-bearing plantar heel and the dorsum of the digits.

In addition to the functions of dermal regulation, tactile sensation, and control of moisture loss, two other important functions of the skin are the inhibition of microorganism invasion and protection against stress from the external environment. Any acute, subacute, or chronic event that violates the integument favors the development of an infection.

INFLAMMATION, INFLAMMATORY MEDIATORS, AND IMMUNOLOGY

Inflammation involves cellular destruction and repair resulting from noxious stimuli. The stimuli may include bacterial, viral, or fungal organisms as well as thermal, mechanical, chemical, or ionizing radiation sources. The inflammatory process purges the site of irritation by facilitating the removal of the offending substance. This process is accelerated through the release of by-products of cellular necrosis.

On a cellular level, inflammation is dependent upon the non–immune compromised host's ability to recognize foreign bacterial surface structures. For example, bacteria initiate the traditional complement (19 different plasma proteins) cascade via IgG and IgM antibodies, and the characteristic sequence of an inflammatory response involves vascular dilation with acceleration of the blood passing through arterioles, capillaries, and venules. The alternative complement cascade (IgG, IgM, IgA, and IgE antibodies) is activated by gram-negative endotoxins, proteases, polysaccharides, and lipopolysaccharides. As permeability increases, leukocytes migrate from the vessel wall toward the nidus of irritation.[8] The invasion of PMNLs typifies the early phase of inflammation, most notably when a bacterial etiology is responsible. Sticky (chemotactic) substances (C5a, C5a des-Arg, and leukotriene B_4) are then released from mast cells and neutrophils, which adhere to microbial surfaces and facilitate the attachment of invaders for destruction by C3b and IgG antibodies (opsonization). This process is augmented by oxidative and nonoxidative neutrophilic antimicrobial proteins (BPFs [bactericidal permeability factors]), cathepsin G, defensins, lactoferrin, and lysozyme, through the process of hydrolysis.[4] As the process advances, a barrage of mononuclear cells enters the region and predominates. These include monocytes, macrophages, lymphocytes, and plasma cells. Therefore, an acute inflammation, by definition, requires vasodilation, exudation of inflammation fluid, and localization of leukocytes.[8]

The initial host defense to bacterial infections involves phagocytosis. Phagocytosis is the engulfment of foreign matter and is accomplished by the PMNLs and monocytes. To facilitate the process of phagocytosis, both gamma globulin and C3, the third component of complement, opsonize the foreign matter. Degranulation occurs subsequent to phagocytosis of the opsonized matter. Peroxidation, the release of hydrogen peroxide, is ultimately responsible for destruction of the foreign matter in the case of invading microorganisms.

BACTERIAL, FUNGAL, AND VIRAL INFECTIONS OF PEDAL SKIN

A plethora of microorganisms are capable of producing a cutaneous infection in the susceptible host skin under appropriate conditions. A review of different disease conditions and the responsible organisms follows.

Bacterial infections of the pedal skin

Cutaneous infections of bacterial etiology include carbuncles, cellulitis, ecthyma, erysipelas, erythrasma, impetigo, intertrigo, paronychia, pitted keratolysis, scalded skin syndrome, and toxic shock syndrome. The features of each relevant to the foot will be addressed individually.

A *carbuncle* is an infection deep within adjacent follicles, typically caused by *Staphylococcus pyogenes*. Although the nape of the neck and shoulders are common locations, the buttocks, thighs, feet, ankles, and legs may be affected. In general, middle-aged or elderly males develop the lesions, especially those in the diabetic or immunosuppressed populations. A carbuncle begins as an exquisitely tender, indurated, erythematous papule progressing to a diameter of several centimeters over 3 to 5 days. Intense localized inflammation of the nearby dermal and subcutaneous structures accompanies the lesion. After several days, pus exudes from the follicular openings on the free surface of the skin. A deep depression, caused by tissue necrosis, occurs within the nodule, covered by a yellow-colored crust. Fever, chills, and malaise frequently accompany the lesion. Oral or parenteral empiric antibiotic therapy with excellent gram-positive coverage should be initiated, pending the sensitivity report. Hyperosmolar warm compresses with Epsom salt or similar agents offer a useful adjunctive modality.

Cellulitis is a skin and subcutaneous infection that generally represents a clinical, rather than cultural, diagnosis. It consists of either a local variety, with intense redness, or an ascending variety, along the path of another anatomic structure (e.g., tendon or lymph chain). Thus, the latter is a more urgent phenomenon, as it can lead to contamination of vital lower-extremity structures. Staphylococci and group B streptococci are typical etiologic agents in the adult, and systemic signs or symptoms are not usually noted. Since localized interstitial tissue volume increases, from both exudates and transudates across capillary membranes, radiographs may demonstrate an increased soft tissue density and volume, in severe cases. Soft tissue planes may also become obliterated (Togard's triangle), yet no radiographic finding is diagnostic of cellulitis. Empiric treatment with nafcillin or penicillin G is often curative. In children, *Haemophilus influenzae* (type b), group A streptococci (traumatically induced), and *S. aureus* are usual pathogens, and systemic chills, fever, and positive blood cultures are often seen. A lumbar puncture may be necessary, in severe cases, to rule out meningitis. Mild cases are treated with cefaclor, while more serious cases are treated with either cefuroxime, cefotaxime, or ceftriaxone.

Ecthyma involves a cutaneous pyogenic infection. The lower extremity represents the most frequent site, with involvement ranging from the gluteal region to the malleoli. Malnutrition, lack of proper hygiene, and superficial insults to the integument predispose an individual to the condition.[2] Although more common among children and adolescents, a person of any age may be afflicted. Cultures from lesions of ecthyma may reveal staphylococci, streptococci, or both microorganisms. The clinical presentation consists of a firmly adherent scab or crust overlying an erythematous, indurated base. Treatment includes debridement of the adherent crust, after hydration to facilitate removal. Topical antibiotic preparations with gentamicin, erythromycin, polymyxin-bacitracin combination, and other agents can be empirically initiated pending laboratory reports and modified as necessary. In addition, if clinically indicated,

nutritional support with a multivitamin-zinc compound may be a useful adjunct.

Erythrasma is a commonly overlooked cause of infective interdigital dermatologic disease. The condition, caused by *Corynebacterium minutissimum,* presents as a superficial, distinctly marginated region of xerotic skin. Frequently the infection is chronic and occasionally it is pruritic. The dark moist environment of a shoe favors the development of erythrasma almost as much as it does tinea pedis. Under Wood's light examination, erythrasma fluoresces coral-red. Coexistent erythrasma and interdigital tinea pedis is not uncommon, and clinical distinction concerning the class of microorganisms responsible for the physical findings provides a formidable challenge. Erythromycin is the current mainstay of therapy. The usual adult dose is 1 g per day in divided doses. The topical use of 2% erythromycin solution is an excellent adjunct to primary oral therapy. The topical solution can be especially helpful in limiting recurrences if used on a maintenance basis. Antibacterial soaps may extend the same benefit.

Erysipelas represents a virulent streptococcal infection in the compromised host, creating systemic manifestations. It differs from the typical streptococcal cellulitis in the otherwise healthy host by the exaggeration of findings evident upon physical examination. In the "noncomplicated" streptococcal cellulitis, a local marginated region of erythema, hyperthermia, and edema exists with limited constitutional symptoms. In contrast to erysipelas, an acute onset of high fever, prostration, and headache coincide with the cutaneous manifestations. In general, the *S. pyogenes* enters through a defect in the integumentary barrier, through hematogenous spread, while seeding of a traumatized area can provide an alternative mechanism. Lymphedema or venous stasis favors the initial development of erysipelas and tends to increase the likelihood of recurrent bouts. Recurrence may develop subsequent to appropriate treatment even without apparent reinoculation of the causative microorganism. Approximately one half of the cases involve the lower leg and foot in the adult population.[2] Treatment consists of parenteral antibiotics with gram-positive coverage pending culture and sensitivity studies of the aspirate recovered from the advancing margin of the infection. Evaluation of the affected limb, antipyretics, nutritional enhancement, and supportive measures may also prove beneficial.

Impetigo (pyoderma) is a contagious skin infection with two morphologic presentations, either bullous impetigo or impetigo contagiosa. Bullous impetigo may involve plantar and palmar surfaces, in addition to other locations. Although the face predominates, the lesions of impetigo contagiosa may appear at any site except the plantar and palmar surfaces. Staphylococci are responsible for bullous impetigo, whereas impetigo contagiosa is of streptococcal or mixed origin.[2] In general, bullous impetigo affects older children and adults, with impetigo contagiosa confined to children of elementary school age. Both bullous impetigo and impetigo contagiosa begin with fluid-filled sacs. In the former case, the lesion approaches a 1- to 2-cm diameter prior to spontaneous rupture. In the latter instance, a thin vesicle ruptures rapidly. A brown-colored crust covers an underlying area of central healing in the bullous variety. A honey-colored crust covers a nonhealed central zone with radial extension, allowing coalescence of nearby lesions, in the contagious variety. Treatment may require the gentle removal of the crusts through either mechanical debridement or soaking. If constitutional symptoms or regional lymphadenopathy accompanies the disease, systemic antibiotics (penicillin V or dicloxacillin, erythromycin, cephalexin, and clindamycin) are clearly indicated. Otherwise, topical therapy with mupirocin may be satisfactory.

Intertrigo develops when epidermal surfaces exist in close juxtaposition, favoring repetitive friction. Numerous examples of this arrangement occur on the body (inframammary folds, gluteal creases, axillae), and one of the best examples is the interdigital spaces or clefts of the foot. A chronic bacterial colonization or infection is more responsible for perpetrating the condition than for actually causing it. Mild cases of intertrigo are typified by faint erythema, minimal maceration, and variable pruritus. A full-blown expression of intertrigo demonstrates oozing or weeping from epidermal erosions, intense erythema, persistent pruritus, and malodor caused by degeneration of the integument. Secondary cellulitis with possible lymphangitis can develop from entrance of microorganisms through associated fissures. Treatment requires a multifaceted approach. Elimination or reduction of friction can be accompanied by looser-fitting shoegear, avoidance of nylon hose, and cotton balls between the toes.

In mild cases with intact skin, drying of the moisture can be effected by talc or baby powder, use of an electric fan, or application of alcohol. Topical corticosteroids and oral or injectable antihistamines may control the pruritus. Topical antibiotic creams and solutions are beneficial in mild cases. Secondary bacterial infections of clinical significance require oral or parenteral antimicrobial therapy.

Paronychia is a skin infection of the ungual labia or nail fold. It represents the most common skin infection observed on the human foot.[9] A cryptotic, deformed, or ingrowing nail typically accompanies, and frequently initiates, the condition. As the nail punctures the nail groove, bacterial microorganisms have a portal of entrance (POE). In addition, a foreign-body reaction develops peripheral to the imbedded nail. The conventional teaching that paronychia is caused only by staphylococcal and streptococcal organisms is erroneous, as a review of cultural data implicates a veritable multitude of commensal and transient microorganisms. These include *Pseudomonas aeruginosa, Escherichia coli, Pseudomonas* sp., *Klebsiella* sp., various dermatophytes (*Trichophyton* sp., *Epidermophyton* sp., and *Microsporum* sp.), and the candidiasis more commonly seen in chronic paronychia. Nondermatophytes, such as the opportunistic

saprophytic organism *Scopulariopsis brevicaulis,* may also produce a paronychia.

Treatment requires establishing a portal of drainage by resection of the offending nail portion. Hyperosmolar astringent soaks or compresses are important adjuncts. The topical application of antibiotic solutions or creams, rather than occlusive ointments, which inhibit necessary drainage, generally remains the only antimicrobial treatment necessary in a healthy host. Oral antibiotics are seldom indicated.

When paronychia is accompanied by an ingrown toenail (IGTN), it may be necessary to remove the offending toenail side(s). Three stages of clinical onychocryptosis are seen. The first may be treated conservatively, while the second and third may require surgery, by any of the usual methods.

Stage I: IGTN with little edema, mild pain, and maceration.

Stage II: IGTN imbrication with granulation tissue production. The toe is painful, swollen, and draining, with or without odor. An abscess may be recognized.

Stage III: IGTN with signs and symptoms more severe than above, and exuberant granulation tissue (proud flesh) or abscess formation. A sinus tract or subungual exostosis may be present. Osteomyelitis is a likely consideration.

Pitted keratolysis typically appears as an incidental finding on physical examination and rarely prompts a patient to seek treatment. The clinical presentation permits the practitioner to establish the diagnosis prima vista. Numerous tiny, circular, discrete superficial erosions with a visible dell or depression characterize the condition. The base of the defect often demonstrates a dirty green to brown color. The superficial infection involves *Corynebacterium.* Most lesions are asymptomatic, and patients frequently will decline offers of treatment. As hyperhidrosis is often a concomitant finding, therapy should address this component as well. Specific treatment includes oral and topical erythromycin.

Scalded skin syndrome (SSS) is usually of *S. aureus* origin, through the production of exfoliatin, an epidermolytic toxin. A severe systemic variant in the newborn, Reiter's disease, appears reminiscent of an acute thermal burn and has a high degree of morbidity and mortality. In the slightly older patient, an erythematous scarlatinaform eruption may be seen with positive Nikolsky sign. In milder localized cases, infected bullous lesions may be seen. Treatment is with dicloxacillin or cephalexin.

Toxic shock syndrome (TSS) is a toxin-mediated disease with multisystem organ involvement, without a rapidly available test to identify the toxin. Relative to localized surgical foot wounds, TSS usually presents with a dearth of inflammatory changes and a high rate of recurrence. Surgical wounds, in most patients with TSS, should be explored even in the absence of significant localized signs of infection.

Whirlpools, jacuzzi hot tubs, and public showers may induce skin, subcutaneous, and soft tissue infections caused by *Pseudomonas aeruginosa.* Medicinal tubs are best disinfected to reduce the likelihood of contamination from one patient to another. Although rare, serious infections may occur with the use of these physical therapy modalities.

Superficial fungal infections of the pedal skin

Cutaneous infections of dermatophyte, fungal, and yeast origins include tinea pedis and onychomycosis. The features of each will be addressed separately.

Tinea pedis represents a cutaneous fungal infection confined to the feet. The condition reportedly appears with greater frequency than any other mycosis.[19] True tinea pedis is a condition caused by dermatophytic fungi. The colloquial term "athlete's foot" denotes cutaneous disease from a plethora of causes acting independently in a microbial interrelationship. They include dermatophytic fungi, saprophytic fungi, *Candida* species, and bacteria. A bilateral symmetrical presentation typifies the clinical picture, although cases of unilateral involvement are not uncommon. Three morphologic subtypes exist: (1) interdigital tinea pedis, with maceration, exfoliation, pruritis, and variable scaling in the toe clefts; (2) vesiculobullous tinea pedis, with acute individual or coalescing lesions of intensely pruritic character on the plantar surface; and (3) hyperkeratotic tinea pedis, with chronic thickening of the stratum corneum, classically in a moccasin distribution, frequently asymptomatic. The most common microorganisms responsible for tinea pedis are classified as dermatophytes.[19]

The list includes *Trichophyton rubrum* (especially with chronic or hyperkeratotic tinea pedis), *T. mentagrophytes* (especially with inflammatory or vesiculobullous tinea pedis), *Epidermophyton floccosum,* and occasionally *T. tonsurans* (especially in children with coexistent tinea capitis). Yeasts, specifically *Candida albicans,* as well as saprophytic fungi, specifically *Scytalidium dimidiatum* (alternatively classified as *Hendersonula toruloidea*), and *S. hyalinum,* can cause tinea pedis. A host of topical creams, gels, solutions, and powders are available for treatment. Some are strictly antifungal, while others possess anticandidal properties, as well. The imidazole derivatives have been workhorses of topical antifungal treatment for two decades. Newer classes of agents, the allylamines and the triazoles, hold promise. Oral treatment, with griseofulvin or ketoconazole, is generally reserved for severe cases of tinea pedis. Other hygienic measures, such as regular bathing, drying between the digits, avoidance of constrictive hosiery or shoegear, regularly changing footwear, and the use of sandals in public pools, locker rooms, and showers, aid in the control of the disease and lessen the probability of reinfection.

Onychomycosis is a fungal or yeast infection of the toenail plate. There may be variable involvement of adjacent structures, including the hyponychium and matrix complex. The nail plate becomes thickened, dystrophic, and opaque and loses its normal texture secondary to the keratinoid degeneration that accompanies advancing infiltration of the microorganism into the substance of the nail plate proper. Aside from pressure-induced discomfort, from wearing closed shoes or attempting to ambulate, onychomycosis of fungal etiology causes few symptoms, although unsightliness is a frequent concern of patients affected with the disorder. Periungual inflammation commonly accompanies onychomycoses of yeast etiology. *T. rubrum* and *T. mentagrophytes* are the dermatophytes usually responsible. *C. albicans* may cause onychomycosis. Debridement is an effective mechanism for control and lessening of symptoms. Because of poor penetration properties, topical therapy (even when assisted by frequent debridement) rarely eliminates the causative organisms. Despite the high recurrence rate and potential systemic side effects associated with extended treatment, oral agents remain the treatment of choice when cure of infection is the goal. For chronic therapy, the manual debridement of fungus- and bacteria-infected toenails may be augmented with the use of high-torque low-speed power drills with appropriate burrs. Unfortunately, this leads to the generation of fungi- and bacteria-laden nail dust (0.1 to 100 μm "fines") particles, often with the organism *T. rubrum* (IgG precipitin antibodies). Since it has been estimated that 25% of all nail and foot infections are induced by dermatophytes, 50% by saprophytic molds and 25% by bacteria, this constitutes a hazard to the clinician. Allergic-immunologic symptoms of exposure to this chronic occupational hazard include conjunctivitis, rhinitis, eyelid pruritus and eczema, and lung contamination. Since the true pathologic consequences of these conditions are not totally known or understood, it behooves the prudent practitioner to take precautions against daily exposure, in the form of masks and ventilator exhaust systems. Surgical ablation may still be needed.

Subcutaneous and deep fungal infections

Sporotrichosis is a granulomatous infection of skin and subcutaneous tissue. The organism is found on vegetables and dirt and may spread along lymphatic channels. The condition presents as raised erythematous plaque-like lesions. A chancre will develop at a site of entry, and patients rarely show systemic signs of infection. Treatment for the hematogenous condition is amphotericin B.

Blastomycosis begins as a papular lesion, which ulcerates and spreads with a pustular border. Diagnosis is through bacteriologic confirmation. Treatment includes local excision of the early lesion or the drug 2-hydroxystilbamidine for chronic cases.

Mycetoma is a chronic granulomatous infection of soft tissue and bone. It requires the triad of indurated swollen lesions, draining sinus, and unilateral presentation, for the clinical diagnosis. The condition is seen in endemic proportions in some Third World nations, and a patient's recent immigration may increase clinical suspicions.

The condition known as *Madura foot* may be either fungal (*Madurella mycetomi, Pertriellidium,* or *Allescheria boydii*) or bacterial (*Actinomyces, Nocardia, Streptomyces,* or *Achnomadura*). Diagnosis is made by Gram stain, KOH slide mount, or culture and sensitivity testing with Sabouraud's agar (fungal) or blood agar (bacterial). Radiographic evaluation in long-standing infections will produce multiple osteolytic lesions in bone. Treatment is through sulfonamides, local wound care, or debridement or amputation in severe cases.

Viral infections of the pedal skin

Verrucae develop from cutaneous infection of the human papillomavirus, a member of the papovavirus family of deoxyribonucleic acid (DNA) viruses. On the foot, the morphologic variants of verrucae include verruca plantaris, verruca vulgaris, and verruca plantae. Statistically, lesions of the plantar variety predominate. The typical presentation features a solitary lesion (although mosaic and disseminated distributions are not infrequent) with a well-defined peripheral margin, an irregular hyperkeratotic cover, pain elicited on lateral compression, and pinpoint hemorrhage on sharp sterile transection during debridement. On the weight-bearing surface of the plantar foot, the lesion exhibits minimal, if any, elevation from the surrounding integument. On regions not involved with locomotion, lesions tend to be elevated. Numerous therapeutic modalities exist, indicating that no option is universally successful. The more frequently employed options include surgical excision, laser ablation, electrosurgery, antimetabolites, cryotherapeutics, and chemical cautery.[12-15] Recurrence rates are high, regardless of the therapeutic route taken.

Molluscum contagiosum results from a viral infection by an unassigned member of the poxvirus family.[16] It is the largest virus to invoke human disease. The typical lesion is a smooth, dome-shaped papule with a central depression at the vertex. The lesion progresses from firm and flesh colored to soft and whitish at maturation. A caseous-texture substance is readily expressible from the center of a mature lesion with a comedone extractor. Although more common at other locations, the lesion may occur anywhere on the lower extremity, including the plantar foot.[17] Molluscum contagiosum is a self-limiting condition. Individual untreated lesions remain for about 2 months, while the untreated disease may last from 6 to 36 months. Treatment options include incision and decompression, curettage, cryotherapy, and topical caustics.

Herpes zoster develops when the varicella-zoster virus becomes reactivated during a period of immunocompromise. The varicella-zoster virus belongs to the herpesvirus family. The virus is responsible for both varicella ("chickenpox") and zoster ("shingles"). Varicella presents with a disseminated eruption; zoster with an eruption restricted to the dermatome innervated by the affected dorsal root ganglion. The individual lesion of either varicella or zoster is a translucent demispherical vesicle on an erythematous base.[18] Treatment of both acute varicella and herpes zoster is primarily supportive with antipruritics, mild analgesics, and protection. Postherpetic complications, particularly neuralgia, may require extended treatment.

CELLULITIS AND SUBCUTANEOUS FOOT INFECTIONS

Cellulitis, an inflammation with or without the attendant infection of connective tissue, primarily involves the reticular dermis. Clinical distinction between the entities frequently proves impossible because of the overlap of symptoms common to both and the inherent tendency of a septic or inflammatory process to violate tissue planes. Consequently, the two conditions shall be reviewed jointly.

The physical examination may reveal the classic or cardinal signs of inflammation, described earlier. Lymphangitis, the proximal linear to serpiginous streaking of red coloration along the route of lymphatic drainage, may be variably present. Regional lymphadenopathy, tender palpable indurated enlargements of the lymphatic nodes, may be occasionally evident. Systemic manifestations of infection include hyperthermia, tachycardia, lethargy, shaking chills, and nausea. Systemic features are usually absent with infections of an aerobic etiology. Ecchymosis, diffuse bluish discoloration, crepitation with palpation or motion, and accumulation of gas evident on radiographs suggest an anaerobic etiology. If vesiculation or bulla formation accompanies the infection, the contents may be sterilely aspirated and recovered for microbiologic cultures.

The injection of sterile saline with subsequent aspiration "washings," from the advancing margin (leading edge) of the infection, can sometimes recover the causative microorganism, but is a controversial technique. Another suggested site is midway between the leading edge and the center of the cellulitis ("midpoint aspiration"). Typically, a 22-, 25-, or 27-gauge needle is used, with a 3-cc syringe and 0.5 to 1.0 cc sterile water or bacteriostatic saline. Positive cultures range from 4% to 6% and are even lower in younger patients. Because of the associated discomfort, patient tolerance of the procedure is poor.

If surgical exploration and debridement are necessary, an opportunity exists to acquire specimens for analysis likely to contain the responsible pathogens. Ideally, a culture specimen will be obtained prior to initiation of antibiotics. Routine laboratory evaluation for moderate to severe infections includes a complete blood count (CBC) with differential and erythrocyte sedimentation rate (ESR) or C-reactive protein, in addition to the standard chemistry panels, urinalysis, and other parameters. Blood cultures are especially indicated in the presence of a high fever. Because of the significant differences between aerobic and anaerobic cellulitis, each will be addressed independently.[20]

ABSCESS FORMATION

A well-defined collection of neutrophils, bacteria, and other debris constitutes an abscess. The accumulation may exist in a distinct anatomic structure or arise as the host attempts to contain the infection. Abscess formation may accompany any pyogenic (pus-producing) infection. Superficial abscesses demonstrate visible evidence of purulent accumulation. The mature lesion may "point," or appear ready to expel its contents. Peripheral erythema accompanies the centrally located abscess. Variable amounts of edema may coexist. Localized hyperthermia is evident. Constitutional symptoms of infection are generally absent. Gram-positive aerobic organisms account for the majority of superficial abscesses; *S. aureus, S. epidermidis,* and *S. pyogenes* are common agents. An abscess represents a surgical condition requiring incision for treatment. Adequate skin antisepsis favors recovering the causative organism, rather than clinically irrelevant normal or transient microflora, during the procedure. Local measures include elevation, moist heat, hyperosmolar compresses or soaks, and antimicrobial agents. Although surgical decompression provides the mainstay of treatment, antibiotics may or may not be employed.

Deep abscesses usually develop after the inoculation of microorganisms into the tissues with a penetrating injury. Puncture wounds are especially likely to create deep abscesses when adequate numbers of a sufficiently virulent pathogen are introduced into a susceptible host, although ulcers, sinus tracts, fistulae, and other integumentary violations may beget the condition. Erythema, ecchymotic discoloration, and mild to marked cutaneous hyperthermia may signal an underlying deep abscess. The site may be fluctuant with palpation or crepitant with motion. A deep dull aching sensation may accompany the condition. Lymphatic streaking, regional lymphadenopathy, tachycardia, hyperpyrexia, shaking chills, malaise, and diaphoresis are more likely with a deep, rather than a superficial, abscess and are related to osteomyelitis.

Deep abscesses may fester between osseofascial barriers or other anatomic boundaries. In the pedal appendage, plantar space abscesses involve the distinct compartments. A diversity of microorganisms can produce a deep abscess. Some of the bacteria commonly isolated are *Staphylococcus, Streptococcus, Enterobacter, Pseudomonas, Serratia, Bacteroides,* and *Peptococcus.*[21] Adequate treatment of a suspected deep abscess involves incision and exploration of the site to effect drainage and obtain specimens for bacteriologic studies. The surgical wound is left open, or closed by secondary or tertiary intention. Broad-spectrum antimicrobials should be selected empirically and employed until microbiologic data become available. In most instances, parenteral antibiotics are appropriate in the management of deep abscesses, whether they are administered in the hospital, on an outpatient basis, or by a home health agency. Local measures, including whirlpool, wet-to-dry dressings with packing of the cavitation, elevation or dependency, and rest, are beneficial.

BURSAL SAC AND TENDON INFECTIONS

Bursae may be anatomic (developmental) or adventitious (reactive) in etiology. Regardless of the mechanism of formation, infections can develop within the structure. Infection follows invasion of the structure by pyogenic organisms, typically as a result of direct trauma. Either accidental (puncture, penetrating foreign body, laceration) or iatrogenic (diagnostic or therapeutic injection) events may be responsible. Alternatively, a tendon-sheath or intraarticular infection may communicate with a bursa, causing spread into the bursal sac. Bursae possess a poor vascular supply. Consequently, hematogenous seeding is an infrequent cause of infectious bursitis. In the foot, the retrocalcaneal bursa is most frequently involved.[20] Edema within and adjacent to the bursa is a clinical feature. Associated with swelling are increased local temperature, erythema, and deep dull aching discomfort with palpation or motion. Drainage may be present if a sinus tract or fistula communicates with the external environment from the bursa. Aspiration of the bursal contents, under aseptic conditions, will provide a specimen for bacteriologic studies. Plain film radiographs may demonstrate an increase in the soft tissue density in the region of the bursa but are not specific.

Magnetic resonance imaging (MRI) is perhaps the best noninvasive diagnostic modality, although ultrasound techniques hold promise. As a closed bursal sac infection is essentially a deep abscess, the treatment closely parallels what has been described. Incision and drainage are paramount. Because of the relatively poor blood supply, antibiotic penetration is diminished. Nonetheless, empiric agents for the most probable pathogens should be initiated. Modifications in the antimicrobial regimen may be necessary after noting of clinical response to current therapy and receipt of in vitro sensitivity studies. Excision of the bursa offers an option for the treatment of infectious bursitis but is generally reserved for recurrent infections.

Septic tenosynovitis is the spread of infection within tendon sheaths. The tendon proper is variably involved. Infection follows invasion of the sheath by pyogenic organisms. Accidental (laceration, penetrating foreign body, puncture) or iatrogenic traumatic events may be responsible. Another common origin for a tendon sheath infection is an undermining ulceration that erodes the sheath, permitting entrance of the microorganisms. Alternatively, infections of the soft tissue, if not treated aggressively or rapidly enough, can contaminate and inoculate the neighboring tendon sheaths. Once the infection enters the sheath, its spread is relatively unimpeded as it dissects toward the myotendonious origin proximally or to the insertion distally. The intensity of the clinical appearance of the infectious tenosynovitis varies by site. The features are more easily apparent when the involved tendon is relatively superficial (i.e., manifestations will be easier to recognize in extensor, rather than flexor tendons). In the lower extremity, the extensor tendons are most frequently involved.[20]

Linear or diffuse edema, erythema, and hyperthermia along a tendon route suggest the diagnosis. Fluctuance and crepitation with palpation and motion may be present. Palpation is uncomfortable. Drainage may be present if a sinus tract communicates with the external environment from the tendon sheath. With aseptic technique, tenosynovial contents can be aspirated to retrieve a specimen for bacteriologic studies. Radiographs offer little diagnostic information, as the finding of an increased soft tissue silhouette is nonspecific. Xeroradiography is superior to conventional radiography because of soft tissue enhancement. Magnetic resonance imaging (MRI) is ideal in delineating the magnitude and extent of involvement. New techniques in diagnostic ultrasound may be helpful. Tenography must not be attempted in the presence of suspected infection. Treatment consists of evaluation, rest, moist heat, and antibiotics. In severe cases, surgical decompression of the tendon sheath will facilitate drainage and permit direct inspection of the tendon proper. Tenosynovectomy may be indicated in the presence of significant adhesions after resolution of the septic process.

BURN INFECTIONS

Necrosis is a common denominator to all burn wounds, which are thus at an increased risk for infection. Signs of infection include the development of fibrous, escharotic, or hemorrhagic tissue or the formation of yellow vesicular lesion(s). The eventual infection is a function of surface area (large surface areas are infection prone), age (older wounds are infection prone), and depth of injury (full-thickness wounds are infection prone). In general, it is best to keep burn wound bacterial colonization below 10^2 CFUs/cm^2, since burn wound sepsis is seen at levels greater than 10^5 CFUs/cm^2. Typically, bacterial colonization is from pathogens such as *Acinetobacter, Enterobacter, E. coli, Klebsiella, Pseudomonas aeruginosa, Proteus, Serratia,* and MRSA (methicillin-resistant *S. aureus*). Increasingly, *Candida, Mucor,* and *Aspergillus* are fungal agents of contamination. Immunocompromised burn patients may even become contaminated with herpes zoster, herpes simplex, and cytomegalovirus.

Topical agents to reduce wound colony counts include 0.5% silver nitrate (broad spectrum, painless, bacteriostatic), silver sulfadiazine (broad spectrum, painless, bacteriostatic), 11% mafenide acetate (broad spectrum, bacteriostatic), and polymyxin-bacitracin-neomycin ointment. Prophylactic systemic antibiotics include penicillin G, cefazolin, vancomycin (MRSA), acyclovir, and various aminoglycosides.[21-24]

CONCLUSION

The integument is a mechanical, chemical, and physiological barrier between the environment and the underlying soft tissue, tendinous, muscular, and bony structures. It is the barrier between the "milieu interieur" and the "milieu exterieur" of Claude Bernard. In the foot, it is both anatomically unique and uniquely susceptible to infectious contamination from all sorts of bacterial, viral, and fungal pathologic contaminants.[25] Many of the more common infectious processes of the pedal skin and underlying subcutaneous tissues have been presented in this chapter. A high index of suspicion will alert the practitioner and encourage both prompt diagnosis and effective treatment of these conditions.

REFERENCES

1. Marples RR: Bacterial infections. Moschella SL, Pillsbury M, Hurley HJ Jr, eds: *Dermatology,* Philadelphia, 1975, WB Saunders, pp 482-491.
2. Rook A, Roberts SOB: Bacterial infections. In Rook A, Wilkinson DS, Ebling FJC, eds: *Textbook of Dermatology,* London, 1972, Blackwell Scientific Publications, pp 475-538.
3. Hoffman AF: Physiological considerations of the skin. In McCarthy DJ, Montgomery R, eds: *Podiatric Dermatology,* Baltimore, 1986, Williams & Wilkins, p. 18.
4. Witkowski J: Pathogenesis of skin infections. In Abramson C, McCarthy DJ, Rupp MJ, eds: *Infectious diseases of the lower extremity,* Baltimore, 1991, Williams & Wilkins.
5. Tachibana DK: Microbiology of the foot, *Ann Rev Microbiol* 30:351-376, 1976.
6. Hoeprich PD: Host-parasite relationships and the pathogenesis of infectious disease. In Hoeprich PD, ed: *Infectious diseases,* Hagerstown, Md., 1972, Harper & Row, pp 36-39.
7. Ryan TJ: Inflammation. In Rook A, Wilkinson DS, Ebling FJG, eds: *Textbook of Dermatology,* London, 1972, Blackwell Scientific Publications, pp 211-218.
8. O'Laughlin JM: Disorders of immunity, hypersensitivity, and inflammation. In Moshella SL, Pillsbury M, Hurley HJ Jr, eds: *Dermatology,* Philadelphia, 1975, WB Saunders, pp 199-218.
9. Brenner MA: Pyodermas. In McCarthy DJ, Montgomery R, eds: *Podiatric dermatology,* Baltimore, 1986, Williams & Wilkins, pp 122-132.
10. Lowberry EJL, Lilly HA: Use of a 4% chlorhexidene detergent solution (Hibiscrub) and other methods of skin disinfection, *Br Med J* 1:510, 1973.
11. Bartolomei FJ, McCarthy DJ, Brandwene SM: Cutaneous manifestation of deoxyribonucleic acid (DNA) virus diseases of the human lower extremity, *Curr Podiatry* 33(6):13-29, 1984.
12. Israel RM: How I treat plantar warts, *Postgrad Med* 46:215, 1969.
13. Borovoy M, Fuller TA, Holtz P: Laser surgery in podiatric medicine—present and future, *J Foot Surg* 22:353, 1983.
14. Bartolomei FJ, Biggs EW: Ultrasonic energy in the treatment of verruca plantaris, *Curr Podiatry* 31(2):16-18, 1982.
15. Lerner K: Management of plantar verruca via excision and curettage, *J Am Podiatry Assoc* 49:11, 1959.
16. Bartolomei FJ, McCarthy DJ, Barndwene SM: Cutaneous manifestations of deoxyribonucleic acid (DNA) virus diseases of the human lower extremity, part 2, *Curr Podiatry* 33(7):14-32, 1984.
17. Cokbett CW: Molluscum contagiosum, *J Foot Surg* 6:3, 1967.
18. Bartolomei FJ, McCarthy DJ, Brandwene SM: Cutaneous manifestations of deoxyribonucleic acid (DNA) virus diseases of the human lower extremity, part 3, *Curr Podiatry* 33(8):11-23, 1984.
19. Page JC, Abramson C, Lee WL: Diagnosis and treatment of tinea pedis, *J Am Podiatr Med Assoc* 81:304, 1991.

20. Oloff LM, Thornton C: The catastrophe of the infected foot. In Marcinko DE, ed: *Medical and surgical therapeutics of the foot and ankle,* Baltimore, 1992, Williams & Wilkins, pp 659-681.

21. Taylor LM, Porter JM: The clinical course of diabetics who require emergent foot surgery because of infections, *Vasc Surg* 6:4 54, 1987.

22. Nikinikoski J, Aho AJ: Combination of hyperbaric oxygen, surgery, and antibiotics in the treatment of clostridial gas gangrene, *Infect Surg* 2:23, 1983.

23. Salisbury R: A burn primer, *Emerg Med* 18:155, 1988.

24. Dinan WA, Talavera, W.: The spectrum of *Mycobacterium* tuberculoses, *The Lower Extremity* 3(1):1-9, 1996.

25. Organ PJ: The role of the podiatric physician in the care of HIV positive patients, *The Lower Extremity* 2(3):55-161, 1995.

ADDITIONAL READINGS

Abramson C: Inhalation of nail dust: a podiatric hazard. In Abramson C, McCarthy DJ, Rupp MJ: *Infectious diseases of the lower extremities,* Baltimore, 1991, Williams & Wilkins.

Abramson C, Fischman GJ: Purification and characterization of the plantar human papilloma virus, *J Am Podiatr Med Assoc* 77:123, 1987.

Abramson C, McCarthy DJ: Athlete's foot infections. In Abramson C, McCarthy DJ, Rupp MJ: *Infectious diseases of the lower extremities,* Baltimore, 1991, Williams & Wilkins.

Arndt KA: *Manual of dermatological therapeutics,* Boston, 1989, Little, Brown.

Baruch K: Pediatric dermatology, *Clin Podiatr Med Surg* 3:399, 1986.

Bauer G: Plantar space infections: anatomical and surgical considerations. In Abramson C, McCarthy DJ, Rupp MJ: *Infectious diseases of the lower extremities,* Baltimore, 1991, Williams & Wilkins.

Dickinson B, Lipkin L: Antimicrobial agents of choice. In Marcinko D, ed: *Medical and surgical therapeutics of the foot and ankle,* Baltimore, 1992, Williams & Wilkins.

Joseph W, LeFrock JL: Infections complicating puncture wounds of the foot, *J Foot Surg* 30S:1, 1987.

9

Infected Ulcerations of the Foot

Thomas M. DeLauro
Rock G. Positano

Medical theory is truly useful, only when its practical results are beneficial. To judge correctly of these results, we must have recourse to the phenomena presented to clinical observers. A. M'Call

Generally speaking, cutaneous ulcerations are full-thickness wounds that fail to heal unless some medical or surgical intervention occurs. Traditionally, their numerous etiologies have been discussed at great length in the medical literature.[1] Although the clinical recognition of cutaneous ulcerations is fairly straightforward, determining when an ulcer has become secondarily infected ("infected") or is of an infectious etiology ("infectious") is not an easy task. The latter requires a high index of suspicion and epidemiologic background, and cultures of ulcers often produce benign, saprophytic microorganisms. The purpose of this chapter, then, is to provide a suggested logical algorithmic approach to these vexing problems.

HISTORICAL REVIEW

In addition to the format espoused in standard physical diagnosis medical textbooks, patients with suspected infected or infectious cutaneous ulcers should be questioned with regard to recent travel, immigration status, immunologic status, vascular status, and change in the ulceration over time. Personal and business travel is so commonplace that infectious diseases endemic to the visited locale may appear stateside. Adventurous patients take their vacations in obscure regions of the world, and may not be familiar with universal precautions regarding health and sanitation. Unless considered, these details may escape the clinician's probe, and lead to a delayed or faulty diagnosis. Immigration carries the same warning, especially when the patient comes from an underdeveloped nation.

In an era of acquired immunodeficiency syndrome (AIDS), resurgent tuberculosis, and widespread chemotherapy use for neoplastic disease, knowledge of the patient's immunologic status is vital to understanding the pathogenesis and treatment of infected and infectious ulcerations. Immunocompromise invites tissue destruction by saprophytes and rarely encountered organisms even in persons who have never traveled outside the country. Immunocompromise also places more responsibility on extrinsic methods for cure, since the patient's own intrinsic systems are either malfunctional or nonfunctional.

Of all the body systems, a patent vascular tree is key to preventing and treating both infected and infectious skin ulcerations. Tissue nutrition, oxygenation, foreign-body phagocytosis, and repair all rely on adequate blood within the macrocirculation and microcirculation. Like immunocompromise, vascular compromise (both arterial and venous) interferes with homeostasis sufficiently to warrant its correction before all other measures. The history should therefore exclude or detect symptoms such as intermittent claudication, rest pain, pedal edema, hyperpigmentation, reactive hyperemia, and coldness of feet.

Duration is the final factor to be considered, but always in relationship to progression. Together, these variables represent the sum total of the body's ability to heal the infected or infectious lesion. An ulcer that has existed for some time without worsening is a sign that, collectively, the host's protective systems are properly functioning, and the pathologic processes are in equilibrium. On the other hand, relentless progression in a short interval carries a grave prognosis, often to the point of replacing continued care of the infected or infectious part with removing it entirely (amputation).

PHYSICAL EXAMINATION

Physical examination of the infected or infectious ulcer should begin with visual inspection. Location is an important etiologic clue (i.e., tips of toes in atherosclerotic ulcers), leading the clinician away from considering an infectious cause. On the other hand, atypical locations may signal the presence of primary infection leading to ulceration. Regardless of the cause, the number of ulcerations is directly proportional to the severity of the pathologic process.

Each ulcer's base should be inspected next. Noninfected and noninfectious ulcers should have clean, moist, granulating bases. Alternatively, atherosclerotic ulcers may have clean but desiccated bases covered by a tenacious eschar. Deeper structures, such as tendon or bone, may be visible. Their ability to resist bacterial colonization is generally considered to be less than that of adjacent soft tissues; hence, the exposure of these structures to the external environment may contribute to the development of infection, necessitating their surgical removal. Exposure of these structures, especially in the absence of other features to be discussed, does not automatically imply that the ulcer is infected or infectious.

In infected or infectious ulcers, the base takes on a different appearance, with tissue necrosis predominating. Such necrosis can be recognized by the gray color of normally white tissues, the watery consistency of usually firm tissues, and an unpleasant, foul odor.[2] Necrotic tissues provide nutrition for invading microorganisms, thereby facilitating the necrotic process. The ulcer base should be probed for deep sinuses, with natural tissue planes and gravity providing clues as to which path the infectious process would most likely take. This discussion of sinus tracts will be continued in greater detail in the next section of this chapter, dealing with sinography.

Once the skin's continuity has been broken, it is normal for tissue fluids to escape. These fluids are usually odorless, and of a serous or serosanguineous quality. If the ulcer's cross-sectional area is large, the amount of drainage can be appreciable. These findings are normal and do not represent infection. True infection presents with purulence of varying color and/or odor. Even anaerobic and streptococcal infections, which are known for their thin, watery discharge (often confused with serous drainage) may be malodorous.

The ulcer border deserves special examination as well. Undermined borders suggest an infectious organism capable of growing at cooler temperatures (i.e., mycobacteria). As a result, the process extends laterally rather than vertically. Necrotizing infections extend laterally because they follow tissue planes. Infected ulcers may also demonstrate undermining in the form of a sinus tract; however, if the host defenses permit such undermining, there is a strong chance that deep, vertical sinuses will be present as well.

Finally, the clinician should take special note of the inflammatory changes in the surrounding skin and soft tissues, such as regional adenopathy, venous cords, and ascending lymphangitis. Although all clinicians are aware of the parameters that constitute inflammation (i.e., warmth, redness, etc.), it is probably safe to assume that few practitioners actually measure or grid the border of each change. This is a little-used, yet invaluable clinical tool,

since it provides some objective assessment as to whether the therapeutic plan is having its desired effect: are borders receding or enlarging? Infected and infectious ulcers will present with marked peri-ulcer changes, including cellulitis, lymphangitis, tissue crepitation, and lymphadenopathy. Noninfected and infected ulcers generally present with little more than a mild erythematous border that remains fairly stabilized. If severe enough, infected and infectious ulcerations will be accompanied by constitutional symptoms and signs (i.e., malaise and fever), while noninfected and noninfectious ulcers will not.

The examination for peri-ulcer changes carries a special warning. The changes discussed above will be seen in patients with uncompromised vascularity. In the case of poor arterial supply, however, infection may cause tissue necrosis without the anticipated host defense responses. There will be little purulence, erythema, or edema. At times, the only changes may be an increase in the diameter of the pain border or the severity of pain. In cases of sensory neuropathy and vascular compromise, progressive tissue necrosis would be recognized as a signal that an infected or infectious ulcer is likely. It may also indicate acute macroarterial or microarterial embolus.

SINOGRAPHY

When sinuses are detected, the extent, depth, and route of the sinus may be visualized through sinography. Simply stated, this procedure involves the instillation of a radiopaque material into the entire course of the sinus, after which some form of imaging (e.g., standard radiograph) is employed. Since the radiopaque dye obscures detail of other tissues in the area, sinography is best employed after images not using the dye are taken. A silver nitrate stick, moistened and inserted into the sinus, may be used instead of the radiopaque dye (personal communication: Dr. Randy Cohen, Staten Island, N.Y., 1997). Although critics of sinography may argue that probing at the bedside or chair side is adequate to map the sinus, sinography may be superior for the initial visualization of tortuous channels and communications with deeper foot compartments. Care must be taken against instilling the radiopaque dye with too much force, since the possibility of opening potential spaces and introducing bacteria exists. Sinography is highly dependent on the skill, enthusiasm, and clinical acumen of the examiner.

CULTURE AND BIOPSY

Microorganisms can be recovered from any ulcer surface (Table 9-1). The organisms collected, however, may not be the true pathogens. Swab cultures are notorious for gathering the "wrong" microbes, and therefore should be used only when deeper methods of culture are contraindicated (i.e., when they would cause harmful extension of the ulcer). Specimens should be collected before antibiotics have been

TABLE 9-1 Most commonly encountered bacteria in diabetic foot ulcerations and infections

Aerobes

Gram-positive cocci
   Staphylococcus aureus
   Staphylococcus epidermidis
   Enterococci (group B streptococci)
Gram-negative bacilli
   Enterobacteriaceae
   Pseudomonas aeruginosa
   Proteus species

Anaerobes

Bacteroides species

Peptococcus species

Peptostreptococcus species

Data from Lipsky BA et al: *Clin Geriatr Med* 6(4):747-769, 1990; Joseph WS: *J Am Podiatr Med Assoc* 82(7):361-369, 1992.

administered or, if possible, after an antibiotic-free period of 48 hours has elapsed.[2]

Purulence (pus), when present, signifies an intact host response to the presence of infection and may or may not provide reliable material for culture. A thin layer of collagen substance usually covers all skin ulcers, and is not to be confused with true purulence. A useful clinical axiom to remember in all culture samplings is that deeper cultures are more reliable cultures. Superficial cultures gather contaminants, and often miss anaerobes (anaerobes thrive centrally). When material from abscesses is to be sampled, anaerobic and aerobic cultures, and a Gram stain should be obtained, in that order.[2] If only fluid is to be obtained, it should be retrieved from the deeper portions of the collection. If tissue from an ulcer base or margins is to be cultured, the tissue should be obtained via curette scrapings of the ulcer base, the margin, or the deepest portions of a sinus. All things considered, tissue biopsies probably form the most reliable cultures, since quantitative assays may be performed on the specimen. Curettage should be gentle, however, and not gouge the wound or result in extensive hemorrhage. Do not rely on sinus cultures if osteomyelitis is suspected (bone cultures are required in these instances), except in the case of *Staphylococcus aureus,* which is recovered in the sinus tract and bone approximately 70% of the time.[4]

Aspiration has been touted as an alternative and controversial culture technique, especially when little purulence is present (such as in an advancing edge of cellulitis). Aspiration cultures are performed by using a large-bore needle (15 or 18 gauge) to gently inject or irrigate the tissue to be cultured with a small amount of nonbacteriostatic sterile water or saline. This fluid is allowed to mix with the adjacent tissues momentarily and then is aspirated through the same needle, hopefully carrying with it the true pathogens. Time has not supported the extensive use of aspiration cultures, since reliable results have been obtained only ten percent of the time.

Up to now, this discussion has focused on aerobic bacteria. Infected and infectious ulcers may also present with and be caused by anaerobes, fungi, acid-fast bacteria, spirochetes, and viruses. If any of these are suspected, special collection containers (although often cumbersome and unreliable) or procedures may become necessary. The microbiology laboratory should be consulted in these instances. When that is not possible, the safest transport system (except for anaerobes) may consist of sterile saline or water. In cases of suspected syphilitic ulceration, serum antibody tests (i.e., VDRL, FTA) take the place of dark-field examinations for the spirochete, since dark-field examinations are nearly impossible to obtain.

Biopsy of infected or infectious ulcers may become necessary when initial therapy is ineffective, or malignant degeneration is suspected. Except for these two instances, biopsy should probably be considered a technique of last resort, since it will always increase the ulcer's size. When necessary, ulcer biopsy should always include a full thickness of the base and/or margin. When the ulcer is problematic and very small, complete excisional biopsy with flap or free graft coverage may be preferred from a diagnostic and therapeutic standpoint. However, small biopsies allow for quantitative cultures, which are possibly one of the more reliable methods to differentiate colonization from infectious contamination.

WOUND CARE

The measure of clinical effectiveness in ulcer and wound care is outcome. Using the inflammatory parameters described earlier, and the wound changes to be presented below, one should be able to quantify steady, progressive improvement. Each redressing should begin with a repeated physical examination. Once the findings have been noted and recorded, attention is next directed to the ulcer surface.

Debridement

The goal in caring for an infected or infectious ulcer is to convert it to one consisting only of clean granulation tissue. Such a surface facilitates epithelialization, or provides a ready receptacle for grafting. The ulcer surface should therefore be debrided of necrotic debris at each and every dressing change. The methods of debridement will vary, depending on the amount and type of necrotic tissue as well as the wound's ability to withstand aggressive therapy. At first presentation, extensive debridement may be necessary, and may or may not require use of a hospital operating room. Nonviable tissue should be removed if (1) it is painful; (2) it provides a nutritional bed for microorganisms, fostering further infection; or (3) it is occluding drainage. Necrotic tissue that is especially tenacious, extremely painful to remove, and fails to meet the other aforementioned tests can often be left in place until a natural liquefaction process occurs beneath it. Some clinicians would disagree with this approach, preferring instead to surgically debride the eschar.

This methodology may or may not be advisable, depending on the specific case under consideration. As long as the above tests are not met, it may be gentler to allow the wound to discharge the necrotic material naturally. This can sometimes be a tedious procedure requiring much more patience, but does not add insult to injury.

As alternatives to sharp, surgical debridement, or after such initial debridement has been performed, one might employ simple curettage, the "gauze curette," wet-to-dry dressings, or topical enzymatic debriding agents. Simple curettage should be performed with a large bone curette, and remove the loose debris that collects between dressing changes. This curettage should extend down to granulation tissue or other normal tissues in the area. Curettage should not gouge the wound or create hemorrhage. The weight of the instrument itself should suffice in terms of gauging how much force to use during debridement.

Normal tissues have a tough, fibrous feel to them, and dragging the curette across the wound will gather very little material.

"Gauze curettage" may be employed in wounds that cannot tolerate surgical debridement or traditional curettage, and involves the use of a dry gauze pad or one that has been moistened with an antiseptic solution. Antiseptic scrubs are not used because they make the gauze pad too slippery, interfering with the mechanical action desired. Once prepared, the gauze pad is rubbed back and forth across the wound, with the pad being exchanged for a new one once the gauze has become saturated with debris.

As another alternative, the wound may be debrided using standard wet-to-dry dressings. Removal of the dried dressing debrides the wound by lifting debris that adheres to the dressing during the drying process. This can sometimes be a painful procedure and should therefore be used only in patients who are not hurt by it.

A variety of topical enzymatic debriding agents exist, and may be selected when more aggressive methods of debridement are not feasible. Ointment-based enzymes should probably not be used in purulent wounds, since the ointment is occlusive and therefore inhibits needed drainage.

Although there is general consensus within the medical community as to the indications for sharp surgical debridement, less agreement is encountered concerning the additional debridement methods just described. One school of thought favors regular wound debridement, while another advocates that this manipulation may be disrupting an immature epithelial layer that is attempting to form.

Many authorities believe that, in a patient whose wound and vascular status can tolerate it, regular, scheduled debridement promotes a clean granulating wound that will rapidly epithelialize or can be covered with an appropriate graft. Extensive collections of debris between redressings indicate that the last debridement was not thorough enough, the wound is deteriorating, or more frequent debridement and dressing changes are required.

Irrigation

Following debridement, the ulcer should be irrigated both to flush away remaining debris and to restore some of the natural moisture that has been lost during debridement. The multiplicity of debridement approaches suggests that no one technique is inherently better than another, and that the critical issues are to remove nonviable tissue, restore viability in marginal tissue (decreasing metabolic demands caused by infection), and promote regeneration of remaining normal tissues. One must keep in mind that ulcers will always drain because the skin's integrity has been lost. This compromise allows normal tissue fluids to escape. Maintenance of a moist wound base is therefore considered necessary for healing of the ulcer. Allowing a wound to desiccate will only promote tissue necrosis.

The choice of irrigant is of less importance than the mechanical benefit to be gained, so simple saline is used in many centers. Nevertheless, clinicians prefer using a microbiostatic or microbicidal agent in the irrigant solution. In large ulcerations with extensive sinuses and undermining, a 1:10,000 potassium permanganate solution (0.01%) provides an inexpensive alternative to dilute povidone-iodine mixtures, and is infinitesimal in cost compared to commonly used aminoglycoside irrigants. Potassium permanganate irrigant can be pharmacy prepared by the gallon, increasing its cost-effectiveness. Whatever the irrigant, it should be applied with a bulb or other syringe (Water-Pik) to permit thorough flushing with a modest amount of pressure.

Caution is important when hydrogen peroxide irrigants are used. Their effervescent quality can create compartment syndrome–like changes if they are employed in small, deep ulcerations with sinuses. This occurs because the gas liberated by the peroxide has nowhere to escape. Such irrigations would therefore be more safely used in broad ulcerations and those with short, relatively straight sinuses and little undermining.

The keratotic ulcer rim

Approximately every 48 hours, the ulcer border becomes covered by a keratotic rim. Since this keratosis interferes with advancing epithelialization, it should be removed by lifting it with surgical forceps and picking it off as though one is opening the top of certain packages. This maneuver may cause some slight bleeding at the wound edge, which should be of little concern as long as the hemorrhage is of minimal degree. Extensive hemorrhage is a sign that more than the keratotic rim has been removed. This is contraindicated, for it causes further injury and the extensive hemorrhage provides a medium for bacterial growth.

Drains

After the ulcer has been debrided, cleansed, and irrigated, drains should be inserted into the depth of every sinus and underneath each undermined border. Sterile packing gauze is adequate, but iodinated gauze packing may be used, although it may "burn" delicate tissues and has not been shown to be more effective than nonmedicated packing materials. The drains may be numerous at times, depending upon the number of sinuses. The drains not only facilitate drainage and oxygenation but also prevent the maceration that can occur between two granulating surfaces. Drains should be placed, and not packed, into position, since packing will inhibit rather than promote drainage. Each day, sinus depth and ulcer border undermining should decrease if the wound is healing normally.

A principle often employed by thoracic surgeons, but of equal benefit in those caring for draining wounds, is postural drainage. Simply stated, this principle requires that the patient or part be positioned so that gravity will aid in draining the wound as well as prevent spread into deeper regions of the area. The best pictorial analogy to illustrate this concept would be a glass of water that has been left standing upright. In this position, its contents will never drain other than by evaporation. This is the scenario in patients with distal ulcerations who are instructed to remain supine. In this position, fluid will usually dissect proximally and laterally. The lateral migration of fluid occurs because the lower limbs naturally assume an externally rotated position when the body is supine. The glass of water described above will empty only if it is turned on its side or upside down. In like manner, patients with distal, draining wounds should be placed on the appropriate side or in a dependent and prone position.

Another aspect of postural drainage is whether the limb should be held elevated, horizontal, or in a dependent position. Lower extremities held in a dependent position for long periods will soon become edematous, a condition that interferes with normal tissue perfusion. This state becomes exacerbated in patients with venous incompetence. On the other hand, lower extremity elevation may be detrimental in cases of arterial compromise, where an already limited blood supply must not combat the forces of gravity. Given these circumstances, horizontal positioning of the limb may be best advised, for it neither produces edema nor resists arterial inflow. Alternating positions may be an effective compromise.

Finally, measurements of transcutaneous partial oxygen tension (TcPo$_2$) are often helpful in making such decisions. For example, TcPo$_2$ is useful in determining the likelihood of healing, in chronic, infected ulcers, since TcPo$_2$ > 20 mm Hg equates with healing in most cases.

Mobilization of wound margins

As the infected or infectious ulcer becomes more healthy and granulating, the clinician must begin to consider the prospect of accelerating wound closure. Although the topic of grafts and flaps is beyond the scope of this chapter, mobilization of wound margins can greatly decrease the size of the wound to be repaired. On occasion, large defects

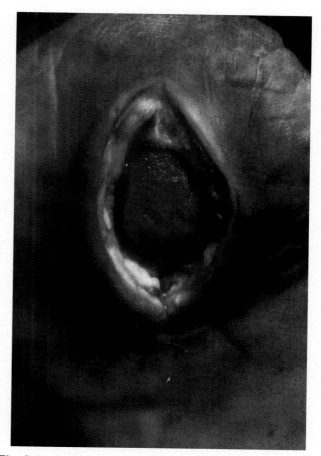

Fig. 9-1 The degree of wound closure that can be accomplished by mobilizing the wound margins.

can be closed primarily without the need for further surgery (Figs. 9-1 and 9-2).

Mobilization of wound margins is made possible by the normal elasticity of soft tissue. Injectable or implantable tissue expanders function on this same principle, which results in the production of additional skin and subcutaneous tissue when those structures are placed on prolonged stretch. Clinically, this effect can be achieved by massaging the wound margins just prior to applying the ulcer dressing. The massage should encompass nearly the entire wound margin, and move toward the center of the wound. In approximately 5 minutes, the available degree of mobilization should have been achieved. Tincture of benzoin or other suitable adhesive is painted on each side of the wound, and the mobilized wound edges are held in place using adhesive tape strips. The placement site of each adhesive strip should be changed to avoid skin maceration. Excessive tension can lead to vascular compromise, and therefore cannot be placed on the mobilized wound margin. Excessive tension can be recognized by blanching, cyanosis, and coolness of the skin in the wound margin itself. At each redressing, the wound margins should be more easily mobilized, and retain more of their new position without the aid of adhesive strips.

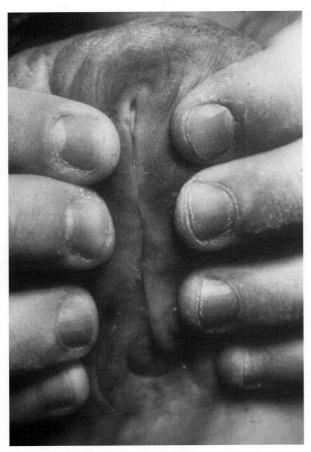

Fig. 9-2 Patient has a deep plantar ulceration following transmetatarsal amputation. (The use of sterile gloves is now considered the standard of care.)

If wound margins are not mobilized at the appropriate time, they will more than likely undergo fibrosis in their existing position. Surgical undermining, larger grafting, or more extensive flaps may therefore become necessary.

Wound dressings

The past decade has witnessed an explosion of wound dressing products. In infected and/or infectious cutaneous ulcerations, the wound dressing should serve several vital functions: (1) it should protect the wound from contamination by microorganisms yet allow cytokines (growth factors) to concentrate beneath it; (2) it should maintain a warm, moist ulcer base to avoid desiccating the wound; (3) it should be absorbent enough to remove excessive drainage that would otherwise cause maceration and foster bacterial growth, but not so absorbent as to cause drying of the wound; (4) removal of the dressing should not cause pain or trauma to the wound; and (5) the dressing should allow gaseous exchange (wound oxygenation). Obviously, no single ulcer dressing can perform each of these functions (some newer products do, however, profess to have "intelligence" (Table 9-2).

Instead, the clinician should be familiar with each of the available dressings, and be prepared to alternate one dressing type with another depending upon the ulcer's condition. Ulcer dressings do not cause healing; they merely facilitate natural reparative processes. Table 9-2 compares most of the wound dressings marketed today. In spite of the wide variety of products available, hydrocolloids and simple saline dressings appear to predominate. Saline dressings supply moisture and are easy for patients to self-administer, but the woven gauze that they are made of does not prevent contamination by microorganisms. Hydrocolloids are also easy to administer, retain wound moisture, are effective barriers against contamination, and may be left in place for long periods, obviating the need for frequent, costly dressing changes. Decades of research have shown that occlusive dressings are superior to permeable ones in noninfected wounds. During infection, however, frequent wound evaluation and redressings are recommended over reliance on biologic dressings or total contact casts, left in place for several days.

Transcutaneous electrical nerve stimulation

Not long after transcutaneous electrical nerve stimulation (TENS) was introduced for pain relief, interest in the effects of electricity on wound healing flourished. Few published reports have indicated any beneficial effect on infected or infectious ulcerations. A recent study however, demonstrated a significant increase in transcutaneous partial oxygen tension in ischemic and pressure ulcers exposed to long-term (up to 9 weeks) alternating current (AC). No significant $TcPo_2$ changes were noted when direct current (DC) was used, or when the exposure to either current was short (not more than 1 hour). The clinician must therefore determine on a case-by-case basis, whether this ancillary modality would aid healing of a noninfected ulcer.

Support surfaces

Since pressure is a well-documented cause of skin breakdown, it is wise to assume that some part of infected or infectious ulcer healing will rely upon removal of pressure from the wound. The most effective way to do this is to have the area suspended in air. In bedridden, compliant patients this is often easily accomplished by simply rotating the patient in bed. Ambulating patients should be nonweightbearing on the affected foot or site. In patients who cannot comply with these requirements (i.e., comatose, mentally incompetent), the clinician must resort to the wide variety of commercial devices designed for this purpose. The therapeutic goal should always be a pressure-free environment, and not just one that is rhythmically alternating but never pressure free. This need was underscored by a recent study comparing rhythmically alternating support surfaces with static-pressure support surfaces.[6] The study did not detect a significant difference in mean skin blood perfusion when normal patients were exposed to either surface for 60 minutes.

TABLE 9-2   Occlusive wound dressings

Semipermeable adhesive transparent polyurethane films
- Change every 1 to 7 days
- Wound can be inspected without removal of the dressing
- Use on shallow wounds with minimal drainage
- Excessive wound drainage may need to be aspirated
- Use skin adherent to protect adjacent skin from maceration

Hydrogel sheets and wafers
- Conform well to wound surface and surrounding skin
- Require a secondary dressing or tape to hold them on
- Absorb a limited amount of wound drainage
- Use on lightly draining wounds
- Usually consist of a polyethylene lattice containing a hydrated cross-linked polymer, e.g., polyethylene oxide
- Retention of any polyethylene film backing makes the dressing occlusive; removal of the backing makes the dressing permeable
- Should be changed every 1 to 3 days
- Will dry out when used with hyperbaric oxygenation, unless the hydrogel is covered with a transparent film dressing
- Must be secured with a secondary dressing
- Suitable for rehydration of dry eschar

Calcium alginates
- Derived from brown seaweed
- High absorbency makes them ideal for wounds with extensive drainage
- Interaction with wound fluid produces a viscous hydrogel
- Available as sheets for shallow wounds, or ropes that can be inserted in cavities (the latter will gel to take on the shape of the wound)
- Are biodegradable, so complete removal is unnecessary
- Change every 1 to 3 days
- Discontinue use once epithelialization has begun (is more cost effective to use a dressing that can be left on for several days)
- Contraindicated in dry wounds

Nonadherent hydrophilic polyurethane foams
- Must be secured with a secondary dressing
- Highly conformable to irregular surfaces
- Variable ability to absorb wound fluid
- Saturated dressings can leak fluid at their lateral margins ("lateral strike-through")

Hydrocolloids (occlusive and wafer dressings)
- Change every 1 to 7 days
- Contain hydrophilic colloidal particles
- Absorb light to medium drainage, but particle swelling may occur
- Fairly comfortable
- Usually adherent but may require secondary dressing
- As wound fluid is absorbed and interacts with dressing, results in the formation of an offensive yellow liquid that can be confused with pus
- Available as powder and paste for deep wounds
- Since most are opaque, the wound cannot be inspected
- Dressing should be changed at least 2 cm beyond wound edges

Moist (saline soaked)
- Change two or three times daily
- Must be secured with secondary dressing
- Gauze is not impermeable to microorganisms
- Easily removed
- Maintenance of moisture is difficult
- Should not be packed or stuffed into wound

Absorptive powders (beads, pastes, gels)
- Contain absorbable material (i.e., starch, pectin)
- Change every 1 to 3 days
- Do not use in patients with dry eschar
- Powders and beads are more absorbent but are difficult to handle and remove
- Unless premixed, preparation may be too dry
- Mixtures may be difficult to confine to wound cavity
- Must be used with a secondary dressing

Paraffin gauze dressing
- Used in noninfected, granulating wounds
- Also useful in pink, epithelialized wounds
- Can be left in place for 7 days

Data from Mulder et al: *Clin Podiatr Med Surg* 7(4): 733-742, 1990; Jeter KF, Tintle TE: *Clin Podiatr Med Surg* 8(4):799-816, 1991; Carver N, Leigh IM: *Int J Dermatol* 20(3):459-465, 1990.

GROWTH FACTORS

During wound repair, the wound is nourished by an exudate of mitogens, chemoattractants, and protein-inducing agents. Collectively, these are known as growth factors. Since these growth factors initiate more than cell proliferation, they are more appropriately referred to as cytokines. In most cases, these cytokines were named after the cells or targets that led to their discovery. As a result, their names are misleading, since they do not describe the full activity of the factor. These cytokines can also induce the transcription of oncogenes, and therefore may be tumorigenic.[7,8] A single growth factor apparently can be either stimulatory or inhibitory, depending upon which other growth factors are present.

Growth factor (cytokine) production and mechanism of action

The cytokines synthesized and released during wound repair may be subdivided into three types: mitogens, chemoattractants, and transforming factors.[9,11] Cytokines are synthesized and secreted in endocrine, paracrine, and autocrine fashions. As polypeptides (proteins), the cytokines do not easily cross cell membranes. Instead, they seem to work by attaching to receptors that sit across the cell membrane. The binding of two or more adjacent receptors to the same growth factor appears to be necessary for activation. Once receptors are activated, a message is sent to the nucleus DNA to create the target proteins that cause cell division, tumorigenicity, and so forth. In experimental animals, cytokines have helped to heal wounds caused by diabetes mellitus, glucocorticoids, irradiation, or chemotherapy.[10]

Mitogens signal cellular proliferation, and can be subdivided into "competence" (cell stimulation to progress from the resting state to a readiness state and finally cell division) types and "progression" (allows continuation of cell cycle after cell division) types. Chemoattractants stimulate cellular migration, and can be subdivided into "chemotactic" (induce the target cell to move in a given direction) and "chemokinetic" (increase the rate of cellular migration) types.

Transforming factors alter cellular phenotypic expression

Growth factors that exist but do not appear in trials for skin wounds (ulcers) include human growth hormone (hGH), insulin-like growth factor-1 (IGF-1), erythropoietin (normally produced in the kidney in response to hypoxia; stimulates bone marrow to increase RBC production), tumor necrosis factor (TNF; cachectin), interleukins, and colony-stimulating factors (CSFs).

Individual growth factors

Fibroblast growth factor (FGF). Two separate subtypes of this peptide exist: basic FGF (bFGF) and acidic FGF (aFGF).[9] Of the two, bFGF is the more useful because of the high number of target cells it can affect. In clinical trials, the effective dose was determined to be 0.5 µg/day in single or multiple doses. Basic FGF appears to "turn itself off" once reepithelialization has occurred. Basic FGF is angiogenic, whereas aFGF is nonangiogenic. Both forms have been isolated from endothelial cells.

Transforming and epidermal growth factors (TGF, EGF). Transforming growth factor exists in an alpha form and a beta form, both of which are angiogenic. The alpha form is more angiogenic than epidermal growth factor and shares the same cell receptor as EGF. Platelets are the most abundant source of the beta form, which seems to regulate the effect of other growth factors so as to control "overproduction." The most important features of epidermal growth factor are its angiogenic properties.

Platelet-derived growth factor (PDGF). PDGF is the major human serum growth factor. It was originally discovered in platelets but has also been found in other cells. Its mitogenic action is dependent on other growth factors, but its chemotactic activity functions independently.

NORMAL WOUND HEALING

Wound repair is a complex multicellular event that begins when a break in the skin occurs and ends when tissue continuity is restored; it consists of cell recruitment, cell proliferation, and protein synthesis.[7] Coagulation for the purpose of hemostasis is the first event, and is made possible by endothelial cells and platelets. The next phase is that of debris removal by leukocytes, and the final result is tissue replacement (i.e., matrix and epidermal regeneration) involving macrophages, endothelial cells, fibroblasts, and epithelial cells (keratinocytes).

Unfortunately, wound repair results in disorganized fibrosis with regenerated epidermis only; adnexal glands and structures are lost. Granulation tissue replaces the injured area, but it is not as good as the original matrix, since granulation consists of small-diameter collagen fibers only. As the wound matures, collagen of different types and diameters is placed, with various and increased linkages designed to restore normal integrity. Granulation tissue facilitates cellular remodeling.

In the initial response to injury (inflammation phase), normal hemostasis and microvascular occlusion during repair cause gradients that worsen as one gets closer to the wound's center. Repair must therefore occur, across a gradient of hypoxia, hyperlactacidemia, and hypoglycemia.

The cooperative ability of hemoglobin to bind oxygen lowers the cardiac output required to bring oxygen to the tissues. Rapidly metabolizing tissues have lower tissue oxygen pressures, so extraction of oxygen from hemoglobin is facilitated by a decreasing pH and the well-known oxyhemoglobin dissociation curve. Therefore, tissues in higher demand have greater access to supply (uninjured tissues). In wounded tissues, however, this gradient is enhanced by the distance away from the capillary source of oxygen, and the presence of fibrin (barrier to oxygen movement).

Arteriolar dilatation and increased capillary permeability are also observed during the initial phase, while at the same time venules constrict. These processes facilitate a pooling of fluids and cells within the area. They also cause edema, increased external pressure on capillaries and a decreasing vascular supply. Injury allows plasma to interact with tissue protein, causing a number of cascades to come into play: the intrinsic/extrinsic clotting cascade, the fibrinolytic cascade, the complement pathway, the kinin system, and prostaglandins.

The clotting cascade leads to thrombin formation, which converts fibrinogen to fibrin. Fibrin is the major coagulation-promoting component, and also plays a role in necrotic tissue removal, chemotaxis, and angiogenesis. Thrombin interacts with platelets to cause the release of platelet-derived growth factor (PGF). Platelets not only plug the vessel tear but also release substances that stimulate cell proliferation, migration, and protein synthesis (alpha granules of platelets release transforming growth factor beta, platelet-derived growth factor, and epidermal growth factor).

The kinin system forms bradykinin, which causes much-needed microvascular dilatation at the wound edge. The complement cascade creates C5a, which attracts neutrophils and monocytes (the first cells to occupy the wound healing space for the first 2 days after injury). Neutrophils and polymorphonuclear leukocytes (PMNLs) primarily neutralize bacteria and begin debridement of the ischemic matrix. Circulating monocytes differentiate into tissue macrophages and lymphocytes, and appear in the wound at 2 days post-injury. While they join neutrophils in bacterial neutralization and debridement, these monocytes also orchestrate granulation tissue formation, especially in an "ischemic" environment (hypoxia and lactate stimulate macrophage secretion of angiogenic factors promoting capillary growth into the repair zone).

The fibrinolytic cascade converts circulating plasminogen (inactive) to plasmin (active), which breaks fibrin clots into fibrin degradation products. The beginning of clot resolution signals the end of the inflammatory phase and the beginning of the repair/regeneration phase of wound healing. Fibrin degradation products are biologically active, functioning as chemoattractants for monocytes (the predominant cell throughout repair) and endothelial cells, as well as collagen synthesis.

Fibrinolysis (blood clot resolution) marks the end of the inflammatory phase and the beginning of the tissue repair phase. Fibroblasts appear in the wound site at 3 days post-injury and onward. They proliferate and migrate into the wound site, synthesizing and secreting collagen. The high lactate–low oxygen character of healing wounds seems to enhance this process.

In addition to collagen formation, angiogenesis and epithelialization are significant and necessary processes of the repair phase of wound healing. Angiogenesis includes capillary endothelial cell migration and proliferation, protease production, and differentiation into tubes. In addition to wound healing, angiogenesis occurs during fetal development, and during tumor growth.[12] Angiogenic growth factors seem to work directly on endothelial cells, or indirectly (macrophages, which can secrete a direct-acting growth factor).[13] In theory, angiogenesis is discontinued as the wound heals, probably in response to the restoration of normal tissue oxygen pressure by a now-normal circulation (tissue macrophages are stimulated by hypoxia and lactate to produce an angiogenesis factor; the absence of hypoxia and lactate will therefore "turn off" the macrophage).

As vascular permeability decreases, growth factors (cytokines) probably decrease because of decreased plasma and cell leakage. Epithelialization and the production of angiogenesis-inhibiting factors may also inhibit angiogenesis factor activity.

PLATELET-DERIVED WOUND HEALING FORMULA (PDWHF)

A partial solution to the problem of wound healing was developed out of the landmark research conducted by Knighton and colleagues, who used a naturally occurring mix of growth factors obtained from the patient's own platelets: PDGF, platelet derived angiogenic factor (PDAF), platelet-derived EGF, transforming growth factor beta, and platelet factor 4 (PF-4).[9] This technology is currently marketed as Procuren, by CuraTech, Inc., Stony Brook, N.Y.

In the first trial by Knighton et al, 49 patients with 95 wounds were studied. The age range of the patients was from 11 to 80 years, and the duration of conventional treatment extended from 1 week to 35 years (mean, 3.8 years). Forty-nine percent of the wounds were attributed to diabetes, 14% to venous stasis, 9% to nondiabetic peripheral vascular disease, 4% to trauma, and 17% to miscellaneous causes. Wounds were categorized according to severity, and subjected to a protocol of debridement, revascularization (where necessary), PDWHF for 12 hours followed by Silvadene or another topical antibiotic for 12 hours, custom-molded shoes, patellar-tendon-bearing prostheses, and instruction in nutrition, blood sugar control, and meticulous wound care. In an average of 7.5 weeks (range, 1 to 22 weeks), complete healing was recorded in 90% of the patients and 97% of the wounds. No harmful side effects, no excessive scarring or connective tissue growth, and no malignant transformation were observed.

Knighton et al next conducted a double-blind, crossover, placebo-controlled trial. The positive group consisted of 13 patients, with 17 of 21 wounds healing in an average of 8.6 weeks. In the placebo group, on the other hand, only 2 of 13 wounds healed in 8 weeks. When crossed over, the remaining 11 wounds healed in an average of 7.1 additional weeks. Knighton and his team believe that PDWHF works by promoting rapid growth of granulation tissue to cover the wound, after which rapid epithelialization will occur.

PDWHF is currently in use in at least 20 wound care centers nationwide. Autologous preparations are expensive; preparations through recombinant DNA technique, impregnation in sutures and bandages, and oral and parenteral administration may all occur in the future. Recombinant DNA techniques make the mass production of growth factors more feasible. In this process, the amino acid sequence of the growth factor in question is identified, from which reverse messenger RNA (mRNA) probes are constructed. These probes screen human DNA for the correct gene, which is then separated out and spliced into bacterial

DNA. The bacteria secrete the factor into culture media, which are then harvested. A human DNA gene is not always required; some growth factors are not species specific and therefore may be isolated from other mammals.[14]

Some barriers to these advances exist, however, and include (1) the chemically unstable nature of these compounds, (2) potential degradation of cytokines by the proteolytic factors found in normal wounds, and (3) uncertainty regarding optimal dosage levels, since different amounts can be either suppressive or stimulatory.

To review the process of wound healing, the first response to injury is coagulation to limit the loss of blood. Platelets participate in this effort, and release EGF, PDGF, TGF-alpha, TGF-beta, and IGF-1 from their alpha granules. These growth factors have chemotactic and mitogenic qualities. Inflammation follows this stage, with neutrophils (PMNs) and macrophages infiltrating the wound. Macrophages secrete TGF-alpha, TGF-beta, PDGF, bFGF, and interleukin-1. These chemotactic factors and other chemotactic factors (C5a, bacterial products) cause fibroblast migration into the wound. Fibroblasts secrete growth factors that produce extracellular matrix components (i.e., proteoglycans, fibronectin, collagen), and are most likely the source of endothelial cell migration and proliferation. Endothelial cells establish blood supply and secrete PDGF and bFGF.

Finally, remodeling processes such as collagen synthesis, collagenase synthesis, and collagen cross-linking reestablish the architecture of the wound.

Alterations in the above system can lead to impaired healing or excessive deposition of connective tissue with fibrosis. Once the infected or infectious ulceration has been brought under control, various platelet-derived wound-healing formulas may play a future role in promoting wound healing and closure.

CULTURED EPITHELIAL AUTOGRAFTS (CEAU) AND ALLOGRAFTS (CEAL)

These grafts are prepared in vitro after a sample has been harvested from the donor.[15] In the case of autografts, the donor and graft recipient (host) are the same person; allografts come from a different person. While in culture, the grafts have a mucoid consistency, are transparent, and consist only of an undifferentiated epidermal layer. Within a week of application of the graft to a granulating bed, however, it assumes the macroscopic and histologic characteristics of normal epidermis. Even more remarkably, the dermal layer underlying the CEAU transforms from a scarlike appearance to one with a normal bilaminar arrangement (i.e., papillary and reticular dermis) of collagen fibrils. CEAUs also seem to possess the unprecedented feature of site-specificity—that is, the ability to generate the same type of skin (epidermis and dermis) found at the donor site regardless of where the graft is placed. CEAUs obtained from the sole of the foot will therefore recreate plantar skin wherever they are placed.

Although cutaneous adnexa (hair, glands) are not recreated by the CEAU, dermal development is clearly directed by the epidermis. This finding disproved the prior belief that the dermis directed events within the epidermis. The epidermis' ability to perform these incredible functions has been attributed to epidermal cytokines, including acidic and basic TGF, which has already led researchers to consider CEAUs as favored wound dressings and natural vehicles for the administration of growth factors. Allografts (CEALs) are more easily obtained but are rejected soon after their application. As a result, they do not survive long enough to demonstrate the dermal remodeling and site-specific changes witnessed with autografts. Nevertheless, they stimulate reepithelialization until the time of rejection.

INFECTIOUS ULCERATIONS

Although the factors discussed above apply to infected and infectious ulcers equally, there comes a time when the infected ulcer may not respond to conventional therapy. A truly infectious etiology should then be considered, especially in patients who are immunosuppressed (e.g., corticosteroids or chemotherapeutic agents) or immunocompromised (e.g., lymphoma patients, patients who are HIV positive). Culture and/or biopsy with staining for fungi, viruses, acid-fast bacteria, and parasites are therefore recommended as the next step in care. The recent literature has documented the following etiologies for infectious cutaneous ulceration.

Amoebae

Four genera of amoebae are pathogenic in humans (*Entamoeba, Naegleria, Acanthamoeba,* and *Vahlkampfia*), and must be considered as etiologic agents in HIV-positive patients who present with papulonodules and ulcerations.[16] The correct diagnosis is usually made after cultures and stains for fungi and bacteria are negative and a skin biopsy is performed. In such cases, the skin biopsy reveals amoebic double-walled cysts (often mistaken for macrophages) and trophozoites. *Naegleria fowleri* is the only amoeba sensitive to antimicrobial therapy in vivo (amphotericin B). All other amoebae demonstrate in vitro susceptibility only (*Acanthamoeba* has shown such susceptibility in vitro to ketoconazole, sulfadiazine, flucytosine, pentamidine, and polymixin B). Amoebae enter through the nasopharynx and then disseminate hematogenously to the central nervous system and the skin. In the central nervous system, encephalitis is the result[17] (Fig. 9-3).

Nocardia

Three species, all found in soil, account for nearly all human infections: *N. asteroides, N. brasiliensis,* and *N. caviae*.[18] Of the three, *N. asteroides* accounts for most nocardial infections. Over 80% of patients present with lung involvement initially, followed by cutaneous dissemination. Only 10% of patients exhibit lung involvement without skin changes.

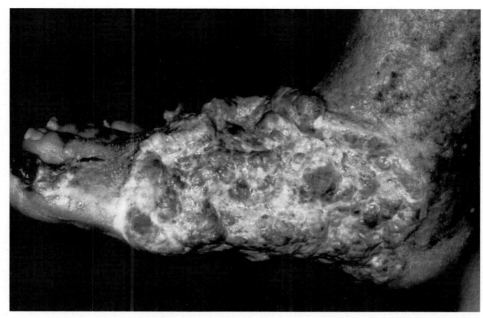

Fig. 9-3 A 63-year-old white male with history of Kaposi's sarcoma. Note extensive involvement of entire foot and ankle. *(Courtesy Dr. Charles J. Gudas, University of Chicago.)*

Primary cutaneous nocardiosis usually requires a history of local trauma to the extremity, followed by cellulitis, pustule formation, ulceration, or a lymphocutaneous syndrome resembling sporotrichosis. Disseminated nocardiosis to the skin usually occurs in an immunocompromised host, whereas primary cutaneous nocardiosis more often occurs in patients without immunocompromise. Nocardiosis responds to 2 g of sulfadiazine administered every 6 hours. Some cases require as long as 2 months for resolution.

Fusobacterium

Sports-induced abrasions can sometimes break down to form shallow, painless ulcers with indurated borders.[19] These lesions occur secondary to a spirochete-fusobacterial gram-negative anaerobic rod *(Fusobacterium ulcerans)* infection, although anaerobes are less frequently isolated from ulcers greater than 6 weeks in duration. This etiology should also be considered in patients with indolent ulcers who are returning from the tropics; hence the term "tropical ulcer." Generally, *F. ulcerans* is more common in cattle, rare in humans, and usually synergistic with *F. nucleatum*. In either case, penicillin or co-trimoxazole may be effective, whereas flucloxacillin is ineffective. Other important species include *F. fusiforme, F. gonidiaformans, F. mortiferum, F. necrophorum, F. prausnitzii,* and *F. varium.*[20]

Mycobacteria

In addition to the ulcerations witnessed in Hansen's disease patients *(Mycobacterium leprae),* a number of other mycobacterial species may cause cutaneous ulceration. *Mycobacterium haemophilum* has reportedly caused skin ulceration in immunocompromised patients.[21] Sources of immunocom-

promise have included renal transplant, AIDS, lymphocytic lymphoma, and Hodgkin's disease, and there have been a small number of idiopathic (immunocompetent) cases in children. Clinically, *M. haemophilum* ulceration begins as an erythematous or violaceous nodule that may progress to form first an abscess, and secondarily an ulcer. The ulceration seems to have a predilection for the extremities, limiting itself to the skin and underlying tissues. The fact that the organism restricts its own spread to these borders indicates the organism's preference for growth in cooler climates. *Mycobacterium ulcerans* infection causes its own variety of skin ulceration.[22] First described in Uganda in 1887, a cluster of cases was discovered in a Ugandan area known as Buruli, in the 1960s; hence, the lesion is often referred to as the Buruli ulcer. The lesion begins as a subcutaneous nodule that becomes attached to the skin or as an intradermal pustule. Over the course of weeks to months, the lesion progresses to a necrotizing panniculitis with ulcerations, the latter having a wood-hard necrotic base with extensive undermining of the wound edges. The surrounding skin is shiny and hyperpigmented. The lesion is relatively pain free and not warm as would be expected in bacterial infection. When the ulceration heals, it does so with a deeply sunken scar caused by the loss of subcutaneous tissue, and overhanging borders of normal skin.

Four clinical stages of the Buruli ulcer exist: I, subcutaneous nodule; II, panniculitis; III, ulceration; and IV, Buruli scar. *M. ulcerans* grows at 32° to 33° C, explaining its preference for the subcutaneous tissue layer, at body temperature, like other mycobacteria. *M. ulcerans* is different, however, in that it produces an immunosuppressive/cytotoxic substance that is heat labile. It is this toxin that

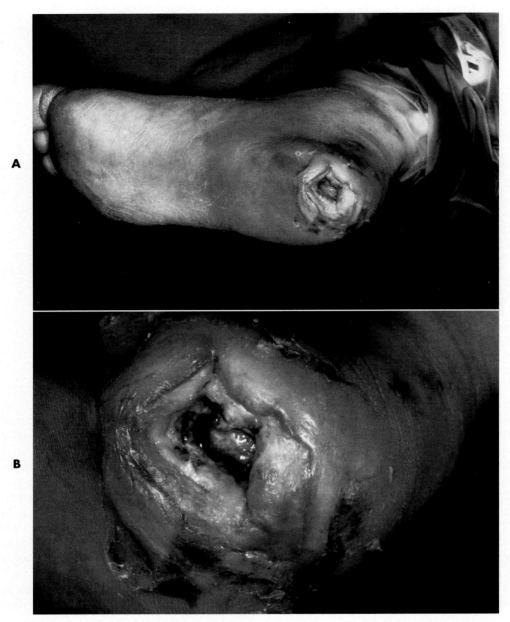

Fig. 9-4 A, A 38-year-old white female with an 8-month history of bilateral heel decubitus ulcers. Patient had neuropathic feet, secondary to long-standing insulin-dependent diabetes mellitus. She was 2 years post–kidney-pancreas transplant and is presently not taking insulin, but is on immunosuppressive therapy. **B,** Erythematous heel with a large Wagner grade III ulceration extending to the calcaneus, which can be visualized in the central portion of the ulcer, following initial bedside debridement.

causes tissue destruction, rather than host defenses. The natural habitat of *M. ulcerans* is unknown, but it seems to occur where large bodies of water exist. Infection can occur at all ages, but children (usually between the ages of 5 and 15 years) are more commonly affected. Ulceration occurs most frequently on the limbs (sparing the palms and soles), but has also been described on the head, neck, or trunk. Despite extensive ulceration, little constitutional change occurs. Clinicians must remember that the Buruli ulcer is not

a disease limited to the poor and malnourished, as it can pose a significant new threat to HIV-positive patients. Case-to-case transmission is unusual, even among family members sharing the same environment. It has been reported in Africa, South America, Southeast Asia, and the Central Pacific (Australia).[24] To date, there is no effective treatment for the Buruli ulcer other than supportive measures, preventing superinfection, and allowing the disease to run its natural course. Antibiotics, ulcer excision and grafting, heat treat-

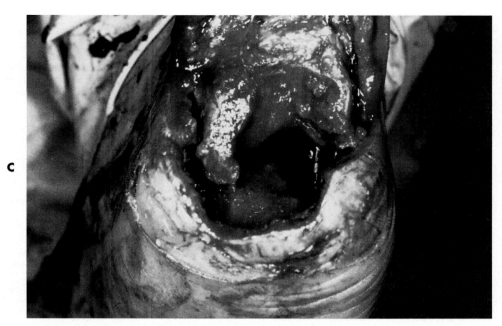

C

Fig. 9-4, cont'd. C, After intraoperative debridement of necrotic soft tissue and intracalcaneal bone, she sustained an intraoperative fracture, and a large Steinman pin was used to hold the fracture open for local wound care. A below-knee amputation was ultimately needed because of extensive microvascular disease, not amenable to vascular reconstruction, with large tissue and bone loss. *(Courtesy Dr. Charles J. Gudas, University of Chicago.)*

ments, and hyperbaric oxygenation have all been used, with mixed results.

Other important species include *M. tuberculosis, M. avium, M. bovis, M. chelonei, M. fortuitum, M. intracellulare, M. kansasii, M. marinum, M. scrofulaceum,* and *M. microti.*[25]

Pseudomonas putrefaciens

Infection with this organism can apparently present as one of two syndromes: benign disease in chronic ulceration, and fulminant disease resembling gram-negative septicemia.[26] It is because of this latter presentation that *P. putrefaciens* ulceration is included in the "infectious" category, since its septic shock–like syndrome (mental obtundation, hypotension) in the absence of demonstrable bacteremia suggests exotoxin production. Exotoxin could possibly account for spread of the ulceration and cellulitis. In this reported case, cellulitis began after an ulceration of the lateral malleolus.

Epithelioid angiomatosis (cat-scratch disease)

In immunocompetent individuals, this disease presents with usually no more than a papule at the site of inoculation, regional lymphadenopathy, fever, myalgias, and arthralgias.[27-30] Recovery is usually spontaneous and occurs within 2 to 4 months, although morbidity may last as long as 2 years. Antibiosis is not of much benefit. In immunocompromised patients, however, the disease is more widespread and fulminating, with cutaneous ulceration necrosis as well as a poorer prognosis. Also, immuno-

compromised hosts may improve with antibiotic usage. Criteria for clinical diagnosis include a history of cat scratch, regional lymphadenopathy in the absence of other causes for lymphadenopathy, characteristic histopathologic changes in a biopsied lymph node, and a positive cat-scratch disease (CSD) skin test (or histologic diagnosis demonstrating the cat-scratch bacillus using Warthin-Starry silver impregnation staining). The organism has been recorded as sensitive to cefotetan, cefotaxime, gentamicin, amikacin, tobramycin, netilmicin, mezlocillin, and ciprofloxacin. Cat-scratch disease should be added to the list of possible infectious ulcerations occurring in immunocompromised (e.g., AIDS) patients.

NEUROPATHIC FOOT ULCERATIONS

Altered pedal sensation allows ambulation beyond the normal shearing tolerance of plantar skin and soft tissue structures. Excessive pressure may create superficial or deep lesions, which may ultimately lead to bone contamination. These may occur in diabetes mellitus, alcoholism, heavy metal poisoning, leprosy (Hansen's disease), myelomeningocele, syringomyelia, spina bifida, or tabes dorsalis (tertiary syphilis) (Fig. 9-4).

HYPERBARIC OXYGENATION

First popularized in burn patients, hyperbaric oxygenation (HBO) of wounds was widely utilized in a variety of nonburn wounds. The successes reported in the early years

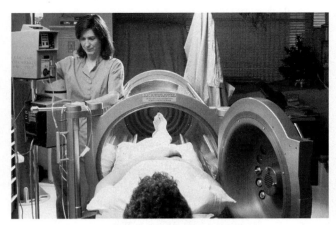

Fig. 9-5 Whole-body hyperbaric oxygenation.

of its use in these circumstances have now waned, regardless of whether whole-body or more-readily-available extremity chambers are employed. Presently, an adequate vascular supply is considered more beneficial than hyperbaric oxygenation. Removal of necrotic debris, drainage of abscesses, copious use of hydrogen peroxide, and exposure of deep wound recesses to room air are more reliable in eliminating anaerobic growth (Fig. 9-5). Patients with infected ulcers in documented sickle-cell disease or other conditions made worse by hypoxia may benefit from hyperbaric oxygenation.[31,32]

CONCLUSION

The purpose of this chapter has been to review the definition, diagnosis, etiology, and treatment methods for infected cutaneous ulcerations of the human foot. New concepts in wound healing and tissue stimulation have also been discussed. Finally, logical algorithmic approaches to this frustrating problem have been presented.

REFERENCES

1. DeLauro TM, Positano RG: Lower extremity ulcerations. In Marcinko DE, ed: *Medical and surgical therapeutics of the foot and ankle,* Baltimore, 1992, Williams & Wilkins.
2. Joseph WS: *Handbook of lower extremity infections,* Philadelphia, 1990, Churchill Livingstone.
3. King MS: Specialized infections. In Abramson C, McCarthy DJ, Rupp MJ, eds: *Infectious diseases of the lower extremity,* Baltimore, 1991, Williams & Wilkins.
4. Bartolomei FJ: Subcutaneous infections. In Abramson C, McCarthy DJ, Rupp MJ, eds: *Infectious diseases of the lower extremity,* Baltimore, 1991, Williams & Wilkins.
5. Likar B, Poredos P, Preseren M, Vodovnik D, Klesnik M: Effects of electric current on partial oxygen tension in skin surrounding wounds, *Wounds* 5(1):32-36, 1993.
6. Mayrovitz HN, Regan MB, Larsen PB: Effects of rhythmically alternating and static pressure support surfaces on skin microvascular perfusion, *Wounds* 5(1):47-55, 1993.
7. Skover GR: Cellular and biochemical dynamics of wound repair: wound environment in collagen regeneration, *Clin Podiatr Med Surg* 8(4):723-756, 1991.
8. Ehrlichman RJ, Seckel BR, Bryan DJ: Common complications of wound healing: prevention and management, *Surg Clin North Am* 71(6):1323-1351, 1991.
9. Knighton DR, Ciresi K, Figel D: Stimulation of repair in chronic, nonhealing, cutaneous ulcers using platelet-:derived wound healing formula, *Surg Gynecol Obstet* 170(1):56-60, 1990.
10. Kingsworth AN, Slavin J: Peptide growth factors and wound healing, *Br J Surg* 78:1286-1290, 1991.
11. Herndon DN, Hayward PG, Rutan RL: Growth hormones and factors in surgical patients, *Adv Surg* 25:65-97, 1992.
12. Heldin CH, Usuki K, Miyazono K: Platelet-derived endothelial cell growth factor, *J Cell Biochem* 47(3):208-210, 1991.
13. Hom DB, Maisel RH: Angiogenic growth factors: their effects and potential in soft tissue wound healing, *Ann Otol Rhinol Laryngol* 101(4):349-354, 1992.
14. Blitstein-Willinger E: The role of growth factors in wound healing, *Skin Pharmacol* 4(3):175-182, 1992.
15. Compton CC: Wound healing potential of cultured epithelium, *Wounds* 5(2);97-111, 1993.
16. May LP, Sidhu GS, Buchness MR: Diagnosis of *Acanthamoeba* infection by cutaneous manifestations in a man seropositive to HIV, *J Am Acad Dermatol:* 352-355, 1992.
17. Wilson DC, Werth SG, King LE: Ulcerative lesions and herpes simplex virus type 2 in a patient with Evan syndrome, *South Med J* 83(12):1484-1486, 1990.
18. Boixeda P, Espana A, Suarez J: Cutaneous nocardiosis and human immunodeficiency virus infection, *Int J Dermatol* 30(11):804-805, 1991.
19. Webb J, Murdoch DA: Tropical ulcers after sports injuries (letter), *Lancet* 339:129-130, 1992.
20. Sharma VK, Sharma R, Kumar B: Ulcerative secondary syphilis, *Int J Dermatol* 29(8):585-586, 1990.
21. Kristjansson M, Bieluch VM, Byeff PD: *Mycobacterium haemophilum* infection in immunocompromised patients: case report and review of the literature, *Rev Infect Dis* 13(5):906-910, 1991.
22. Muelder K: Wounds that will not heal: the Buruli ulcer, *Int J Dermatol* 31(1):25-26, 1992.
23. Endeley EML, Enwerem EO, Holcome C, Patel RV: Buruli ulcer, *J Indian Med Assoc* 88(9):260-261, 1990.
24. Muelder K, Nourou M, Al-Najjar AA, Harrington CI, Slater DN: Angiosarcoma: a complication of varicose leg ulcerations, *Acta Derm Venereol* 6:167, 1986.
25. Hur W, Ahn SK, Lee SH, Kang WH: Cutaneous reaction induced by retained bee stinger, *J Dermatol* 18(12):736-739, 1991.
26. Chen SCA, Lawrence RH, Packham DR: Cellulitis due to *Pseudomonas* putrification: possible product of endotoxins, *Rev Infect Dis* 13(4):642-643, 1991.
27. DeMarco MJ, Soroko TA, Kirsh S, Smith L: Epithelioid angiomatosis, *J Foot Ankle Surg* 32(1):20-26, 1993.
28. Lipsky BA, Pecoraro RE, Ahroni JH: Foot ulceration and infection in elderly diabetics, *Clin Geriatr Med* 6(4):747-769, 1990.
29. Joseph WS: Treatment of lower extremity infections in diabetics, *J Am Pediatr Med Assoc.* 82(7):361-369, 1992.
30. Mulder GD, Mason R, Tepelidis N: Ulceration and osteomyelitis, *Clin Podiatr Med Surg* 7(4):733-742, 1990.
31. Jeter KF, Tintle TE: Wound dressings of the nineties: indications and contraindications, *Clin Podiatr Med Surg* 8(4):799-816, 1991.
32. Carver N, Leigh IM: Synthetic dressings, *Int J Dermatol* 20(3):459-465, 1990.

ADDITIONAL READINGS

Cuzzell JZP: The right way to culture a wound, *Am J Nurs* 5:48, 1993.
Fox HR, Karchmer AW: Management of diabetic foot infections, including the use of home intravenous antibiotic therapy, *Clin Podiatr Med Surg* 13(4):671-682, 1996.
Ganio C, Tenewitz E, Wilson RC, Moyles B: The treatment of chronic non-healing wounds using autologous platelet-derived growth factors, *J Foot Ankle Surg* 32:263, 1993.

Hanna JR, Giacopelli JA: A review of wound healing and wound dressing products, *J Foot Surg* 36(1):2-14, 1997.

Kirsner RS, Falanga V, Eaglstein WH: The biology of skin grafts: skin grafts as pharmacologic agents, *Arch Derm.,* 4:481, 1993.

Loveland LI, McClure LP, Page JC: Living skin equivalents, *The Lower Extremity* 3(4):227-231, 1996.

Oloff L, Thornton C: Catastrophe of the infected foot. In Marcinko D, ed: *Medical and surgical therapeutics of the foot and ankle,* Baltimore, 1992, Williams & Wilkins.

Principato R: Peripheral vascular disease and its evaluation, *The Lower Extremity* 14(2):265-281, 1997.

Servold SA: Growth factor impact on wound healing, *Clin Podiatr Med Surg* 8(4):937-953, 1991.

Unger HD, Lucca M: The role of hyperbaric oxygen therapy in the treatment of diabetic foot ulcers and refractory osteomyelitis, *Clin Podiatr Med Surg* 7:483,1990.

Wattel F, Mathieu D, Coget JM, Billard V: Hyperbaric oxygen therapy in chronic vascular wound management, *Angiology* 1:59, 1990.

10

Traumatic Infections of the Foot and Ankle

O. Kent Mercado

Devouring Famine, Plague, and War, Each able to undo mankind,
Death's servile emissaries are.   Shirley

Traumatically induced infection of the foot and ankle may be a complication more devastating than the original injury. Such infections are the consequence of opportunistic pathogens that damage healthy tissue; their likelihood is proportional to the predilection for infection. Injuries with associated breakage of the integument have a higher infection rate, because of the inoculation of bacteria or other contaminants into the wound. Devitalized and necrotic tissue then acts as a nidus for normal skin flora and externally introduced organisms, which in turn become opportunistic pathogens.

The possible sequelae of traumatic infections include wound sepsis, cellulitis, abscess formation, osteomyelitis, septicemia, and even death. The severity and nature of the instigating trauma are determining factors.

PUNCTURE WOUNDS

Puncture wounds to the plantar aspect of the foot are common injuries. They account for 7.4% of all lower extremity accidents encountered in hospital emergency rooms and physicians' offices. This number may be low because of the seemingly innocuous presentation of the injury and the number of patients who self-treat. Seasonal variations have been noted, with most cases occurring between May and October because of the increase in outdoor activities and the propensity for children to go barefoot.

The majority of all puncture wounds (98%) are from nails. The remaining injuries are from a plethora of sources, including glass, sewing needles, toothpicks, barbecue skewers, plastic spikes, wire coat hangers, gravel, wood, metal objects, bullets, and straw. Despite a seemingly benign presentation, the consequences of a simple puncture wound can include cellulitis, abscess formation, retained foreign bodies, septic arthritis, and osteomyelitis. Therefore, the necessity for proper wound evaluation, historical review, and x-ray interpretation cannot be overemphasized.[1]

The management and complication predictability of puncture wounds are dependent upon, but not limited to, the following factors:

1. The type and condition of the material that punctured the foot (clean, dirty, rusty, etc.)
2. The depth of the wound and its location (e.g., near metatarsal heads, which leads to deeper penetration)
3. The type of shoe gear if any, because of the possibility of foreign body retention in the wound
4. The underlying health status of the patient, such as diabetes mellitus, long-term steroid use, or any other condition that may immunocompromise the patient
5. Tetanus immune status
6. Time of presentation (less than or greater than 24 hours)

Retrospective studies have demonstrated postpuncture infection rates of 8% to 15% for cellulitis and 0.6% to 1.8% for osteomyelitis. Time of presentation is a good predictor of potential for poor outcome. For example, Houston et al related a 10% total infection rate; however, they found that only 51 of 2303 patients (2.2%) who were early presenters (within the first 24 hours) developed an infection and that only one developed osteomyelitis.[2]

Foreign bodies

Foreign body retention, such as pieces of a tennis shoe, sock, wood splinters, glass, or metal, have been found in 3% of all puncture wounds. Broken needles have been the most frequently encountered, at 30%. Foreign bodies introduced through the wound track can lead to infection and have been found in a large majority of unresolved cellulitis cases that did not respond to intravenous antibiotics.[3] Conventional radiographic evaluation can be utilized to rule out foreign bodies, debris from penetrating objects, and the presence of gas in the soft tissues. CT scans, xerography, and ultrasound have been used when a nonmetallic object, such as plastic, glass, or wood, is suspected.

Foreign-body granuloma

A foreign-body granuloma, or epidermal inclusion cyst, is known by several other designations, including inversion cyst and epithelial inclusion cyst. Most are located in the scalp, face, neck, shoulders, back, or scrotum. They are rarely found on the palms and soles and are usually nonpigmented and, unilocular and often the result of trauma, such as in a puncture wound.[3] One of the largest cysts, seen in the lower extremity, was reported by Marcinko and Elleby, in 1986.[4] It occurred in a 27-year-old man who sustained a fractured tibia after a motor vehicle accident.

Classification of puncture wounds

In order to aid the clinician in the management of puncture wounds and to discuss the indications for various medical and surgical treatment, Resnick and Fallat developed a classification scheme for puncture wounds, according to the depth and severity of injury[5-8] (Table 10-1).

Type I: superficial cutaneous penetration. These injuries involve the penetration of the epidermis and/or dermis. They are generally considered clean wounds, which exhibit no clinical signs or symptoms of infection. The area should be cleaned, followed by daily dressing changes. Initial treatment includes avoidance of weight bearing and appropriate padding around the wound if pain persists or if the foot is insensitive. Patients need to be followed closely and are instructed to monitor the wound for any changes that would impede healing.

Type II: subcutaneous or articular joint involvement without signs or symptoms of infection. These injuries involve the penetration of an object into the articular structures and/or the overlying subcutaneous tissues. Type II injuries are considered the most common of all penetrating wounds, accounting for greater than 50% of all puncture wounds. Pain is the predominant symptom, and initial treatment usually requires local anesthesia for adequate examination of the wound. Regional anesthesia is preferred, to avoid inoculation of healthy tissues with possible pathogens. The wound is probed and explored, and foreign bodies are removed. A Gram stain and cultures are taken, and pressure irrigation is used to decrease wound contamination. The wound edges and all necrotic or devitalized tissue are debrided and widened to facilitate drainage. The area is

| **TABLE 10-1 Resnick and Fallat classification of puncture wounds** |

Type I:	Superficial cutaneous penetration
Type II:	Subcutaneous or articular joint involvement without signs or symptoms of infection
Type IIIA:	Established soft tissue infection, including pyarthrosis and retained foreign body
Type IIIB:	Foreign body penetration into bone
Type IV:	Osteomyelitis secondary to puncture wound injury

From Resnick C, Fallat LM: Puncture wounds: therapeutic considerations and a new classification, *J Foot Surg* 29:2, 1990.

packed open and allowed to heal by second intention and to reduce anaerobic activity.

Type IIIA: established soft tissue infection, including pyarthrosis and retained foreign body. These infections are often delayed complications of type II injuries. Patients most frequently present with edema, erythema, and pain. When an infected puncture wound is suspected, the patient should be evaluated for systemic signs and symptoms. A complete blood count should be taken, and the erythrocyte sedimentation rate should be monitored. Aggressive local treatment, along with the appropriate antibiotic therapy, is necessary to avoid dangerous sequelae such as ascending cellulitis and osteomyelitis. Foreign bodies are found in a high percentage of unresolved cellulitis cases and those that do not respond to intravenous antibiotic therapy. Unresolved cellulitis and abscess formation usually require incision, drainage, and retrieval of the foreign object. Rarely, the foreign body may be left in place if it is inert and asymptomatic, does not impede function, and is not within a joint. Materials that are reactive or large, located within a joint, impeding function, or near tendons, nerves, or vessels should be removed.

Radiographs should be ordered in all cases of clinical suspicion of a retained foreign body. Foreign bodies are often difficult to localize. Objects such as wood or plastic are not readily visualized; therefore, indirect evidence such as pseudotumor, joint destruction, periosteal thickening, and lytic areas should be noted in osseous radiographic changes. Fluoroscopy is also useful for localizing and retrieving foreign objects. A three-needle technique is highly effective in localizing objects when fluoroscopy is unavailable. In this three-dimensional translocation process, three needles of different sizes are inserted around an anesthetized puncture wound in a pyramid fashion. A straight hemostat is inserted directly into the center of the wound and is used as a reference point to locate the exact position of the object on a flat-plate x-ray. Computerized tomography, sonography, and xeroradiography have been described as alternative modalities in foreign body localization.

In joint sepsis, repeated aspirations of the joint, away from cellulitic areas, may be beneficial in both diagnosis and treatment. Surgical drainage of a septic joint is usually necessary when fluid rapidly accumulates in the joint. This debridement and drainage will help facilitate the removal of infected accumulated fluids, retained foreign bodies, and debris, which must be removed before the infection can be resolved. Intraoperative wound cultures may be beneficial because they often reveal different pathogens, which must be dealt with before proper antibiotic therapy can be initiated.

Type IIIB: foreign-body penetration into bone. When foreign bodies penetrate bone, immediate attention is imperative because of the potentially devastating consequences of osteomyelitis. Surgical removal of a foreign body and surgical debridement of the infection are necessary. Care is taken to remove all debris, such as shoe gear and the paper wrapping from power nails and retained foreign bodies, which can harbor infections. The wound should be packed open, followed by monitored dressing changes. Deep, superficial, and intraoperative cultures should be taken, and prophylactic intravenous antibiotics initiated. Definitive antibiotic care should be determined by deep and intraoperative antimicrobial sensitivity studies. Nails and sewing needles over bony prominences as well as projectiles (bullets and nail gun injuries) have a higher incidence of bone penetration, and therefore higher rates of osteomyelitis. Expedient removal of the penetrating object, along with aggressive local and systemic management, is imperative.

Type IV: osteomyelitis secondary to puncture wound injury. Osteomyelitis is a rare (0.6% to 1.8%) but potentially severe sequela of any penetrating injury. The clinical presentation of osteomyelitis following a puncture wound (direct extension osteomyelitis) is quite different from the hematogenous osteomyelitis usually found in children. There is a delay of approximately 3 weeks before the onset of symptoms. The patient usually appears to undergo clinical improvement. There is a decrease in cellulitis, pain, and swelling, and the wound may even appear to heal. Then there is a recurrence of pain, swelling, and localized erythema. Serial x-rays and bone scan evaluation can demonstrate changes consistent with osteomyelitis; however, bone cultures are done for definitive diagnosis. Once a diagnosis is tendered, specific therapy must begin.

Green and Bruno observed a pattern of bone infection response and its sequelae. From their studies, they developed a surgical treatment regimen based on the timing of the diagnosis.[9] Their regimen consists of three categories:

Type 1: Early diagnosis with surgical drainage and debridement, along with appropriate antibiotic coverage. This will usually result in complete healing.

Type 2: If there is a 9- to 14-day delay in diagnosis and treatment, the infection can be eradicated with surgical drainage and debridement, along with appropriate antibiotic coverage. However, residual bone and joint destruction may occur.

Type 3: If there is a 3-week or more delay in the diagnosis and treatment, the infection becomes chronic, necessitating bone resection as the final cure.

Therefore, early recognition and prompt aggressive treatment of pedal puncture wounds are essential in the proper management of osteomyelitis. Wound lavage with hexachlorophene should be avoided because of the occult potential, *Pseudomonas* contamination, in this situation.

Finally, needle sticks constitute a special kind of puncture wound, with their potential exposure to the hepatitis B virus (HBV). In hospitalized patients with known HBsAg, the risk is 1:20, while it is much lower in hospitalized patients in general. By comparison, the risk of AIDS contamination by a blood transfusion is 1:28,000, while the incidence of posttransfusion hepatitis is 0.3 to 0.9 per 1000 units of blood.

ZOONOTIC FOOT INFECTIONS

Zoonotic infections are disease states that are transmitted from animals to humans. Direct contact with animals or their products, through topical, percutaneous, or arthropodic vector, is necessary for the transmission of infection.[10]

Zoonotic infections can be divided into two categories: those induced by animal bites or scratches and those transmitted by an arthropod vector. Animal bite infections are most commonly due to *Staphylococcus aureus, Pasteurella multocida,* or alpha-hemolytic streptococci (Table 10-2). Arthropod vectors and fleas are associated with, and can transmit, the plague, tularemia, and Rocky Mountain spotted fever (RMSF).

Animal bites and scratches

More than one million animal bites are reported each year in the United States alone, and this figure may be artificially low as a result of unreported incidents or family wound care. Dogs account for the vast majority of all animal bites (80% to 85%), followed by cats (10%), with the remainder from rodents, rabbits, raccoons, skunks, horses, bats, and a myriad of other domestic and wild animals. Animal bites have been categorized as an unrecognized epidemic.[11] Four types of bite or scratch-wounds are generally encountered: (1) Lacerations with tearing or avulsion tissue defects are commonly caused by dogs and cats. These are usually inflicted when the victim abruptly pulls away with the animal's tooth or claw firmly embedded in a limb. (2) Crush injuries from large animal bites (horses) are of concern because of the tremendous crush injury potential. Large dogs are capable of exerting jaw pressures of 200 to 450 psi, which is enough to puncture a piece of sheet metal. (3) Puncture wounds from cats and rodents, because of their razor-sharp teeth, are potentially the most dangerous and have the highest rates of infection. Because of the small fang or nail opening left, the wound is more likely to close over quickly, allowing for greater potential abscess formation and anaerobic activity. (4) Abrasion injuries are usually caused by large animals, with little breakage of the skin. They are generally the least prone to infection, but because of the possible saliva contamination, should be considered tetanus prone.

Dog bites. Dog bites are the most common of all animal bite wounds. Most are inflicted by animals known to the victim, with 50% occurring on the lower extremity. Ordog noted a 15% infection rate following a dog bite to the lower extremity, despite medical care.[12] Goldstein noted two distinct groups: (1) patients who presented within 8 hours of injury and (2) those who presented after 12 hours postinjury.[13] As in puncture wound management, the time of presentation is an excellent predictor of poor outcome potential. She found that while those in group 1 may have expressed concern over wound care or disfigurement, or believed they needed a tetanus or rabies shot, none had an established infection, as opposed to those in group 2, who

TABLE 10-2 Bacteria isolated from animal bite wounds

Aerobic and Facultative Bacteria

Streptococcus species
    Alpha-hemolytic
    Beta-hemolytic
    Gamma-hemolytic
Staphylococcus aureus
Staphylococcus saprophyticus
Staphylococcus intermedius
Staphylococcus epidermis
Micrococcus species
Micrococcus luteus
Moraxella species
Moraxella phenylpyrovica
Chromobacterium species
Corynebacterium species
Pasteurella species
Pasteurella multocida
Yersinia pestis
Proteus mirabilis
Enterobacter cloacae
Neisseria species
Acinetobacter actinomycetemcomitans
Flavobacterium species
Streptobacillus moniliformis
Spirillum minus
Eikenella corrodens
Haemophilus aphrophilus
M-5, EF-4, II-j, DF-2

Anaerobic Bacteria

Actinomyces species
Bacteroides species
Bacteroides melaninogenicus
Bacteroides asaccharolyticus
Fusobacterium species
Fusobacterium nucleatum
Fusobacterium russii
Peptostreptococcus species
Peptostreptococcus prevotii
Peptostreptococcus magnus
Propionibacterium acnes
Propionibacterium species
Propionibacterium granulosum
Eubacterium species
Leptotrichia buccalis

From Goldstein EJC: Infectious complications and therapy of dog bites, *J Am Podiatr Med Assoc* 79:10, 1989.

sought medical attention 90% of the time because of an established infection.

Dog bite infections commonly proceed to cellulitis and abscess formation. They may, however, lead to septic arthritis or osteomyelitis. The majority of infections are due to the normal oral flora of the biting animal, as opposed to opportunistic environmental pathogens. The infection is usually polymicrobial and commonly includes *S. aureus*, alpha-hemolytic streptococci, *Pasteurella multocida*, and, to a lesser extent, *Pseudomonas*, sp., *Eikenella corrodens*, *Proteus mirabilis, Klebsiella, Bacteroides,* and *Clostridium* sp. Other infections known to be transmitted by dog bite include rabies, tetanus, tularemia, cat-scratch disease, and even the fatal sepsis of asplenic patients that is due to CDC DF-2 (dysgenic fermenter 2).

Cat bites. Cat bites are the second and most common animal bite wound. They have a much higher predilection for infection. Cats typically inflict puncture wounds. The needle-like structure of their teeth or claws easily penetrates the epidermis and dermis. Abscess and cellulitis are more frequent, probably because of the benign presentation and apparent quick "healing" appearance of these deeply inoculated wounds.

Pasteurella multocida, a gram-negative coccobacillus, is the major pathogen in feline-inflicted wounds, but the majority of infections are polymicrobial with a distribution similar to that of dog bites. Because of the unusual grooming behavior of felines, they can inoculate oral flora by scratch wounds. Other diseases known to be transmitted by cat bite wounds are tularemia, plague, rabies, and cat-scratch disease.

Human bites. Human bites, though rare to the lower extremity, are potentially the most dangerous animal bite. Many are "fight bites," sustained when an opponent bites into the extremity during a fight. Since human saliva contains 1×10^8 bacteria per milliliter, with up to 42 different pathogens, human bites have the highest rate of infection and are associated with *Streptococcus viridans,* beta-hemolytic streptococci group A, *Staphyloccus aureus* and *epidermidis, B. fragilis,* and *Eikenella corrodens.* In rare cases they are even associated with the transmission of the blood-borne virus of hepatitis B, HIV, and a host of other diseases.

Cat-scratch disease. Cat-scratch disease is caused by an unnamed gram-negative bacillus. The organism enters the body through a break in the skin, which may result from a bite, a scratch, or a penetrating object (wood, fishhook, thorn), followed by exposure to a cat (handling or cat licking the injury site). Eighty percent of the reported cases are pediatric, and almost all are associated with lymphadenopathy, fever, malaise, or fatigue. They are usually managed with oral tetracycline.

Treatment. As with all traumatically induced wounds, early evaluation and prompt and aggressive therapy are essential. All bite wounds are considered tetanus prone because of the possibility of contamination by soil, ingested feces, or saliva. Therefore tetanus prophylaxis should be given. Superficial bite wounds should be cleansed thoroughly and debrided. *Pasteurella multiocida* has been found in 10% to 20% of infected dog bite wounds and in 30% to 50% of infected cat bite wounds, and its potential for infection should be addressed. Bites or scratches overlying bone, joint spaces, tendons, or neurovascular structures, particularly puncture wounds, are at high risk for infection.

Tendon sheaths, bursae, and joint spaces are not very well vascularized and are easily inoculated with bacteria. The treatment of choice is incision and drainage, with appropriate antibiotic coverage.

Rabies. Rabies is a very rare complication of animal bite wounds. Over the last 50 years the incidence of rabies has declined in most parts of the world, and in the United States only two cases per year are recorded.[14] In July 1993, a 12-year-old girl was the first rabies fatality in New York since 1954. Rabies insemination is possible in racoon (8645 cases in 1992), bat, skunk (2334 cases in 1995), and fox bites, and is not the norm in unprovoked domestic dog and cat bites. If rabies is suspected, the use of rabies vaccine and immunoglobulin should be delayed until state and local health agencies are consulted as to prevalence in a particular area. There are five clinical phases of rabies:

1. Incubation: nine days to years (average 30 to 70 days). Most patients are asymptomatic during this time period; however, the shorter the incubation time, the greater will be the severity of the illness.
2. Prodrome: two to ten days' duration. Symptoms are nonspecific but include generalized malaise, nausea, and vomiting.
3. Acute neurologic phase, with two classic presentations:
   a. Furious presentation: hyperactivity, disorientation, and periods of excitement are followed by hydrophobia, painful contractions of the pharynx, aspiration, coughing, and choking.
   b. Dumb presentation: paralytic usually near the bite, or entry wound. Occasionally symptoms include Guillain-Barré–type flaccid ascending paralysis.
4. Coma phase: supportive care is needed.
5. Death or recovery: only three recoveries have been documented.

Diagnosis is by rabies antigen and pathologic examination (Negri bodies) of brain tissue. If rabies is suspected, the identified animal should be observed or sacrificed. Aggressive local wound care, including copious irrigation with 1% benzalkonium chloride, and tetanus prophylaxis are essential. Rabies is relatively rare, and prophylaxis with human diploid cell vaccine (HDCV) and human rabies immune globulin (HRIG) should be initiated only under accepted guidelines.

Sylvatic vectors

Many bacteria, viruses, and protozoa utilize lower animals as reservoirs and then transmit their disease states to humans by arthropod vectors, including mosquitoes, ticks, and mites. Most arthropod-borne zoonoses are transmitted out of doors, but direct contact with animal reservoirs is not necessary. Ticks and fleas are the most common vectors; lice are very host specific and are very unlikely vectors. Some of the more frequently transmitted vector diseases include Lyme disease, tularemia, Rocky Mountain spotted fever, and plague (Table 10-3).

TABLE 10-3   Arthropod-borne zoonoses

Vector	Disease
Hard tick	Lyme disease, babesiosis, Rocky Mountain spotted fever, and tularemia
Mite	Rickettsialpox
Flea	Plague, tularemia, and murine typhus
Tse-tse fly	African trypanosomiasis
Sandfly	Leishmaniasis
Reduvid bug	Chagas' disease

Lyme disease. Originally reported in Old Lyme, Connecticut, Lyme disease is now the most commonly reported tick-borne disease in the United States. Frequency increases during the summer months and near river valleys, lake shores, and coastal areas. The causative agent of Lyme borreliosis is *Borrelia burgdorferi,* a spirochete transmitted by a tick vector.[15] There are three clinical phases: erythema chronicum migrans, neurologic and cardiac involvement, and arthralgia.

1. Erythema chronicum migrans (ECM) is an expanding annular erythematous lesion with central clearing, which is characteristic of Lyme disease. ECM usually develops within 1 day to 4 weeks after the tick bite.
2. Neurologic or cardiac involvement develops within the first few weeks after a tick bite. Neurologic manifestations (15%) include generalized weakness or fatigue, but may lead to meningitis, cranial neuritis, and painful radiculopathy. Cardiac manifestations (8%) include pericarditis and atrioventricular blockage.
3. Arthritic-type pain can develop in 60% of the untreated Lyme disease patients within the first few months. The arthritis is usually monarticular, affects large joints (e.g., knee), and is without associated swelling.

Diagnosis is by increased antibody titer to *Borrelia burgdorferi.* The treatment includes local wound care, oral tetracycline or erythromycin for adults, and penicillin for children.

Tularemia. Tularemia, a plague-like disease, was found to be prevalent in the hare, rodent, and squirrel populations near Tulare, California. The disease was first described in Japan, and was known as "wild hare" disease, since it was a generalized systemic infection following the ingestion of wild hares. It is an acute infectious disease caused by the aerobic gram-negative coccobacillus *Francisella tularensis.* The disease is transmitted by vectors such as the tick from wild animals, particularly rabbits, hares, squirrels, moles, muskrats, and beavers.[16]

There are six clinical manifestations of tularemia, which include (1) ulcero-glandular, (2) glandular, (3) oculo-glandular, (4) typhoidal, (5) oral-pharyngeal, and (6) pneumonic diseases. The most common two presentations are:

1. Ulcero-glandular disease: up to 85% of tularemia patients present with small painful pustules, which

later ulcerate and have an associated lymph node involvement.

2. Glandular disease: most of the remaining patients present with enlargement of the lymph nodes without an associated ulcerative lesion.

Diagnosis is by serologic titers of greater than 1:160. Treatment is usually with streptomycin.

Plague. Although relatively rare in modern times in North America, the plague had devastating effects throughout Europe in a series of historic outbreaks, which were responsible for the deaths of millions of people. The plague is an infection of rodents, caused by the gram-negative coccobacillus *Yersinia pestis.* It is transmitted to humans via a flea vector. Clinical presentation is acute and often fatal. Symptoms of bubonic plague include generalized weakness, fever, shaking chills, enlarged regional lymph nodes (buboes) that drain the area of inoculation, and plague pneumonia. Therapy is usually with streptomycin, but does include isolation because of the contagiousness of plague pneumonia.

Rocky Mountain spotted fever. Rocky Mountain spotted fever (RMSF) is an arthropod-borne disease characterized by fever, petechial rash of the palms and soles, vasculitis, and a purpuric rash of the legs secondary to intravascular coagulation. RMSF is an infection caused by the spirochete *rickettsia rickettsii;* it is transmitted via tick vector. Diagnosis is usually clinical but can be confirmed by serologic tests. Treatment consists of various tetracyclines or streptomycin in adults, and chloramphenicol in children.[17]

Scabies. Scabies is an infectious disease caused by the parasitic mite *Sarcoptes scabiei.* The mite penetrates and burrows into the upper layer of skin. The fertilized females lay eggs and feed on the epidermal skin. The affected area is an intense source of irritation. Scratching and rubbing of the area produce vesicular eruptions with intense pruritis, which is often followed by a secondary infection of *S. pyrogenes.* Diagnosis is from microscopic evaluation of pathologic scrapings, which demonstrates the mites. The newly infected, unexcoriated papules are the best sites for finding mites. Treatment includes the use of antipruritics, sulfur compounds, and appropriate antibiotic care.[18]

Spider bites

Arachnid bites are relatively common zoonoses, and as with insect bites, they should be cared for immediately. They can lead to painful irritation, allergic reaction, possible secondary infection, and in rare cases necrotizing lesions. Very few species in the United States can cause necrotizing lesions; these include *Loxosceles reclusa* (brown recluse) and *Latrodectus mactans* (black widow). The necrotic lesions are primarily caused by venoms and are not infectious in nature. As with all necrotic lesions, however, they can serve as a nidus for infection.

The brown recluse, *Loxsceles reclusa,* is a small spider, 8 to 12 mm in size, with a brown violin-shaped marking on its back. It is typically found in the central and southern

states and produces venom. The venomous bite contains at least eight different components, including hyaluronidase, protease, esterase, and an isolated portion with dermonecrotic properties. Spider venom decreases in potency with age, and only intradermal venom can cause destruction.

Necrotic arachnidism. In necrotic cutaneous arachnidism, the spider bite is marked by an immediate area of hyperemia and the development of a papule containing a central zone of ischemic pallor surrounded by an erythematous halo. As the edema subsides, the zone takes on the appearance of a dry, demarcated, and necrotic eschar. The eschar is sterile and its edges separate in 3 weeks, leaving a superficial ulceration.

A more serious, but rare, consequence of spider bites is viscerocutaneous arachnidism. This begins in the same manner as the localized form but leads to systemic involvement. Malaise, restlessness, vertigo, tachycardia, fever, nausea, and vomiting are the presenting symptoms. These can lead to jaundice and hematuria within the first 12 to 24 hours. In small children, convulsions may occur. As the disease progresses, dyspnea, cyanosis, deepening jaundice, hypotension, coma, and death may occur.

Acute manifestations are treated with corticosteroids and antihistamines, as well as prophylactic antibiotics. Some authors have suggested the use of low-molecular weight dextran to decrease the blood viscosity and reduce the harmful effects of cutaneous necrosis. Local surgical debridement is the definitive treatment for end-stage cutaneous necrosis, followed by appropriate skin grafting as needed.[20]

Marine-borne zoonosis

The majority of marine borne zoonosis is from the secondary infection from trauma or puncture wounds allowing pathogen penetration, with a predominance for *Staphylococcus* and *Streptococcus* species. Many organisms have been described, including *Pseudomonas aeruginosa, Erysipelothrix rhusiopathiae* (cellulitis), *Aeromonas hydrophilia* (cellulitis), and a variety of *Vibrio* species (cellulitis with bullae, and necrotizing fascitis).

SKELETAL FRACTURES AND INFECTIONS

Fractures of the foot, with tissue damage, have a tremendous predilection for infection. Those with associated breakage of the integument system have an even higher infection rate. Devitalized and necrotic tissues can act as a nidus for infection, and normal skin flora and externally induced organisms can become opportunistic pathogens.

Osteomyelitis and delayed bone and/or wound healing are the primary concerns of trauma complication management. Improper or inadequate cleansing of the wound, along with insertion of foreign material (plates or screws for stabilization), can again lead to nidus formation. The importance of proper and adequate wound care led Gustilo and Anderson,

TABLE 10-4 Gustilo-Anderson classification of open wound fractures

Type 1: Clean open fracture with wound less than 1 cm long

Type 2: An open fracture with a laceration more than 1 cm long, without extensive soft tissue damage, flaps, or avulsions

Type 3: Either an open segmental fracture, or open fracture with extensive soft tissue damage or traumatic amputation. Special consideration is given to farm machine injuries and gunshot wounds

TABLE 10-5 Gustilo-Mendoza classification

Type 3A: Open fracture with extensive tissue damage

Type 3B: Open fracture with extensive tissue loss, with periosteal stripping and bone exposure

Type 3C: Open fracture with associated arterial injury

TABLE 10-6 Pozo-Powell-Andrews limb injury scoring system

Tissue	Maximum Points
Skin damage or loss requiring a major graft, or myocutaneous flap	2
Bone injury with marked comminution or bone loss	2
Muscle damage requiring excision of muscle or tendons	2
Vascular damage involving the femoral artery, popliteal artery, or both tibial arteries	2
Nerve damage involving the sciatic or posterior tibial nerve	2
Wound contamination	2

in 1976, to develop their criteria for long bone open fracture management (Table 10-4).[21] It highlights the relationship between soft tissue damage, fracture healing, and complications of long bone healing.

In 1984, Gustilo et al created a new classification of severe open fractures[22] (Table 10-5).

Later, Fisher et al theorized that utilizing early flap coverage for type 3B fractures would reduce infection and delayed union rates. The purpose of their work was to determine the rate of major complications after early, late, or no coverage, in patients who had a type 3B open fracture of the tibial shaft.[23] An infection was noted in only 2 of 11 patients who had early muscle flap coverage, compared with 10 of 19 patients who had open wound management without flap coverage, and 9 of 13 who had delayed coverage. Patients who had bone grafting after complete reepithelization of the wound, regardless of closure method, had a lower infection rate, and an earlier "time to union," than those in whom the wound was not completely closed.

In type III (severe) fractures, the muscles contiguous to the wound were the primary source of vascularity, since the intramedullary blood supply and periosteum were disrupted. The muscle flap, or envelope, was critical for the avoidance of infection. Wounds with vascular flaps therefore neutralized a larger amount of bacteria, and at a faster rate, than those with poor or no muscle coverage. Apparently, a change in the biology of the wound, from contamination to colonization, occurred in the first weeks, with corresponding increased infection rates.

THE TIMING OF AMPUTATION FOR LOWER LIMB TRAUMA

Pozo, Powell, and Andrews theorized the need for a more detailed classification, than Gustilo-Anderson, to improve prognosis for salvage and function[24] (Table 10-6). The severity of Gustilo-Mendoza type 3B and type 3C injuries was analyzed using a point system. One point was awarded for moderate damage and two points for severe damage to each of the five tissue elements and for wound contamination. The maximum possible score was 12 points. A score of 10 or more within the first month would indicate the necessity for an amputation.

BURN WOUNDS AND INFECTIONS

Burn wounds are traumatic injuries with potential for infection. The severity and morbidity of an injury depend upon extent, depth, location, causative agent, and general health status of the patient.

Determination of the extent of a burn is based on the total body surface area (TBSA) system of Lund and Browder.[25] They divided the body into eight major components and estimated the percentage of body area for each of these, in adults and infants. This was later modified into the Rule of Nines, for quick reference: head, 9%, adults and 21% infants; thorax and back, 18% each for adults and infants; arms, 9% each in adults and infants; legs, 18% adults and 12% infants; and genitalia, 1% in adults and infants.

The body surface area of the leg, below the knee, is 7% in adults and in 5% infants, while the feet represent 3.5% in adults and children (Fig. 10-1).

The depth of a burn wound is categorized as partial-thickness or full-thickness, or whole-thickness, skin loss. Burn wounds are further divided into four classes:

1. First degree: superficial tissue destruction involving only the epidermis. May be caused by hot fluids or ultraviolet light.
2. Second degree:
   a. Superficial partial-thickness loss of the epidermis and dermis. Classically appears red and moist with blister formation and usually caused by scalding injuries.
   b. Deep, partial-thickness loss involving the entire epidermis and dermis, leaving only the skin appendages intact. The skin appears mottled and

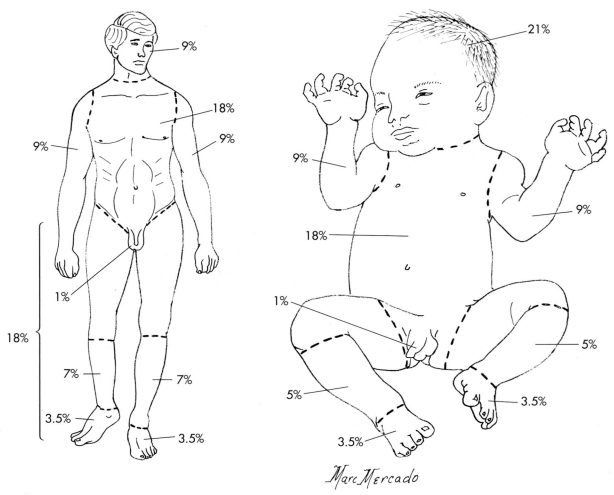

Fig. 10-1 Burn wounds: Rule of Nines for adults and infants.

waxy with a propensity for late hypertrophic scarring.

3. Third degree: Full-thickness burns; involve destruction of the epidermis, dermis, and the underlying subcutaneous structures. They have a dry and leathery appearance and may be painless because of nerve damage. They may be caused by flames, chemicals, or prolonged contact with any heat source. Skin grafts are needed.

4. Fourth degree: destroy fascia, fat, ligament, muscle, and/or bone.

The American Burn Association combines depth, body surface area, and location into its classification of major, moderate, and minor burn wounds.

1. Major burn injury: a second degree burn of greater than 25% BSA or 20% in children; or any third-degree burn of 10% or greater BSA or involving the hand, face, eyes, perineum, or feet

2. Moderate burn injury: a second degree burn of 15% to 25% BSA in adults (10% to 20% in children); or less than a 10% third-degree burn that does not involve the hands, face, eyes, ears, perineum, or feet

3. Minor burn injury: a second-degree burn involving less than 15% BSA (10% in children) or less than a 2% third-degree burn.

Burns to the anterior tibial region are of concern because of the proximity of the tibial crest and associated bony periosteum. If the periosteum is left intact, a skin graft may be attached. If it is damaged, a fat or primary free muscle flap may be needed for coverage. Thermal injuries to the heel cord, anterior ankle, and top of the foot are of concern because of the superficial tendons and neurovascular structures. Helm noted that the incidence of neurologic deficits and associated drop foot was high in patients with lower-extremity burns.[26] Surgical debridement is typically performed on the top of the foot, although the sole is usually left to heal by second intention.

Wound sepsis

Burn wounds will demonstrate little or no bacterial colonization within the first 24 hours, primarily because of the heat sterilization of surface bacteria. Within the next two or three days, there is a surface proliferation of gram-positive organisms, particularly beta-hemolytic streptococci and group A S. pyogenes, along with *S. aureus* and *S. epidermidis.* By the fourth or fifth day, colonizing cells from the integumentary glands invade the wound (*Escherichia* sp., *Klebsiella* sp., *Pseudomonas* sp., *Proteus* sp., *bacteroides* sp., *Tnerobacter* sp., *Providencia* sp., and *Candida* sp.). An alternative source of wound contamination is the external environment. *Pseudomonas* infections are of particular concern. Following initial antibiotic therapy against grampositive organisms, *Pseudomonas* sp., and other gramnegative organisms can act as opportunistic pathogens, with an overall infection rate of about 8%.

All burn wounds should be considered contaminated, especially deep partial-thickness burns or any burn wound with necrotic tissue that can act as a nidus for infection. Necrotic tissue can produce localized immunosuppression whereby a quantity of only 1×10^3 bacteria per gram of tissue can produce an infection. Therefore, wounds should be debrided and prophylactic antibiotics administered, along with topical agents such as silver sulfadiazine, to decrease further bacterial colonization and wound sepsis. Long-term treatment may include skin grafting, skin flaps, or other plastic surgical techniques. Unfortunately, beta-hemolytic streptococci produce the protein fibrinolysin, which inhibits binding and melts away skin grafts.

CONCLUSION

Traumatically induced infections of the foot may ultimately prove more calamitous than the original offense, since they are the consequences of the etiologic event along with the opportunistic pathogens that have a predilection for that event. The potential sequelae of such episodes include soft tissue infections, osteomyelitis, disfigurement, lost function, and even death. Therefore, this chapter has reviewed such traumatic episodes as punctures, zoonotic infections, fractures, and burn wounds. It is hoped that the practitioner will appreciate the catastrophic clinical potential implicit in these injuries.

REFERENCES

1. Chesbro MJ: A complicated nail puncture wound, *J Fam Pract* 27:640-641, 1988.
2. Houston AN, Roy WA, Faust RA: Tetanus prophylaxis in the treatment of puncture wounds on patients in the deep South, *J Trauma* 2:439-450, 1962.
3. Cooke RA: Foreign bodies. In Scurran BL, ed: *Foot and ankle trauma,* New York, 1994, Churchill Livingstone.
4. Marcinko DE, Elleby DH, Read JM: Cysticus cruris giganticus, *J Foot Surg* 25:204, 1986.
5. Joseph JS, LeFrock JL: Infections complicating puncture wounds of the foot, *J Foot Surg* 26:530, 1987.
6. Minnefor AB, Olson MI, Carver PH: *Pseudomonas* osteomyelitis following puncture wounds of the foot, *J Pediatr* 47:598, 1971.
7. Mahan KT, Kalish SR: Complications following puncture wounds of the foot, *J Am Podiatry Assoc* 72:497, 1982.
8. Fisher GW: Acute arterial injuries treated by the U.S. Army Medical Services in Vietnam, *J Trauma* 7:844-855, 1967.
9. Green N, Bruno J: *Pseudomonas* infections of the foot after puncture wounds, *South Med J* 73:146, 1980.
10. Verdile VP, Freed HA, Gerard J: Puncture wounds of the foot, *J Emerg Med* 7:193, 1989.
11. Feder HM, Shanley JD, Barbera JA: Review of 59 patients hospitalized with animal bites, *Pediatr Infect Dis* 6:24, 1987.
12. Ordog GJ: The bacteriology of dog bites on initial presentation, *Ann Emerg Med* 15:1324, 1986.
13. Goldstein EJC: Infectious complications and therapy of dog bites, *J Am Podiatr Med Assoc* 79:10, 1989.
14. Lakhanpal V, Sharma RC: An epidemiological study of 177 cases of human rabies, *Int J Epidemiol* 14:614, 1985.
15. Notari M, Mittler B: Lyme disease: a review and case report with symptoms, *J Am Podiatr Med Assoc* 79:244, 1989.
16. Markowitz LE, Haynes NA, de la Cruz O: Tick borne tularemia, *JAMA* 254:2922, 1985.
17. Walker DH: Spotted fevers. In Hoeprich PD, ed: *Infectious diseases,* New York, 1989, Harper & Row, pp 961-967.
18. Arlian LG: Biology, host relations and epidemiology of *Sarcoptes* scabies, *Ann Rev Entomol* 34:139, 1989.
19. Marcinko DE, Rappaport MJ: Cutaneous necrotic arachnidism: a case report, *J Foot Surg* 76:2, 1986.
20. Andersen PC: Necrotizing spider bites, *Am Fam Physician* 26:198, 1982.
21. Gustilo RB, Anderson JT: Prevention of infection in the treatment of one thousand and twenty-five open fractures of long bones, *J Bone Joint Surg* 58A:453-458, 1976.
22. Gustilo RB, Mendoza RM, Williams DN: Problems in the management of type III (severe) open fractures: a new classification of type III open fractures, *J Trauma* 24:742-746, 1984.
23. Fisher MD, Gustilo RB, Varecka TF: The timing of flap coverage, bone grafting and intramedullary nailing in patients who have a fracture of the tibial shaft with extensive soft tissue injury, *J Bone Joint Surg* 73A:1318-1322, 1991.
24. Pozo JL, Powell B, Andrews BG: The timing of amputation for lower limb trauma, *J Bone Joint Surg* 72B:288-292, 1990.
25. Lund LC, Browder NC: The estimation of areas of burns, *Surg Gynecol Obstet* 79:352, 1944.
26. Helm P: Peripheral neurologic problems in the acute burn patient, New York, 1984, Raven Press.

ADDITIONAL READINGS

Born CT, Tahernia AD: Imaging of calcaneal fractures, 14(2):337-357, 1997.

Fox IM, Collier D: Imaging of injuries to the tarsometatarsal joint complex, *Clin Podiatr Med Surg* 14(2):357-371, 1997.

Giorgini RJ, Bernard RL: Traumatic wound infections. In Abramson C, McCarthy DJ, Rupp MJ, eds: *Infectious diseases of the lower extremity,* Baltimore, 1991, Williams & Wilkins.

Mammone JF: MR imaging of tendon injuries about the foot and ankle, *Clin Podiatr Med Surg* 14(2):313-337, 1997.

Port M, Bartolomei FJ: Integumentary system and related disorders. In Marcinko DE, ed: *Medical and surgical therapeutics of the foot and ankle,* Baltimore, 1992, Williams & Wilkins.

Potter EK: General principles of pathology. In Marcinko DE, ed: *Medical and surgical therapeutics of the foot and ankle,* Baltimore, 1992, Williams & Wilkins.

11

Osteomyelitis of the Foot and Ankle

Alan R. Catanzariti
Nicki Dowdy Nigro
Jason K. Pearson
Kenneth Y. Rosenthal

All fell prostrate at Cloaca's shrine". Molière

Bone and joint infection, with its attendant disastrous disability, can present a difficult situation in the lower extremity. Despite recent advances in antibiotic therapy, wound physiology, radionuclide imaging, magnetic resonance imaging, and surgery, osteomyelitis continues to be a difficult disease to diagnose and treat in the foot and ankle. Surgical procedures involving bone grafting, joint replacement, fixation devices, and reconstructive surgery have contributed to the expanding scope of the disease. New antibiotic treatment regimens are continuously being examined that emphasize early initiation of antibiotic therapy. The broad spectrum of signs and symptoms produced by this disease in the lower extremity is altered by the precipitating etiologic event, organism, and site of involvement, as well as the acute and chronic sequelae that may develop.

DEFINITIONS

Nealton initially used the term "osteomyelitis" to describe an infection of bone and bone marrow.[1] The infecting agent may be bacterial, fungal, viral, or parasitic in origin.[2-4] Osteomyelitis may be defined by the bone involved, by the site of infection within the bone (i.e., metaphyseal, diaphyseal), by the causative organism, or by the histopathologic appearance. Two other terms should be mentioned: "suppurative" or "infectious" osteitis describes suppuration of bone cortex without marrow extension[5]; "infectious" or "suppurative" periostitis describes contamination of the periosteum alone.[6] Osteomyelitis is described as an infection involving the marrow cavity or growth plate, whereas osteitis is described as an infection of bone tissue that does not penetrate the medullary cavity or involve the growth plate.[7] Nonetheless, these terms have been used interchangeably throughout the literature.

Currently, popular classification systems include those of Waldvogel et al,[8] Kelly and colleagues,[9] Cierny and Mader,[10] Peterson,[11] and Buckholz.[7] These classification systems will be described later in this chapter.

Osteomyelitis can be defined on the basis of clinical course (acute, subacute, chronic, and residual) or by the pathogenesis of the lesion (hematogenous osteomyelitis, osteomyelitis secondary to a contiguous focus infection, and osteomyelitis associated with peripheral vascular disease).[8] It can be difficult to distinguish between acute and chronic osteomyelitis on a clinical basis alone. In addition, histologic changes may not be consistent with clinical course. As a result, the various terms and definitions can be ambiguous and confusing.

PATHOPHYSIOLOGY

A complete understanding of the pathophysiology of osteomyelitis is essential for the clinician engaged in the management of the disease process. The establishment and progression of infection within bone are dependent upon the interaction between an infectious agent and a susceptible host.[12] An understanding of this interaction is the key to preventing the establishment and ultimate sequelae of osteomyelitis.

The establishment of an infectious agent within bone occurs through one of two basic mechanisms: either hematogenous spread or spread from an external or contiguous source. Hematogenous osteomyelitis develops as a result of seeding of bacteria through the bloodstream from a distant source. Some common distant sources of hematogenous osteomyelitis include the gastrointestinal (GI) tract, genitourinary (GU) system, cardiovascular (CV) system, and upper respiratory (UR) tract. This form of osteomyelitis is the most common form of acute osteomyelitis; however, it is relatively rare in the foot. A study performed by Waldvogel et al reported 8% of 62 cases showing pedal involvement of hematogenous osteomyelitis.[8] Most cases of hematogenous osteomyelitis occur in children under the age of 16 years, and in adults 50 to 70 years old.[13]

In children, the metaphyseal regions of rapidly growing long bones are usually involved, while adult hematogenous osteomyelitis commonly involves the vertebrae. The anatomy of metaphyseal bone plays an important role in its susceptibility to the establishment of hematogenous osteomyelitis. The nutrient capillaries within metaphyseal bone form sharp loops near the epiphyseal plates and merge into a system of sinusoidal veins. Blood flow in this metaphyseal region of bone becomes considerably slower and more turbulent allowing the seeding of hematogenous bacteria.

Hematogenous osteomyelitis is usually a single-organism infection, with certain organisms common to specific types of patients. By far, *Staphylococcus aureus* is the primary organism causing hematogenous osteomyelitis; therefore, empiric therapy should be directed toward treating a *S. aureus* infection.[14] Group B *Streptococcus* is the predominant organism found in neonatal hematogenous osteomyelitis.[15] Children under the age of 2 years also exhibit *Haemophilus influenzae* as a common pathogen.[16] Intravenous (IV) drug abusers commonly exhibit *Pseudomonas* infections, and patients with sickle cell disease tend toward *Salmonella* osteomyelitis.[17,18] Plasma cell osteomyelitis is a primary chronic form of hematogenous osteomyelitis, with insidious involvement of the metaphyses of long bones. In this infection, granulation tissue is located centrally, with a predominating plasma cell infiltrate. *S. aureus* is the primary pathogen (Fig. 11-1).

The second manner in which infectious agents are introduced into bone is through direct extension from an external or contiguous source. This form of osteomyelitis is the most common type that develops in the lower extremity.[8] Osteomyelitis within the foot is usually a result of contiguous spread from adjoining soft tissue infection in the form of: infected ulcerations, abscesses, sinus tracts, or paronychia. Direct implementation of bacteria also results from traumatic injury, such as puncture wounds, open fractures, crush injuries, infected burns, and postoperative wounds. As a general rule, osteomyelitis that develops from direct extension is often a mixed infection of gram-positive, gram-negative, and anaerobic organisms.[19]

Once bacteria have been established and colonized within bone, whether by a hematogenous route or through direct extension, a distinct pattern of pathogenesis ensues. The earliest destructive changes noted with the progression of osteomyelitis are a destruction of trabeculae and degeneration of bone matrix at the site of infection. This early loss of trabeculae and bone matrix results in a radiolucency on plain film radiographs.[20] As the osteomyelitis progresses, it begins to spread from the original site of colonization. The infection spreads both through the spongy medullary bone and through the haversian systems of cortical bone. In growing bones, the epiphyseal growth plates act as a natural barrier against the spread of infection. The spread of the infectious process of osteomyelitis results in vascular compromise to the involved portion of bone, with a resultant ischemic necrosis of those involved segments of bone.[21]

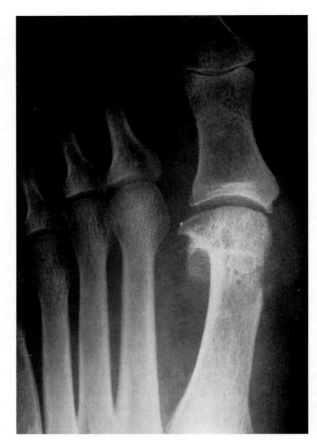

Fig. 11-1 Incipient *Pseudomonas* osteomyelitis of the first metatarsal head, following surgery. Note osteopenic bone with loss of trabeculation and early osteolysis.

Over time, as the infectious process of osteomyelitis progresses, one begins to see the classic signs of chronic osteomyelitis. As the infection within bone expands, segments of devitalized necrotic bone become isolated from viable bone. These isolations of dead bone are called sequestra and are evident on radiographs as dense sclerotic segments of bone.[21] Eventually, the outer cortex of an involved bone will be violated and infection will spread on the outer surface of the cortical bone. This spread of infection can result in septic arthritis if near a joint, or the infection may spread subperiosteally. The elevation of periosteum from its cortical base results in a stimulation of new bone formation from the involved periosteum. This proliferation of new bone formation results in a "walling off" of the site of infection and gives the classic radiographic sign of "involucrum."[22] Eventually, the infective process may violate the involucrum and overlying periosteum with an extrusion of the suppurative material into adjacent soft tissues. This breach in the involucrum is classically known as a cloaca formation.[22] Subsequently, following the formation of a cloaca, abscess and sinus tracts may develop. In some cases, chronic osteomyelitis may result in the formation of a Brodie's abscess. A Brodie's abscess consists of an

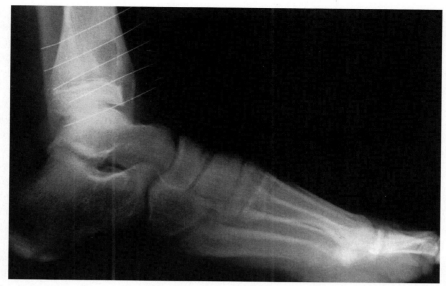

Fig. 11-2 Brodie's abscess: lateral radiograph demonstrating a well-defined lytic lesion with surrounding sclerosis extending to tibial epiphyseal plate. This abscess, secondary to hematogenous osteomyelitis, is mapped for incisional placement utilizing off-horizontal wire.

TABLE 11-1 Waldvogel classification

Acute (initial episode)
  Hematogenous osteomyelitis
  Osteomyelitis secondary to a contiguous focus
  Osteomyelitis associated with vascular insufficiency
Chronic (recurrent)

TABLE 11-2 Kelly classification

Chronic hematogenous osteomyelitis
Osteomyelitis with fracture union
Osteomyelitis with fracture nonunion
Posttraumatic or postoperative osteomyelitis
Vertebral osteomyelitis
Osteomyelitis involving the small bones of the foot
Osteomyelitis involving the skull, facial bones, or phalanges of the foot or hand

TABLE 11-3 Weiland classification

Drainage duration:
  <6 months
  >6 months
Type I: Open exposed bone without evidence of osseous infection, but with evidence of soft tissue infection
Type II: Circumferential, cortical, and endosteal infection with radiographic evidence
Type III: Cortical and endosteal infection with an associated segmental bone defect

area of smoldering infection surrounded by and walled off by dense, sclerotic, sequestered dead bone (Fig. 11-2).

CLASSIFICATION

Several different classification systems have been associated with osteomyelitis. Generally, these have evolved in order to help gain a better understanding of the pathogenicity and, thereby, treatment protocol for this entity (Tables 11-1 through 11-6).

Historically, osteomyelitis has been defined as being either acute or chronic. The distinction between the two was dependent upon the clinical course or the histologic findings.[8] These groupings have fallen short in their ability to accurately and consistently describe the disease process. Clinical presentations of acute and chronic osteomyelitis may frequently have great overlap. Histologic findings have also been found not to correlate accurately with clinical staging. Waldvogel and colleagues found that a more reliable way of clinically classifying osteomyelitis as acute or chronic was to examine the patient's history for a previous admission for the same disease (Table 11-1). The patient population could then be divided into initial episodes and recurrences.[8] They further classified the disease on the basis of pathogenicity.[8,23,24] The patient could be placed into one of three categories: (1) hematogenous osteomyelitis, (2) osteomyelitis secondary to a contiguous focus of infection, and (3) osteomyelitis associated with vascular insufficiency.

TABLE 11-4   Gordon and Chiu classification

Type A: Tibial defect and nonunion without significant segmental loss

Type B: Tibial defect greater than 3 cm long with an intact fibula

Type C: Tibial defect greater than 3 cm long that involves both the tibia and the fibula

TABLE 11-5   Cierny and Mader classification

Anatomic type:
  Type I: Medullary osteomyelitis
  Type II: Superficial osteomyelitis
  Type III: Localized osteomyelitis
  Type IV: Diffuse osteomyelitis
Physiologic class:
  A-Host: Good immune system and delivery
  B-Host: Compromised locally (BL) or systemically (BS)
  C-Host: Requires suppressive or no treatment; treatment is worse than disease itself
Clinical stage:
  Type + Class = Clinical stage

TABLE 11-6   Buckholz classification

Type I: Wound induced
  IA: Open fracture
  IB: Penetrating wounds
  IC: Postsurgical infections
Type II: Mechanogenic infection
  IIA: Joint prosthesis and stable fixation devices
  IIB: Implant instability
Type III: Physeal osteomyelitis
Type IV: Ischemic limb disease
Type V: Combinations of types I to IV
Type VI: Osteitis with septic arthritis
Type VII: Chronic osteitis with osteomyelitis

Hematogenous osteomyelitis

Hematogenous osteomyelitis results from a seeding of bacteria through the bloodstream from a distant site of origination to the bone.[25] This is classically found in children and more commonly seen in males. It is, however, also being seen with increasing frequency in adults over the age of 50.[13,26] The condition is thought to occur most commonly with children because of the microanatomy of the metaphyseal area.

Many theories have been postulated as to the exact mechanism for bacterial deposition in metaphyseal vessels. Trueta suggests the concept of sluggish blood flow occurring in the tortuous sinusoidal arterial loops in the juvenile metaphysis.[27] Some newer studies offer evidence that the metaphyseal blood flow rate may not be as slow as previously believed.[28] Other contributing factors, such as the lack of phagocytic lining cells in the afferent metaphyseal vessels of children and possible hydrophobic interactions between bacterial cells and a passive substrate such as degenerative physeal cartilage, may also play a part in pathogenesis.[29,30] Local trauma has been found to be associated with hematogenous osteomyelitis.[13] However, there is no evidence to suggest that local trauma preceding hematogenous osteomyelitis occurs with any greater frequency than in the general community at risk.

The bones involved in hematogenous osteomyelitis are most commonly the long bones of the lower extremity, in particular the femoral and tibial metaphyses.[8] In adults, hematogenous osteomyelitis often occurs in the vertebrae.[8,25,26] The infecting organism is usually a single pathogen, and the condition is rarely polymicrobic.[8,26] Although the specific infecting bacterium tends to vary with the age group of the patient, *Staphylococcus aureus* accounts for the majority of cases.[8] In addition to *S. aureus,* group B streptococci and *Escherichia coli* are frequently seen with hematogenous osteomyelitis in infants.[31] *Streptococcus pyogenes* and *Haemophilus influenzae* are commonly isolated in children over 1 year of age.[31]

Certain patient populations lend themselves to unusual pathogens presenting in hematogenous osteomyelitis. Patients with sickle cell disease frequently have *Salmonella* species as the infecting organism. *S. aureus, Streptococcus pneumoniae,* and *Haemophilus influenzae* are also common.[32] Intravenous drug addicts are predominantly infected with *S. aureus. Pseudomonas aeruginosa,* other gram-negative bacilli, and yeasts are also common principal isolates.[17] While *S. aureus* is the predominant organism in hematogenous osteomyelitis with hemodialysis patients, *S. epidermidis* and *Mycobacterium tuberculosis* are commonly seen.[33]

Osteomyelitis secondary to a contiguous focus of infection

Osteomyelitis can occur as a result of an extension of an adjacent infected focus from an area outside the body to the bone. Examples would include osteomyelitis that occurred secondary to a long-standing paronychia or secondary to a puncture wound. Waldvogel et al related that 79 of 96 postoperative infections in their study had open reduction of fractures.[23] A large percentage of these occurred after open reduction with internal fixation (ORIF) of hips and femoral and tibial shafts. Norden noted that this particular type of osteomyelitis is commonly seen in patients over the age of 50 years.[26] He further proposed that this probably occurs because patients in this age group may be predisposed to events such as hip fractures.

It is logical to assume that any type of soft tissue infection may progress to an eventual osteomyelitis. This would be more likely to occur in a compromised patient. It could occur

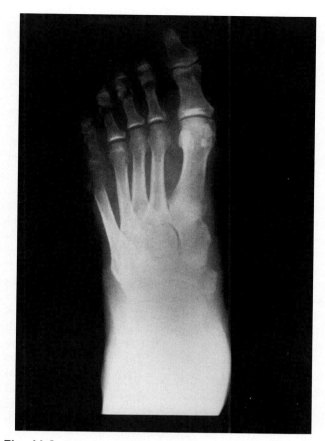

Fig. 11-3 Soft tissue deficit laterally secondary to ulceration leading to direct-extension osteomyelitis. Pathologic fracture at base of the proximal phalanx occurred. There is local osteopenia and loss of cortical bone.

locally or on the systemic level, as in a diabetic patient or a rheumatoid patient on long-standing corticosteroid or immunosuppressant therapy. Postoperatively, the surgical site may be locally impaired in its ability to respond to an impending infection.[25] Anatomic tissue planes, which normally provide a physical barrier to spread of infection, may be disrupted. This, combined with hematoma, foreign bodies (fixation), and disruptions or alterations of blood supply, could transform a local soft tissue infection into an osteomyelitis. Diabetic patients with long-standing neuropathic ulcerations or seemingly minor soft tissue trauma, if left unattended, can progress to deep bone infection. Infections in contiguous-focus osteomyelitis tend to be polymicrobial.[23,31] *S. aureus* is the most common pathogen, but bacteria such as *S. epidermidis, Enterococcus,* gram-negative rods, and anaerobes are all commonly identified[23,31] (Fig. 11-3).

Osteomyelitis associated with vascular insufficiency

Osteomyelitis associated with vascular insufficiency produces a special challenge in regard to its clinical course, prognosis, and treatment.[26] Waldvogel et al chose to include an additional category of osteomyelitis for this group of patients. In their early published literature, almost all of these patients were diabetic. Most of the included patients were between 50 and 70 years of age. It is particularly relevant to note that all of the patients included in their series had infections that involved the bones of the feet.[24] This is not surprising, since vascular insufficiency commonly manifests itself early on in the acral portions of the lower extremity. Trophic changes such as loss of digital hair, onychomycosis, and shiny atrophic skin should clue the physician in to a possible underlying vascular abnormality, even in the presence of palpable pedal pulses.

Kelly and colleagues, in 1975, devised an additional classification (Table 11-2), which elaborated on Waldvogel's original classification. Kelly's classification took into account the anatomic location of osteomyelitis and osteomyelitis with respect to fracture union/nonunion and postoperative sequelae.[9] Kelly later used a limited variation of this classification system to classify 114 patients who underwent treatment for infected nonunions of the tibia and femur.[34]

Other authors have proposed new classifications for use in examining the efficacy of various treatments for osteomyelitis. Weiland and associates, in 1984, examined the use of free tissue transfer in the treatment of osteomyelitis in 33 patients[35] (Table 11-3). The overwhelming majority of the infections occurred in the tibia. The classification was used for two patients who had pedal infections and was composed of two parts. The first part examined the duration and used 6 months as a cutoff point for drainage. Wounds with exposed bone that cultured positive drainage for less than 6 months were not considered to be chronic. A similar wound that had drained for more than 6 months was considered to be chronic. The second part of their classification centered around the severity of the infection, based upon the extent of the tissue involvement. Three types of bone lesions were described. Type I represented exposed bone with evidence of soft tissue infection without bone infection. Type II was characterized by circumferential, cortical, and endosteal infection. Type III represented a cortical and endosteal bone infection that had an associated segmental osseous defect.

Gordon and Chiu, in 1988, devised a classification system (Table 11-4) while examining infected nonunion and segmental defects of the tibia that were treated with muscle transplantation and bone grafting.[36] Patients were categorized into one of three types, which deal with the degree of osseous defect and provide insight into prognosis and treatment. Type A problems represent tibial defects and nonunion without a significant segmental loss. Type B problems are tibial defects that are greater than 3 cm in length with an intact fibula. Type C includes patients with defects greater than 3 cm in length involving both the tibia and fibula.

Cierny and Mader, in 1984, presented what has probably been the most thorough classification with respect to prognosis, treatment, and possibility for a degree of consistency with future clinical studies.[10] This classification encompasses four anatomic types of osseous involvement, which are ordered "according to the complexity of the disease and/or its treatment," and three physiologic classes, which describe the host.[37] These parameters combine to form twelve different clinical stages for adult osteomyelitis. Anatomic type I, or medullary osteomyelitis, refers to osseous necrosis that is limited to medullary contents and endosteal regions. The etiology of this is often hematogenous. Type II, or superficial osteomyelitis, occurs when the pathology is limited to the exposed surface of the bone. This represents a contiguous focus–centered etiology. In both type I and type II, there is a common underlying facet of soft tissue compromise. Type III, or localized osteomyelitis, pertains to bone that contains a full-thickness, well-marginated center of dead cortical bone. Since the area of sequestration is discrete, the affected segment is considered to be stable both before and after surgical debridement. This condition usually is precipitated by trauma but may also occur as a progression from types I and II.[37] Type IV, or diffuse osteomyelitis, is a more extensive, through and through involvement, which encompasses a circumferential portion of bone.[37] This category refers to segments that are inherently unstable before or after debridement. Examples include infected nonunions.

The physiologic classification takes into account the host's condition and the degree of disability produced by the disease.[10,37] The A-host will mount a normal physiologic response to infection or surgical intervention with respect to immune system and metabolism. The B-host will be compromised either locally (BL) or systemically (BS), or combined (BL, BS), in its wound healing capabilities. The C-host is one in which the results of treatment or the treatment itself would be more detrimental to the patient's well-being than the disease itself. This classification takes into account four factors that Cierny et al have found to influence the treatment of adult osteomyelitis. The condition of the host, patient functional disability caused by the disease, the osseous location, and extent of the involvement of necrosis are included so that treatment protocols can be more effectively compared.[37] In 1985, Cierny et al published the results of a study that utilized a treatment protocol based on their classification.[37] They evaluated 425 patients and used specific treatment algorithms to address the earlier mentioned clinical stages. The UTMB (University of Texas Medical Branch) staging system, as it is referred to, was found to be useful in selecting adjunctive therapies and for providing comparison of treatment protocols between different institutions. They concluded that there is a positive correlation between the clinical disease stage and the treatment and prognosis in adult osteomyelitis.[37]

Buckholz, in 1987, proposed an additional classification, with special emphasis on the surgical management of osteomyelitis.[7] This scheme further defined osteomyelitis to include thalamic osteomyelitis and physeal osteomyelitis. Thalamic osteomyelitis refers to an infection involving the medullary cavity in adults and children. Physeal osteomyelitis refers to an infection of the epiphyseal plate, which can occur only in children and adolescents. Osteitis refers to a bone infection that spares the medullary cavity; however, Buckholz included thalamic osteomyelitis within the term "osteitis."[7]

The seven types of bone infection that Buckholz described are based upon pathophysiology. Each type is explained in terms of etiology, along with proposed treatment options. The emphasis of this classification is on surgical intervention. Type I refers to wound-induced infections. This is further broken down into IA, in which osteitis occurs secondary to an open fracture; IB, osteitis following puncture wounds; and IC, which involves postsurgical infections (excluding implant surgery). Type II, or mechanogenic infections, are divided into IIA, which occur with stable implants, and IIB, which occur with instability in implanted devices. The infectious process in both IIA and IIB occurs as a result of a mechanical interference with local vascularity. Type III, or physeal osteomyelitis, refers to osteomyelitis of the growth plate in children. Type IV, or ischemic limb disease, occurs with inadequate circulatory perfusion. Type V represents combinations of types I through IV that occur concomitantly. Type VI consists of coexisting osteitis and septic arthritis. Type VII is chronic osteitis with osteomyelitis. Although this classification is not currently widely recognized, it appears to be a very thorough means of evaluating the pathology, and thus the treatment, of the patient from a pedal standpoint.[7]

PREDISPOSING FACTORS

In order for an infective organism to establish itself in bone, the normal defense mechanisms of the host must be compromised. Several predisposing factors can leave a host susceptible to the establishment of bone infection. Host compromises can be categorized as systemic factors, local factors, and postoperative factors. Systemic factors that can leave an individual susceptible to osteomyelitis include immune deficiency, diabetes mellitus, chronic steroid therapy, malignancy, extremes of age, malnutrition, renal or liver failure, alcohol abuse, and tobacco abuse.[38] Important local factors that can contribute to the establishment of osteomyelitis include arterial compromise, chronic venous stasis, chronic lymphedema, and radiation fibrosis.[38] Finally, some special factors in the postoperative patient allow the individual to become susceptible to the development of osteomyelitis; these factors include focal insult to bone, focal point of ischemia, foreign body or implanted material, hematoma formation, and extensive scarring.[38] It is imperative that the surgeon be conscious of all of these predisposing factors when planning any procedure for a patient who may be compromised and susceptible to the development of osteomyelitis.

INFECTING MICROORGANISMS

Osteomyelitis caused by gram-positive organisms

Gram-positive cocci represent the most common bacteria associated with both hematogenous and direct-extension osteomyelitis. The gram-positive organisms *S. aureus, S. epidermidis,* and *Streptococcus* account for up to 73% of osteomyelitis that develops following musculoskeletal surgery.[39] Because of the high incidence of infection by gram-positive organisms, compared to other infective agents, both surgical prophylaxis and empiric therapy for osteomyelitis are targeted at these organisms.

Osteomyelitis caused by gram-negative organisms

Osteomyelitis secondary to gram-negative organisms presents a particular challenge because of its recalcitrant nature and the fact that the minimum inhibitory concentration (MIC) of antibiotics required to treat gram-negative osteomyelitis is higher than the MIC required for gram-positive osteomyelitis.[40] Some common gram-negative organisms that cause osteomyelitis include *Pseudomonas aeruginosa, Proteus, E. coli, Salmonella,* and *Klebsiella.*[41] Patients who develop gram-negative osteomyelitis usually have underlying diseases such as diabetes mellitus, malignancy, or alcoholism.[42] Gram-negative osteomyelitis rarely develops hematogenously and is more commonly associated with some break in the skin, such as chronic ulceration, open fractures, crush injury, or puncture wounds.[41] Puncture wounds of the foot especially tend toward the development of *Pseudomonas* osteomyelitis.[42,43]

Osteomyelitis caused by anaerobic organisms

Anaerobic organisms are found fairly frequently in osteomyelitis and would probably be recovered more often if not for the fact that they are often missed during standard laboratory isolation techniques. One should suspect anaerobes when a Gram stain from infected bone shows organisms but a clinical specimen fails to grow organisms.[44] As in gram-negative osteomyelitis, the patient population that develops osteomyelitis with anaerobic organisms tends to be older with systemic compromise of normal defense mechanisms.[45] Classically, anaerobic organisms tend to be members of a polymicrobial osteomyelitis along with gram-positive and gram-negative organisms.[46] Some common anaerobic organisms isolated from osteomyelitis include *Bacteroides fragilis* and *Bacteroides melanogenicus.* Some common predisposing factors for the development of anaerobic osteomyelitis include diabetes mellitus, previous fractures, and human bites.[44]

Osteomyelitis caused by fungi

Osteomyelitis secondary to fungi is primarily due to hematogenous spread of a systemic fungal infection. Systemic fungal infections, including blastomycosis, coccidioidomycosis, mycetoma, and sporotrichosis; all have the potential to establish themselves in bone.[44] Though rare, *Candida* osteomyelitis may also develop following candidemia.

Osteomyelitis caused by mycobacteria (tuberculous arthritis)

Skeletal tuberculosis is a fairly common sequela of a systemic tuberculosis infection. The tuberculosis bacillus establishes itself in bone via the hematogenous route or through lymphatic drainage from adjacent infected tissue such as the pleura. Tuberculous osteomyelitis is usually associated with weight-bearing joints and often results in a septic arthritis.[47] The vertebral column is the most common site for tuberculous osteomyelitis (Pott's disease), followed by the large joints of the lower extremity.[44] Osteomyelitis secondary to tuberculosis may also establish itself within the ribs. Though rare, nontuberculosis mycobacterial osteomyelitis may develop secondary to infection by *M. marinum, M. avium-intracellulare, M. fortuitum,* and *M. Gordonae.*[48]

Viral osteomyelitis

The concept of viral osteomyelitis is not a certain one. However, it does seem plausible when osteomyelitis is associated with smallpox, rubella, or cytomegalovirus.

DIAGNOSIS AND CLINICAL FEATURES OF OSTEOMYELITIS

Hematogenous osteomyelitis

The classic presentation of acute hematogenous osteomyelitis in children consists of an abrupt onset of high fever, systemic toxicity, and physical findings of local suppuration about the involved bone.[49] It is not uncommon for these children to guard the affected extremity and to have an antalgic gait. Localization of a coexisting infection at a site remote from the foot or ankle may be achieved through history, physical examination, and appropriate diagnostic studies. Identifying the possible source of infection may suggest a likely pathogen involved. A previous history of trauma to the involved area is reported in 30% to 50% of the cases.[50,51]

In adults, the classic presentation of abrupt onset, high fever, and toxicity is less frequently seen. About one half of the patients may have symptoms of pain, swelling, chills, and fever for less than 3 weeks before admission to a hospital. Other patients may have had symptoms for 1 or 2 months with few constitutional complaints.[52] The major complaint is usually pain in the involved foot or ankle. Drainage is an infrequent occurrence.

The subtle presentation of hematogenous osteomyelitis in the elderly can make diagnosis quite difficult. This is especially true in patients with peripheral vascular disease, in whom the inflammatory response to infection may be impaired. Patients with diabetes mellitus and coexisting peripheral neuropathy and peripheral vascular disease present a special problem. Signs and symptoms may be minimal or absent because of the inability to perceive pain, combined with lower arterial disease.

Hematogenous osteomyelitis can result in bone infection at the site of fixation devices or a joint prosthesis. Typically, an increase in discomfort or local inflammatory findings may occur at the site of a previously asymptomatic implant. In this situation, it becomes difficult to differentiate osteomyelitis from loosening of the implant, implant rejection, or reactive synovitis. Loading pain is frequently consistent with a loosened device. Nonetheless, these clinical presentations can be indistinguishable.[6] .

Osteomyelitis secondary to a contiguous focus of infection

In the initial episodes, fever, edema, and erythema are seen in approximately one half of all cases of osteomyelitis secondary to a contiguous source of infection. Sinus formation and drainage are the two major presenting signs usually seen during recurrences. Patients generally show fewer systemic signs of recurrences than initial episodes. Purulent exudate or drainage should be noted, along with the consistency, color, and any odor. Open fractures, elective surgery, and puncture wounds of the foot and ankle can develop contiguous osteomyelitis.[53]

Osteomyelitis associated with vascular insufficiency

Local symptoms predominate, with very few patients manifesting any type of systemic signs. Patients may have long-standing, chronic, draining ulcers in the lower extremities or may be admitted because of cellulitis manifested by pain, swelling, and redness of the involved area. Fever and septicemia, however, are quite uncommon. Such patients usually have evidence of long-standing diabetes, with neuropathy, nephropathy, and retinopathy. These patients may have absent pedal pulses, atrophic skin changes, delayed subpapillary venous plexus filling time, dependent rubor, and pallor on elevation. Lower arterial noninvasive vascular examination and transcutaneous oxygen determination may be of some value.[54]

Laboratory studies

With osteomyelitis, laboratory studies are primarily used as a monitoring tool to evaluate the efficacy of therapy. Unlike other disease processes in which laboratory studies help to confirm a diagnosis, a diagnosis of osteomyelitis is dependent upon biopsy and culture. Important laboratory studies utilized to monitor the treatment of osteomyelitis include complete blood count (CBC) with differential, erythrocyte sedimentation rate (ESR), C-reactive protein (CRP), and blood cultures. Systemic infection is reflected in a CBC by an increase in the white blood cell count, and a differential count will show a classic shift to the left with an increase in immature white cell types. The ESR and CRP are utilized to monitor inflammatory conditions. Though nonspecific, the ESR and CRP are very sensitive for inflammation. Of the two tests, the CRP is the more sensitive test for inflammation and infection; however, this test takes 24 hours to become positive, and delays with laboratory turnover are often encountered. Blood cultures may also be utilized in the febrile patient with bacteremia in an attempt to isolate the causative agent of an underlying osteomyelitis.[55]

Microbiologic studies

Because a precise identification of the causative agent of osteomyelitis cannot be made by any distinctive clinical or radiographic pattern, it is imperative that the clinician employ proper microbiologic studies to identify the agent. A precise identification of the causative agent is imperative, because patients are subjected to prolonged courses of antibiotic therapy to treat this disease process; such a regimen must have a precise and well-identified target in order to be effective.

Indirect attempts to identify the etiologic agent of an underlying osteomyelitis, such as swab culture of sinus tracts or overlying ulcerations, often have a poor correlation with the true etiologic agent and should, therefore, not be relied upon.[56] Only through direct contact and sampling of bone may a clinician be confident that a true representation of the causative agent has been obtained. Such direct-contact evaluation of suspicious bone includes open culture and biopsy, needle aspiration or biopsy, and bone washing and aspiration with nonbacteriostatic saline. Careful planning of surgical dissection or the needle pathway must be employed to avoid passing through overlying soft tissue inflammation and infection, if possible.[57]

Careful preoperative planning will ensure a true biopsy and prevent seeding of bone with bacteria from overlying soft tissue infection. To ensure a definitive identification of the causative organism of an underlying osteomyelitis, a portion of suspicious bone should be obtained for histologic evaluation and a second portion should be obtained for Gram stains and culture and sensitivity studies for aerobic and anaerobic bacteria, fungi, and mycobacteria.[58] Though not entirely reliable, blood cultures may also be employed in an attempt to identify the causative agent of osteomyelitis. Blood cultures, however, fall way short when compared to the accuracy of direct biopsy of suspicious bone.

Radiographic interpretation

Upon suspicion of soft tissue or osseous infection, conventional radiographs should be obtained (Fig. 11-5). They are easy and inexpensive to obtain. Three views of the involved area are necessary, and comparative views of the contralateral extremity are recommended when open growth plates are present. Although radiographs are the least specific of the advanced imaging modalities available today in the detection

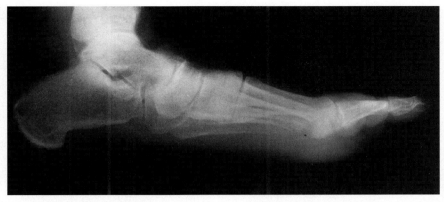

Fig. 11-4 Lateral radiograph showing increased soft tissue density with obliteration of soft tissue planes of forefoot. Also visible is gas within tissues plantar to hallux.

of early osteomyelitis, radiolucency may be visualized within 10 to 14 days after the onset of infection.[59] This is particularly true when baseline or previous radiographs have been obtained. Actual bone loss or osteomyelitis will not be apparent until at least 30% to 60% of bone is resorbed or destroyed.[60] These radiographic changes lag about 2 weeks behind clinical findings.[60] It is the role of the physician to recognize early, subtle changes on the radiograph in the presence of clinically suspected osseous involvement. The following are hallmark signs of infectious involvement of bone:

1. Rarefaction: Rarefaction is generally one of the earliest findings of bone infection and is seen as a localized loss of bone density, producing radiolucency.
2. Osteolysis: Osteolysis is caused by hyperemia and appears as a ground glass–like darkened region (Fig. 11-1). This represents decreased bone density with loss of trabeculations.
3. Sclerosis: Sclerosis produces a radioopacity indicating periosteal changes in the advanced stage of bone repair or the reverse, dead bone.
4. Sequestration: Sequestration is generally indicative of active infection. Impaired or eliminated blood supply to bone will result in necrotic bone. This may fragment, and the density is either normal or increased relative to the surrounding bone.
5. Involucrum: Involucrum is viable new bone laid down around an area of necrosis. This is especially seen in cases of chronic osteomyelitis.
6. Cloaca: A cloaca is an opening along the cortex of bone for discharge of pus or debris. This usually applies to hematogenous infection of bone and is seen as an area of decreased density at the bone-periosteal interface.
7. Sinus: A sinus, synonymous with tract or fistula, forms a passageway for pus from the soft tissues to the bone.
8. Subperiosteal calcification: Calcification occurring between elevated periosteum and bone is termed subperiosteal calcification.

TABLE 11-7 Radiographic characteristics of hematogenous osteomyelitis

Inside soft tissue edema to obliteration of soft tissue planes
Outside regional osteoporosis
Sclerosis
Periosteal elevation and calcification
Sequestrum
Involucrum
Cloaca
Gross structural change

9. Brodie's abscess: This is a bone abscess of localized infection that develops several years after initial trauma. It is a painful lesion, represented by a radiolucency surrounded by a diffuse, ill-defined sclerotic border and typically seen in the metaphyseal area of tubular bones. (See Figs. 11-2 and 11-6.)

Hematogenous osteomyelitis. Hematogenous osteomyelitis is most commonly a disease of children and infants in which bacteria transported through the bloodstream typically affect the metaphyseal or cancellous bone. The disease is relatively uncommon in the foot compared to other sites; 5% to 11% of pediatric patients and 8% of adult patients have involvement of the foot bones.[3] The calcaneus is most frequently involved (51%), followed by the metatarsals (23%), tarsal bones (10%), talus (9%), and phalanges (7%).[61] The ankle may also be involved. Radiographic appearance of hematogenous osteomyelitis may lag weeks behind the clinical picture. Abnormalities appear 3 to 4 weeks after onset of symptoms in 90% of patients.[61] The earliest findings are deep soft tissue edema adjacent to the involved area and obliteration of soft tissue planes. These findings are followed by regional osteoporosis in response to inflammation.[62] Depending on the virulence of the organism, the radiographic findings (Table 11-7) may vary from a purely lytic process to a small area of destruction surrounded by sclerosis [63] (Fig. 11-2). Subperiosteal elevation with or

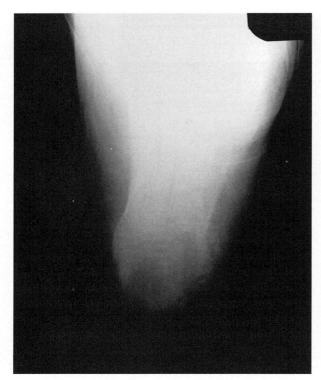

Fig. 11-5 Loss of cortical bone can be appreciated in this calcaneal axial view.

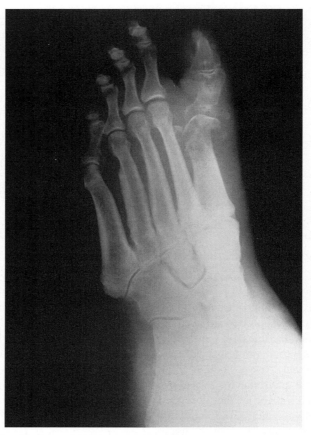

Fig. 11-6 Medial oblique view showing extensive destruction of the first metatarsophalangeal joint. Increased soft tissue density. Rarefaction, osteolysis, loss of cortex, and bony proliferation are noted.

TABLE 11-8	**Radiographic characteristics of direct-extension osteomyelitis**
Uninterrupted infection	Progressive increased soft tissue density
	Loss of definition of soft tissue planes
Outside to inside	Rarefaction
	Periosteal elevation and subperiosteal new bone formation
	Cortical erosion
	Osteolysis and marrow involvement
	Sequestration and sclerosis
	Involucrum

without calcification, sequestrum, cloaca, and involucrum may follow if the infection is allowed to continue.

Direct-extension osteomyelitis. The most common form of osteomyelitis in adults is direct-extension osteomyelitis. Infecting organisms are introduced from the outside and make their way to the inside, affecting the periosteum, cortex, and marrow (Fig. 11-3). The radiographic findings, then, will follow a logical sequence[62] (Table 11-8).

Increased soft tissue density and volume are usually the initial radiographic findings in soft tissue infection. Obliteration of soft tissue planes occurs as a result of the increased soft tissue density and volume[60,62] (Fig. 11-4). Rarefaction, followed by periosteal elevation and new bone formation, is produced by purulent exudate lifting up the periosteal membrane. This is called infectious periostitis.[60] On x-rays,

it will appear as a thin parallel line of increasing density, irregular and limited in area.[64] This is generally solid, but may present as lamellated or interrupted.[60] Infectious osteitis will follow if infection is allowed to progress, and cortical erosions will appear (Fig. 11-5). Osteomyelitis involves both the marrow and the cortex; eventual sequestration, sclerosis, and involucrum are findings suggestive of necrotic bone and marrow death (Fig. 11-6).

Chronic osteomyelitis. Chronic osteomyelitis may evolve from hematogenous seeding, direct inoculation, or contiguous spread. Distinctive findings such as grossly remodeled bone, osteoporosis, and Brodie's abscess are identifiable on radiographs. The hallmark of chronic osteomyelitis is infected dead bone within a compromised soft tissue envelope. This may remain dormant for years.[60,65] The presence of sequestra is highly suggestive of active infection.[60] However, Tumeh and associates found that radiographs detected only 5 of 15 cases of sequestra that were present intraoperatively. The sensitivity of radiographs to predict sequestra formation in this study was 33%, compared to 50% obtained by others.[66]

Chronic osteomyelitis involving a pin tract has an incidence of 0% to 4%.[61] A classic ring sequestrum, a zone

TABLE 11-9 Radiographic findings in less frequently encountered osteomyelitis

Tuberculous Osteomyelitis

Hematogenous

Combination of osteomyelitis and arthritis

Predilection for cancellous epiphyseal areas

Fusiform soft-tissue edema

Osteopenia

Cystic lesion, well demarcated *or* aggressive spread and destruction of diaphysis, sinus formation

"Moth-eaten," "spina-venosa," "tuberculosis dactylitis," "cold abscesses"

Coccidioidomycosis Osteomyelitis

Hematogenous

Multiple bone lesions

Tendency for bony prominence, calcaneus and diaphyseal bones of the foot

Purely lytic

Soft tissue swelling and loss of bone substance

Linear calcifications

Thickening of long bones

Rarely: periosteal new bone and diffuse sclerosis

Congenital Syphilitic Osteomyelitis

Placental transmission

Multiple bones

Wimberger's sign: destruction of the proximal tibial metaphysis

Widening of the epiphyseal plate

Periostitis

Irregular destruction of metaphysis

Expansion of tubular bone, "spina ventosa leutica," "syphilitic dactylitis"

Syphilitic Osteomyelitis

Tertiary stage can extend to bone

Affects marrow of medullary canal

Tibia most commonly affected

Multiple mottled osteolytic lesions

"Saber shin"

Laminated marrow

Subperiosteal calcification and involucrum

Mycetoma (Madura Foot)

Secondary to molds

Traumatic implantation

Dorsum of foot; most common presenting symptom: recurrent drainage

Extensive soft tissue swelling

Multiple lytic lesions

"Hair on end" periostitis, sclerosis, ankylosis

Multiple sinuses

Spotty osteoporosis

Sclerosing Osteomyelitis of Garré

Due to organisms of low virulence

Affects single bone

Shaft of long bones

Fusiform cortical thickening

Sclerotic changes in the spongiosa

Viral Osteomyelitis

Chronic nonsuppurative

Metaphyses of long bones

Osteoporotic changes

Well-defined, transverse zones of bone destruction

Gonococcal Osteomyelitis

Due to gonococcal arthritis

<10% of all cases

Rarefaction

Osteolytic defects

Periosteal reaction leads to hypertrophic changes of bone

---

of radiolucency around the involved pin, and a radiolucent cleft between the bone adjacent to the pin and the surrounding osseous tissue are radiographic findings associated with chronic pin tract infections. These findings are obtained when the x-ray beam is precisely centered on the pin tract parallel to its long axis.[65] Ultimate progression to chronic osteomyelitis is rare, since pin tract infections from surgically implanted K-wires or Steinmann pins is remote (incidence, 0.46%).

Complicating conditions. Osteomyelitis coexisting with fracture, trauma, osteotomy, osteoarthropathy, metabolic disease, frostbite, or trench foot is difficult, at best, to identify by radiographs. The sensitivity and specificity, in the presence of such conditions, fall drastically in the detection of active bone infection. It is for these reasons that advanced imaging modalities, close clinical correlation, and bone biopsy may be employed.

A thorough knowledge of anatomy, physiology, and pathology of bone will enhance the interpretation of the radiographs.[64] Although the role of standard radiographic evaluation and sequential radiographic studies is significant, the diagnosis of osteomyelitis is established by a high index of suspicion, clinical correlation, and bone biopsy.[8,23,24] Reliance on radiographs may delay therapy while the infectious process continues to destroy osseous tissues. However, because radiographs are of low cost and are simple to obtain, they often should be obtained initially in all cases of suspected osteomyelitis. (See Table 11-9.)

Joint sepsis

A septic joint or septic arthritis may most simply be defined as the presence of infection within a joint cavity. The septic joint has also been referred to as pyogenic (suppurative) arthritis or pyarthrosis (pus within a cavity of a joint) (Table 11-10).

The intraarticular infection may be introduced by any route of contamination, including hematogenous spread, direct extension or implantation, or postoperatively. Systemic illness, corticosteroid administration, and trauma are predisposing factors for joint infection.[67] Joint sepsis confined to the foot is uncommon but occurs twice as frequently in children (17%) as in adults (8.5%).[67] Polyarticular involvement is rare.

The clinical presentation involves generalized signs of fever, anorexia, and malaise, along with local signs of pain, erythema, edema, and limitation of joint motion.[67,68] Pain may be out of proportion to the presenting clinical findings and exacerbated with weight bearing. Rest, ice, compression, and elevation incompletely relieve the discomfort.[68]

Acute monarticular arthritis should be assumed to be infection until proven otherwise, and arthrocentesis should be performed immediately. Joint effusions are present in more than 90% of infected joints.[67] The following tests should be performed on the joint fluid: color, clarity, and viscosity,[68] mucin clot test,[69] protein and leukocyte count, glucose level, Gram stain, and aerobic, anaerobic, and fungal cultures.[67,68] In the presence of pyarthrosis, the joint fluid will have an off-white to amber and cloudy appearance with poor viscosity. The mucin clot will be poor. The leukocyte count will be greater than 100,000/mm^3 with 90% polymorphonuclear leukocytes, protein will be elevated, and glucose levels will be lower than 40 mg/dl in joint fluid analysis of pyarthrosis. Microorganisms will appear on the Gram stain in more than one half of the patients, and cultures will present the pathogens[68] (Table 11-11).

A CBC with differential should be obtained, and most commonly a shift "to the left" is noted; however, this varies with disease. Blood cultures are positive in 10% to 60% of adults and 30% of children.[67] Other tests to include are sedimentation rate, C-reactive protein, and liver and kidney profiles.

Radiographs taken early may show soft tissue edema and destruction of the joint capsule. If the disease is allowed to progress, juxtaarticular osteoporosis and decreased joint space caused by rapid loss of cartilage and destruction of articular margins will appear radiographically.[60,69] Gallium soft tissue scans of the joint area usually reveal substantial inflammation, while technetium bone scans document the increased activity of the juxtaarticular bone.[68]

Treatment should be initiated once the diagnosis of joint sepsis is entertained. Oral antibiotics can be started and then adjusted in accordance with the Gram stain and culture. When the diagnosis is established or highly probable, intravenous antibiotics should be considered and chosen on the basis of culture and sensitivity, patient age, and hepatic and renal function. Bacterial joint infections require 2 to 3 weeks of antibiotic therapy unless the infection has spread to the adjacent bone. Adequate drainage is essential. This may be done through daily needle aspirations and flushing irrigation or a closed suction-irrigation and drainage system (Fig. 11-7).

In the presence of persistent fever, continuance of pus from the joint aspirate, or an inaccessible joint, open surgical decompression may be employed. This includes synovec-

TABLE 11-10 Most likely pathogen causing joint sepsis

Patient's Age	Causative Organism(s)
Neonates <1 month	Group B streptococci
	Gram-negative rods
	S. aureus
1 month to 2 years	Haemophilus influenzae
2 years to adulthood	S. aureus
	Group A streptococci
Adults <30 years of age	Neisseria gonorrhoeae
Adults >30 years of age	S. aureus
	Streptococci
	Gram-negative rods
	Streptococcus pneumoniae

TABLE 11-11 Joint fluid examination

Characteristic	Noninflammatory	Noninfectious	Infectious
Color	Colorless/pale yellow	Yellow	Yellow
Turbidity	Clear/slightly turbid	Turbid	Turbid, purulent
Viscosity	Nonreduced	Reduced	Reduced
Mucin clot	Nonfriable	Friable	Friable
Cell count (white cells/mm^3)	200-1000	1000-10,000	10,000-100,000
Cell type	Mononuclear	PMNLs	PMNLs
Glucose (mg/dl)	0.8-1.0	0.5-0.8	<0.5
Gram stain	No organism	No organism	Positive
Culture	Negative	Negative	Positive

From McCarty DJ: *Arthritis and allied conditions,* Philadelphia, 1988, Lea & Febiger.

tomy, exposure of the joint, joint irrigation, removal of necrotic tissue, and excision of any sinus.

Joint sepsis may result in extensive damage and permanent disability. This should be considered a medical emergency and treatment initiated rapidly. Deformities may require surgical intervention, including arthroplasties, fusions, or joint replacement. An infection-free interval of at least 6 months to 1 year should elapse prior to elective surgical joint replacement.[68]

Growth plate involvement

Growth disturbances and epiphyseal arrest may occur as a result of pyogenic disruption of the physeal plate. Infections involving the epiphysis develop by spread of infection from the metaphysis or septic joint, as a sequela of bacteremia (hematogenous), or by external introduction of organisms (open fracture).[70] Closed epiphyseal infection primarily occurs in neonatal and children less than 2 years of age.[71,72] It is more common in males and usually monarticular.[73]

Germinal and proliferating cells, responsible for growth and expansion, are found within the zone of growth between the epiphysis and the metaphysis. These cells receive nutrients from small terminal arterioles that penetrate and cross the epiphyseal bone plate. If infection

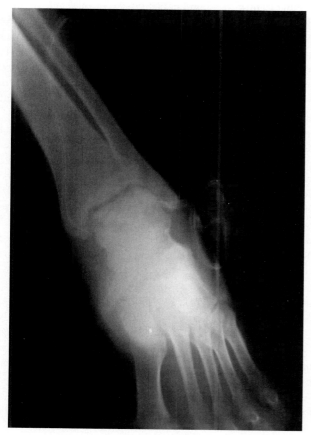

Fig. 11-7 Closed suction-irrigation utilized in joint sepsis of the ankle.

involves these terminal arterioles, rapid destruction of the epiphysis with serious consequences for growth and function will occur.

Between 6 and 20 months of age, depending on the bone, the ossific nucleus forms with its own blood supply. The arterioles now end beneath the epiphyseal bone plate, which leaves it relatively avascular. This now forms a temporary barrier against spread of infection into the epiphysis.[70,71] However, the distal lateral part of the tibial metaphysis is intraarticular and is not safe from infection spreading from a contiguous focus.[70]

Rapid diagnosis and treatment decrease the chances of significant morbidity and permanent disability. The goal is to make the diagnosis within 72 hours of the onset of symptoms.[70] The child is usually febrile, irritable, and apprehensive. The newborn may be afebrile.[74] There will be localized swelling of the affected joint with painful range of motion. The child will hold the affected limb in the most comfortable position (pseudoparalysis).[73,74]

The diagnostic workup includes a complete blood count, erythrocyte sedimentation rate, blood cultures, and radiographs (Table 11-12). Joint aspiration is perhaps the most valuable test. It confirms the inflammatory nature of the pathology, leads to organism identification, and aids in determining the treatment.[70] Bone scanning has been advocated when precise localization is difficult to achieve clinically.[72] Remember, however, if infarction has occurred in the area, the scan may be "cold."[70] Gram stain and culture of the joint aspirate will allow antibiotic therapy to be initiated and then specifically directed to the causative organism. Throat, urine, wound, and urethral cultures may also be indicated.[70] Overall, suspect inflammation, locate the involved area, and seek to identify the organism[70,74] (Table 11-8).

The treatment is aimed at selecting the correct antibiotic(s) for the identified organism(s) and surgically debriding any necrotic bone or destroyed synovial recesses, when indicated. In children under 2 years of age, *H. influenzae* is the predominant causative organism. *Staphylococcus* is the most frequent causative organism in children over 2 years of age. Other common organisms include groups A and B streptococci, gram-negative bacilli, *N. gonorrhoeae, Salmonella, Pseudomonas aeruginosa,* and *Mycobacterium tuberculosis.*[70,71,74] Surgical intervention should be employed if a soft tissue or subperiosteal abscess is identified or an inadequate response to initial therapy has occurred.[72] If after 24 hours from the onset of antibiotics and supportive treatment(s) the local signs have increased, surgical exploration is justified.[72] Surgery should include pneumatic tourniquet of the affected limb, incision and drainage of abscess, debridement of necrotic tissue, closure of skin only, and suction drainage.[72]

Complications of delayed or inadequate treatment include involvement of an adjacent joint, local extension into adjacent soft tissues, fracture, recurrent or chronic infection, aberration of growth, and, in extreme cases, death from overwhelming septicemia.[72,73,75]

TABLE 11-12	Diagnostic workup for possible growth plate involvement

Test	Findings
CBC	Leukocytosis
ESR	Increased
Blood culture	Organism identification
Aspiration of joint with Gram stain and culture	Organism identification
Joint fluid analysis	White cells >50,000/mm^3
Radiographs	Periarticular soft tissue
	Edema
	Distension of joint capsule
	Increased density
Bone scan	Increased blood flow and pool phases
	Reactive bone formation
	"Hot" spot—delayed phase

Implants

Implants play an integral part in foot and ankle surgery. Implantable materials such as internal fixation devices and prosthetic joint replacements raise special challenges when dealing with osteomyelitis. In order to gain a therapeutic foothold on this situation, one must first be familiar with the properties that enable bacteria to overcome the host's defense mechanisms. Most of the specific mechanisms concerning implant infection have only recently been uncovered.[76] The majority of this information stems from investigation into the response of bacteria and tissue to foreign bodies.[76] Complex interactions occur between implants and bacterial and tissue cells.

Integral to bacterial colonization of a substrate is the process of adhesion or adherence.[76] Bacterial adherence has been divided into four phases: (1) transport of bacteria to a substrate by diffusion or convection; (2) initial contact and binding of bacteria to a substrate; (3) attachment to the substrate, which is mediated by special anchoring structures such as fibrils; (4) colonization, which is a product of newly formed cells that aggregate to form a biofilm.[77,78] Under normal circumstances, this bacterial colonization would be overcome by the host's defenses. There are certain instances in which invading organisms can overcome the host's defenses. These conditions are described by Gristina et al: (1) the inoculum size of the bacteria exceeds the threshold levels; (2) impairment of the host's defense; (3) trauma to tissue surfaces (such as occurs in a postoperative setting); (4) the presence of a foreign body; (5) the substrate is acellular or inanimate. When nonliving implants are placed into the recipient host's tissues, they may function as a nidus for bacterial colonization.[79]

The presence of pili and exopolysaccharide production by colonizing bacteria provide a mechanism for bacteria to adhere to their substrate.[80] The formation of a glycocalyx occurs when biofilms consisting of proliferative colonies of bacteria begin production of extracapsular polysaccharide or capsular slime.[78,81] These exopolysaccharide polymers may function to sequester nutrients and enable the resident bacteria to maintain nutrition by acting as an ion-exchange material.[80] Studies have shown that greater levels of antibiotics are needed to maintain MIC and MBC when biofilms are present, as opposed to the situation with free-floating organisms.[82,83] Current literature suggests that resistance to antibiotics increases after bacteria adhere to biomaterials.[84-86] This increased resistance may not be due to a physical barrier, as earlier theories suggested, but to alterations in metabolism and phenotypic expressions.[76,84,86-88] By similar mechanisms, bacteria that adhere to biomaterials will also adhere to the host's tissues. Gristina et al describe a "race for the surface" that occurs when the host's normal tissue cells compete with transient bacteria for a binding or receptor site on the newly implanted material.[76] Ideally, the host's tissues will bind to the implant and produce their exopolysaccharide coat before bacteria can colonize on the implant. There is evidence that a stable tissue-implant interface will resist bacterial colonization.[89,90] Bone provides an optimum substratum for bacterial adherence. It is unusual in that it is mostly or completely acellular, particularly bone that has been traumatized by surgical intervention.[76] Bone that has been compromised by altered blood supply or by bacterial glycocalyx adhesion can function as a foreign body nidus for infection.[86]

Functioning in a similar fashion to an infected implant, compromised or colonized host bone will not be protected by the host's normal resistance mechanisms. The presence of an implant, such as a total joint or an internal fixation device, in contact with surgically traumatized soft tissue and bone can greatly increase susceptibility to infection.[79] There is evidence that bone in proximity to a colonized biomaterial may itself become secondarily infected.[79,91,92]

Implant-associated infection produces a situation that inhibits or impedes the host's underlying combative response. Infections, particularly osteomyelitis, that evolve around an infective biomaterial require removal of the biomaterial for effective treatment.[76] Likewise, osteomyelitis, with possibly the exception of acute hematogenous osteomyelitis, mandates surgical debridement for cure.[76] Joint implants must be removed if an implant-based infection is suspected. It is logical to assume, however, that some postoperative infections in which total joint arthroplasty was performed are not necessarily implant based. Jacobs and Oloff describe an "imminent osteomyelitis" and the simple soft tissue infection that does not necessarily require implant removal.[6] Clinically the distinction between a superficial infection and a deep implant-based infection may be difficult. There is evidence to suggest that most implant-related infections follow a delayed or late pattern.[93] A classification for infection following joint replacement has been described by the Mayo Clinic group.[94] This classification presents three stages, which represent chronologic criteria and offer possible origins for infection.[95] Stage 1 represents infections that occur in the first 3 months after

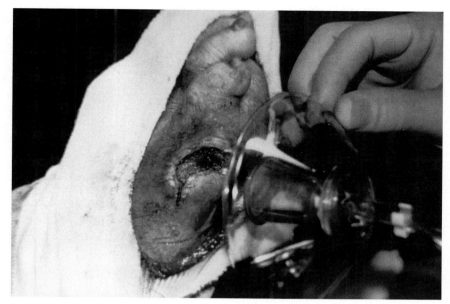

Fig. 11-8 Debridement of fifth metatarsal head followed by jet-pulse high-pressure lavage.

surgery. It may be possible during this phase to discern between a superficial and a deep infection. Stage 2 represents infections that occur between 3 months and 2 years postoperatively. The majority are believed to stem from organisms that become implanted at the time of surgery. Stage 3, or late, infections present after 2 years following surgery. These are often secondary to hematogenous organism seeding.

Internal fixation materials in the presence of osteomyelitis do not necessarily have to be removed. Implants that are loose and nonfunctional in terms of providing stability should be removed. Other means of achieving stability, such as the use of external fixation, can be employed. Internal fixation devices that are functioning to maintain osseous stability with fractures or osteotomies may be tightened following debridement and left in place. Implants that function to provide stability should help maintain or establish vascularity to the affected site.[96]

SURGICAL TREATMENT OF OSTEOMYELITIS

Surgical debridement

Surgery plays a key role in the treatment of osteomyelitis. Surgery is indicated when an abscess forms in a fistulous tract, in the subperiosteal space, or within the bone marrow. The appearance of necrotic bone and sequestra is another undisputed indication for surgery. Rapid decompression of an abscess provides the best protection against extensive bone necrosis.[23] Adequate drainage is essential. Generally, surgery is indicated in acute osteomyelitis when there has been no response after 48 to 72 hours of vigorous antibiotic treatment.[97] Acute osteomyelitis will require incision and drainage if a subperiosteal abscess is present, regardless of

clinical course. Ditch et al recommend immediate needle aspiration whenever acute osteomyelitis is suspected. If subperiosteal pus is not obtained, the needle is inserted into the bone and, if any amount of pus is obtained, the patient is taken to surgery for drainage.[98]

Surgical management of chronic osteomyelitis should include removal of grossly infected and devitalized tissue, obliteration of the dead spaces, skin coverage, and treatment of nonunion if present[99] (Fig. 11-8).

The removal of infected and diseased tissue to the point of good vascular supply is mandatory in the treatment of osteomyelitis. Exercise of judgment is critical because excessive removal of osseous tissue could lead to mechanical compromise or pathologic fracture, and because bone is a rigid structure that cannot collapse, a dead space in which hematoma may collect. The incisional approach for bone biopsy and debridement is planned carefully to accommodate potential future reconstructive alternatives. The surgical approach should be direct and atraumatic, and should minimize the devitalization of the surrounding bone and soft tissues. The debridement should be aggressive and predictable from preoperative evaluation.[100] The surgeon should keep dissection and vigorous retraction to a minimum. An intravenous injection of disulphine blue dye administered 1 hour prior to debridement will stain viable bone. This will decrease the risk of overly aggressive debridement of viable bone at the time of surgery.[101,102] If extensive debridement of bone is necessary and mechanical stability is threatened, external fixation and/or a bypass graft may be required prior to or during surgical debridement.[38] The debridement of not only bone but also soft tissue should be aggressive. Necrotic soft tissue serves to sequester the bacteria, allowing progression of the disease as well as recurrence. Superficial osteomyelitis and medullary (diaphyseal) osteomyelitis may

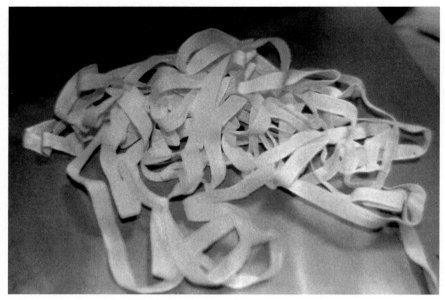

Fig. 11-9 Gauze packing (¼ inch) suitable for open wound packing.

be debrided by decortication or diaphyseal reaming.[103,104] Medullary contents, however, must be exposed. Any type of subperiosteal abscess must be drained. The saucerization or unroofing of medullary contents should be generous. Following debridement, all cortical and cancellous bone remaining in the wound must bleed uniformly. This is known as the "paprika" sign.[105]

The clinical management of the remaining dead space may proceed following debridement (Fig. 11-9). Coverage and filling in of the remaining defect may be achieved by one of the following methods:

1. Packing the wound open and allowing epithelialization from surrounding skin to cover the cavity gradually[106,107] (Figs. 11-8 to 11-11)
2. Delayed application of split-thickness skin grafts following formation of clean granulation within the saucerized cavity[108-111]
3. Insertion of bone grafts to obliterate dead space, followed by immediate skin closure[112,113]
4. Transfer of a pedicle of skeletal muscle into the saucerized cavity and immediate skin closure[99,114,115]
5. Implantation of antibiotic-impregnated polymethyl methacrylate bone cement, followed by primary closure[116-118]
6. Use of closed suction irrigation, followed by primary closure[119-124]

Patients presenting with osteomyelitis and underlying peripheral vascular disease present a special problem. These patients must have preoperative evaluation of their lower arterial status prior to any surgical intervention for osteomyelitis. Local debridement is contraindicated in the presence of lower arterial compromise. If possible, vascular reconstruction should be performed. Once revascularization has been performed, debridement may then take place. If the infected part is beyond vascular reconstruction, then amputation or disarticulation should be given serious consideration. However, even if vascular status seems adequate, but the infection is difficult to control, then amputation is indicated.[125,126]

Postoperative management should include a course of systemic antibiotics for 6 weeks following the last major debridement. Antibiotics augment the host response, protect the grafts, and suppress bacterial proliferation onto the debridement surfaces. Subsequent surgeries on the debrided segment routinely require preoperative antibiotics based on the previous culture and sensitivity studies.[38]

The decision to remove a fixation device necessary for bone stabilization is difficult. Infection after consolidation of an arthrodesis site, osteotomy site, or fracture site is an indication for removal of fixation devices. These patients should be treated with 6 weeks of parenteral antibiotic therapy. If the implant has not provided adequate fixation, it should be immediately removed and stability restored. In this respect, external fixation devices have become increasingly more popular. Infected osteotomy, arthrodesis, or fracture sites can often unite if stable internal fixation is provided. Thus, immediate removal of a stable but infected implant is not mandatory. The primary goal is to achieve union, despite sepsis. If this can be achieved, antibiotic treatment and removal of the fixation devices can follow accordingly.[126]

Wound closure

One of the major dilemmas the foot and ankle surgeon encounters during sequestresectomy and necrectomy is the timing of wound closure.

Secondary wound closure is indicated after operative debridement alone. The wound is usually packed open with gauze and is covered with a dry sterile dressing. The packing

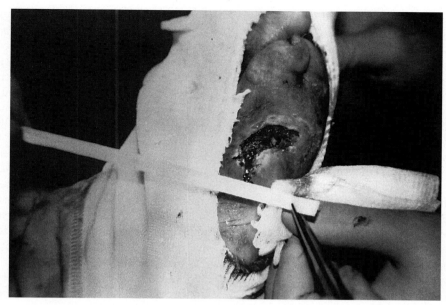

Fig. 11-10 Packing of gauze into remaining void following debridement.

is then removed on a daily basis, and fresh packing and dressing are applied. This process is repeated daily until enough granulation tissue is present to support a skin graft, or the wound may continue to granulate until epithelialization provides complete coverage.[127]

Delayed primary closure is similar to secondary wound closure, with the exception that the wound apposition will take place a number of days following debridement. The wound is usually packed with gauze following debridement. Sutures are placed approximately 1 to 2 cm apart and at least 1 cm away from the incision line. These sutures are left untied. A sterile dressing will follow. The wound is inspected and packing replaced on a daily basis until all signs of inflammation have subsided and the wound borders are vital. The sutures can then be tied and left in until the wound edges are well coated[128,129] (Fig. 11-10).

Immediate primary closure is also an option following osteomyelitis debridement. However, a certain number of criteria must be met, which have been described by Heppenstal.[127] Immediate primary closure is usually advocated in conjunction with closed suction-irrigation,[119,120] implantation of antibiotic-impregnated polymethyl methacrylate beads,[118] or bone grafting,[112] as reviewed below.

Closed suction-irrigation systems

Wound irrigation in the management of osteomyelitis dates back at least to 1917.[130] Closure of wounds with irrigation and drainage utilizing vitallium tubes was first recorded in 1945.[131] In 1956, Mitra and Grace reported 95 cases of chronic osteomyelitis treated by installation of penicillin and a detergent through catheters into the wound for 10 postsurgical days.[132] Goldman and associates, in 1960, and McElvenay, in 1961, discussed a method of closed irrigation and suction, as did Willenegger and Roth in 1962.[133-135]

Compère and his associates, in 1962, recommended the addition of tyloxapol through irrigation fluid.[136] They believed that such an addition would inhibit or prevent formation of penicillinase, allow better perfusion, clean the wound by the action of mucolysis, and contribute a mild bacteriostatic property. In 1969, Dilmaghani et al recommended a closed system that permitted reversal of flow of the irrigation fluid without disconnecting the tubing.[137] They felt that this maneuver would protect against secondary invaders.

Dombrowski and Dunn discussed the treatment of osteomyelitis by debridement and closed wound irrigation-suction. They compared 22 closed irrigation patients with 14 open-packing patients.[120] The results indicated a 43% failure rate in patients receiving open-packing, compared with a 22% failure rate for patients receiving closed suction-irrigation. Anderson and Horn, in 1970, utilized closed suction-irrigation as part of their treatment for acute and chronic osteomyelitis.[138] They reported a 68% success rate. Lawyer and Eyring, in 1972, reported on the details of an intermittent suction-irrigation method and provided follow-up reports on 12 cases.[139] They concluded that intermittent irrigations avoided the serious disadvantages of continuous irrigation (maceration, cost, and tube clogging). Iino and Sakurai introduced a method of infusing isotonic solution containing antibiotics into the site of bone infection.[140]

Closed irrigation-suction is not therapeutic in itself; it is only adjunctive. Radical surgical debridement and necrectomy are the primary forms of treatment in osteomyelitis. However, the presence of a flowing irrigation system in a closed wound controls dead space hematoma and prevents cross-infection.

In the treatment of osteomyelitis, the goals of closed suction-irrigation are to provide wound irrigation and to provide an open egress channel in the form of suction. In ideal conditions, the suction acts to eliminate dead space by allowing granulation tissue to obliterate the cavities. If there is no cavity, soft tissue will quickly close in around the tubes, which can then be removed. The irrigation solution not only delivers high levels of antibiotics to the wound site but also prevents the suction system from clogging.

Continuous instillation and intermittent instillation of topical antibiotic solution have been developed. The intermittent irrigation method seems to be as effective as the continuous while at the same time being simpler, neater, and less expensive.[139]

It would seem that the suction-irrigation technique, especially for difficult or recalcitrant cases, is an improvement over the method of extensive saucerization with an open wound. Closed suction-irrigation is successful because of the high concentration of the local antibiotics and continuous drainage of dead space.

Proper functioning of a closed suction-irrigation system requires the following: (1) airtight and watertight wound closure; this prevents skin maceration and allows hydrostatic pressure in the wound to be varied; (2) placement of irrigation tubes where necessary, including the marrow cavity; this keeps isolated and unprotected hematoma formation to a minimum; (3) keeping multiple perforated portions of the tubes short (3 to 4 inches); the fluid is then in motion as a constant falling hydrostatic pressure along the perforations distally; when tubes are long, clots form distally and migrate proximally, ultimately plugging the system; (4) siliconization of tubes, which decreases the problem of fibrin and clot formation; (5) keeping the flow rate of the irrigation solution high; this not only helps to prevent slugging during the irrigation, but also is also noted to be a mechanism essential to proper function; a continued flow rate of 2 to 3 liters per tube per day is desired; during the first few days of irrigation, a flow rate several times this may be necessary.[120]

Irrigation tubes should be positioned in the wound with their nonperforated ends brought out through normal muscle, subcutaneous tissue, and skin and as far away from the wound as possible. Tubes should never exit through the wound itself. This can be easily accomplished with a tubing-placement trocar. The perforated ends of the irrigation and suction tubes are not allowed to fall into place until the wounds have been irrigated free of clots, a good flow of saline is present from the irrigation tubes, and suction is present in the suction tubes. The wound should be closed with a very tight skin closure. Vasoline-impregnated gauze will further seal the skin wound. The irrigation and suction tubes can be secured and anchored to the skin with sutures. However, with the use of a tubing-placement trocar, this is usually not necessary.

Adequate duration of irrigation is critically important. Reliable criteria for ending irrigation have not been developed. Dombrowski and Dunn have concluded that the criterion of three or four consecutive negative cultures of the egress fluid is not a reliable indication for termination of an irrigation system.[120] Cultures usually become negative after a few days of irrigation. The persistence of positive cultures into the third week is an indication of an inadequate debridement. It is recommended that irrigation be continued for 1 week after three consecutive negative cultures have been obtained. Plain saline should be used in the irrigation solution for 24 to 48 hours prior to collection of specimens. However, clinical improvement should be the primary aid in determining discontinuation of closed suction irrigation. It is important to note that negative Gram stains or cultures from the egress fluid are not an absolute necessity for removal, since positive cultures may result from technical breakdown in the system. Upon completion of irrigation, suction tubes are removed at the same time as the irrigation tubes, to avoid inadvertent suction of contaminants into the wound through the irrigation-tube sinus tracts.[120]

A number of side effects and complications can result from a continuous closed suction system. Superinfection and contamination of the wound by the tubing can occur, resulting in bacteria being colonized to the tubing. Seepage of the continuous irrigation fluid into the wound through sites of tubing entrance and exits is not uncommon, as is wound maceration. Sloughing can be avoided with air-tight systems utilizing silicon-rubber buttons.[141] Problems such as blockage must be recognized immediately. Multiple sets of irrigation tubes can be utilized to avoid this problem.

Antibiotic-impregnated polymethyl methacrylate beads

The mainstay in the treatment of osteomyelitis is still considered to be surgical debridement followed by IV, or a combination of IV and oral, antibiotics.[31,34] There are certain instances, however, when this course of treatment may not be feasible (Figs. 11-11 and 11-12). Complete debridement of necrotic tissues is generally considered to be a necessary step in the treatment of osteomyelitis. This may not be possible when there is extensive involvement of the medullary canal, or with adjacent intraarticular infection. Local antibiotic delivery systems have been devised for use in these situations.[142] These systems are designed to provide high local levels of antibiotics. Many different vehicles have been studied to provide a local release of therapeutic agents, including bioabsorbable materials such as lactic acid oligomer and collagen sponge. Very little, if any, evidence is available to support the efficacy of these vehicles at this time.[143,144]

In 1970, Buckholz and Engelbrecht described the mixing of antibiotic with bone cement, which was used as a luting agent in orthopedic joint replacement surgery.[116] Klemm used gentamicin-impregnated polymethyl methacrylate beads on chains for the local administration of antibiotics as an adjunctive treatment for chronic bone infection.[117,145]

These beads are advantageous in that extremely high local levels of antibiotics may be achieved with very little

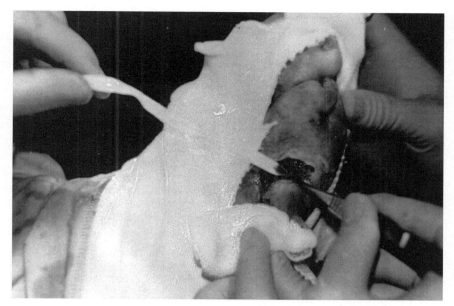

Fig. 11-11 Packing of gauze into remaining void following debridement.

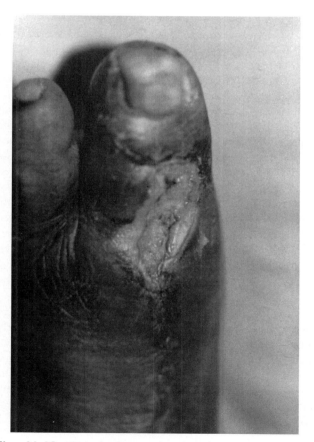

Fig. 11-12 Clinical photograph of patient who underwent revisional first ray surgery, which included plantarflexory wedge osteotomy and hallux interphalangeal joint fusion with AO fixation. This patient presented approximately 2 weeks postoperatively with wound dehiscence and clinical signs of infection.

detectable serum concentration.[146] Although concomitant use of IV antibiosis may still be indicated, depending upon the surgeon's experience, gentamicin beads have been shown to be of use without additional parenteral antibiotics.[147] This may be helpful in the management of osteomyelitis in patients with severely impaired renal or hepatic function. Other advantages include a low incidence of allergic reactions associated with gentamicin, prompt pain relief from surgical decompression and infection control, and the possibility of a cost-effective treatment regimen.[148]

Following surgical debridement of all necrotic or marginally viable tissues, antibiotic-impregnated PMMA beads can be used as an effective adjunct in dead space management. This method can provide a means of sterilizing the cavity until a definitive procedure such as bone grafting can be performed.[37]

Gentamicin has been the most commonly used antibiotic at the present time. The eluted gentamicin has been shown to penetrate 7 mm of dead bone.[146] Antibiotic concentrations ranging from 10 to 100 times those of systemic methods have been achieved in wounds with gentamicin beads.[146]

Stabile and Jacobs suggest that sensitivity and resistance of organisms may need to be redefined with respect to local antibiotic usage.[118] Minimum inhibitory concentrations are defined in terms of parenteral antibiotics. The extremely high local concentrations that can be achieved with methyl methacrylate beads may, in theory, provide effective antibiotic coverage for bacteria that would normally be resistant to regular therapeutic levels of the same drug.[146] The one exception to this is anaerobes, which will still be resistant to gentamicin.

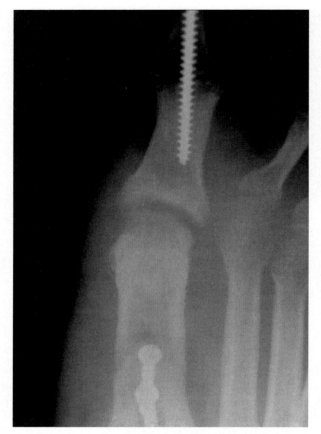

Fig. 11-13 X-ray of same patient at approximately 4 weeks after surgery. A strong suspicion of underlying osseus infection must be raised. Evidence of bone destruction can be seen about the first metatarsophalangeal joint.

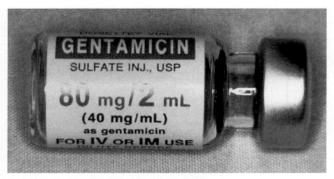

Fig. 11-14 Gentamicin antibiotic added to polymer-monomer polymethyl methacrylate mixture.

Many other antibiotics have been used with PMMA beads. Tomczak, Dowdy, and Storm have shown that ceftazidime-impregnated PMMA beads may be an effective alternative to gentamicin in treating *Pseudomonas aeruginosa* osteomyelitis.[149] One advantage of gentamicin is that it is heat stabile. Other aminoglycosides, penicillins, and cephalosporins are also heat stabile and function effectively in this setting.[150] Tetracycline and chloramphenicol are not effective, because of their lack of heat stability. This has been thought to be important, since an exothermic reaction takes place with hardening of the PMMA. Some authors feel that if the beads are formed during the dough phase, their "surface-to-mass ratio" will allow for low enough core temperatures to maintain antibiotic activity.[151] Recent evidence has shown that clindamycin, vancomycin, and tobramycin possess good elution characteristics from PMMA beads in vitro and in vivo. These also have exhibited high concentrations in bone and granulation tissue.[151] Clindamycin has been found to be the best overall antibiotic used in terms of pharmacologic characteristics.[151] It may be a useful adjunct to gentamicin. In addition to being effective against anaerobes (which gentamicin lacks coverage of), clindamy-

cin is effective against *S. aureus, S. epidermidis,* and many streptococcal species.[152]

The use of antibiotic-impregnated PMMA beads generally requires a thorough surgical debridement. Appropriate cultures, Gram stains, and histologic specimens should be obtained. Implants and any osteosynthesis material not providing osseous stability should be removed. The antibiotic beads on the stainless steel wire should be placed into the wound cavity so that no kinks occur, which would impede removal of the chain. Tight wound coverage is required in order that hematoma or seroma may provide a fluid environment, which is necessary for the antibiotic to elute from the PMMA beads. The tail of the chain can be left extending from the wound to facilitate removal. If a well-apposed incision is not possible, a synthetic skin barrier may be used to prevent fluid leakage.[118] Patients should be kept non-weight-bearing to prevent wound dehiscence secondary to increased tension. Clinical progress of the site should be evaluated periodically. Any evidence of increased or unresolved infection should alert the physician to the possibility of inadequate debridement. Beads are generally removed at 10 to 14 days, although they may be left in place for months to years until a definitive procedure is performed.[118] After approximately 14 days, removal may be difficult because of ingrowth of granulation tissue. Removal can be performed at bedside, under local anesthesia and on a sterile field.

Antibiotic-impregnated beads provide a useful adjunctive therapy in treating osteomyelitis. They provide a particularly useful means of maintaining a sterile dead space environment until a definitive surgical procedure such as bone grafting or reimplantation can be employed. It should be realized, however, that clinical studies have not consistently shown this modality to be more efficacious than conventional methods of treatment[142] (Figs. 11-13 to 11-22).

Bone grafting

Following surgical debridement of infected osseous tissues, the osseous void needs to be addressed. The debridement surgery, which often involves decortication, saucerization, or sequestrectomy, can leave a structurally weakened bone,

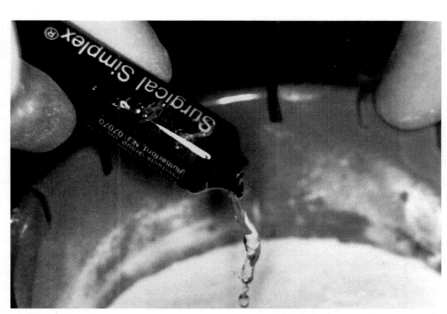

Fig. 11-15 Liquid monomer is added to polymer powder to produce the bone cement.

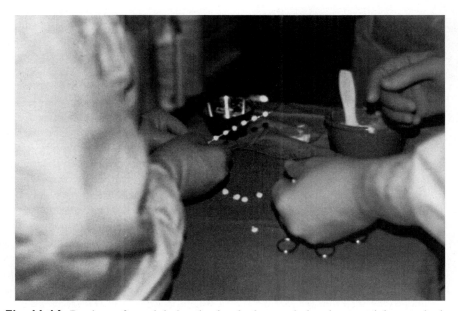

Fig. 11-16 Beads are formed during the dough phase and placed onto stainless steel wire.

which may be subject to pathologic fracture. Cancellous bone grafting can provide an effective method for filling an osseous void and returning stability and function to the affected bone.[153]

Much insight into the use of cancellous bone grafting for treatment of chronically infected bone was gained during World War II. Bone defects with associated osseous infection were frequently encountered following compound fractures or gunshot wounds.[154] Early views on this subject suggested that bone grafting should not be performed while infection was present, regardless of how mild that infection

might be.[155] This treatment was felt to be "surgically unsound."[155]

During approximately the same time period, Coleman and Bateman performed debridement followed by cancellous chip grafting on 52 infected osseous segments. They reported that 48 of these had healed, a 92% success rate.[154] They used autogenous iliac crest graft, which was decorticated and shaved into chips. The recipient site was thoroughly debrided of all infected or necrotic tissue. These bone chips were mixed with penicillin and sulfathiazole powder and placed into the osseous void. In

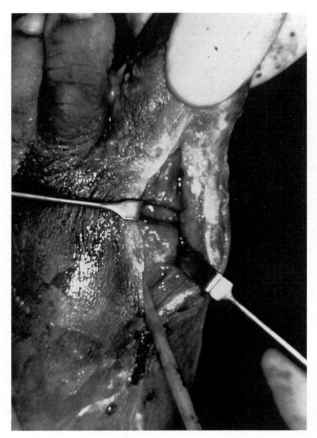

Fig. 11-17 After debriding all necrotic soft tissue, necrotic bone is resected until viable, bleeding bone remains.

these early studies, Coleman and Bateman felt that it was "essential" that all cortical bone be removed, as cortical bone was believed to offer less resistance to infection than cancellous bone.[154]

The use of cancellous bone has been the preferred method of other authors as well.[4] Cancellous bone, because of its increased ability to revascularize when compared to cortical bone, may provide a greater means of combatting any residual infections.[112]

Bone grafting may be considered acceptable today regardless of whether an underlying infection is present.[158] Vascularity of the donor site has been shown to be the major feature in determining the viability of a bone graft.[157] Incorporation can take place in spite of contamination, provided that the graft is revascularized. Cancellous grafts are known to revascularize at significantly shorter intervals following implantation when compared to cortical grafts.[158,159] During the time when the cortical graft is implanted, there will be a significantly longer period of time before it will become vascularized. This cortical implant may function as a foreign body, unable to resist bacterial colonization.[153]

Cancellous bone grafts are implanted beneath local or possibly transferred soft tissues, which provide a local blood supply.[37] Gentamicin-impregnated PMMA beads have also been used for short periods in order to decrease bacterial populations prior to bone grafting.[160] Bone grafting may be performed either in one stage or as part of the initial procedure in a multiple-stage approach.[153] If instability exists prior to grafting, some form of protection to the graft site should be employed until incorporation and remodelling occur. This can be in the form of internal or external fixation, casts, or orthosis.[37]

Autogenous cancellous bone grafting has been shown to be an effective method of filling osseous voids created by debridement of osteomyelitic tissue. It has the benefit of eventually providing stability to restore function to previously unstable bones.

Skin grafts

Utilization of skin grafts is one technique that can be employed for treating defects secondary to radical excision of sequestra and necrectomy for osteomyelitis. In 1922, Reed first suggested the use of skin grafts to cover the defects.[161] Since that time, a number of different authors, including Mowlen, Kelly, and Knight and Wood, have reported success with this technique.[109,113,162-164] Debridement was carried out at one surgical session. A week or more later, when a bed of granulation had developed, a skin graft would be applied to provide coverage.

In 1954, Shannon and Woolhouse published a review of 82 cases of chronic bone infection in which saucerization was combined with immediate split-thickness skin grafting.[165] They reported a 90% success rate. They felt that following traditional treatment for osteomyelitis, dormant pathogens may exist with the potential to exacerbate at a later date. The potential for future abscess formation existed. Poor overlying skin, chronic ulceration, and draining sinuses only complicated the surgical problem further. They excised the unstable skin and scar, damaged and adherent muscle, and all dense, damaged, and sclerotic osseous tissue back to normal bleeding bone. A partial-thickness skin graft was then applied immediately and usually took well where it was apposed to healthy soft tissue and bone. This method ensured that all tissues that would ordinarily support a recurrence of infection were removed along with most of the pathogenic organisms. The saucerization in effect exteriorizes the site of infection so that if recurrence should develop, it would drain early and easily through the split-thickness skin graft.[111]

Flap coverage

Skin coverage is of paramount importance in dealing with osteomyelitis. When the skin has been damaged beyond salvage and extensive debridement is required, skin may need to be brought from another source. The successful treatment of osteomyelitis has recently progressed in conjunction with the ability to achieve coverage of infected wounds. The increased proficiency in using various types of flaps has paved the way for a more radical approach to

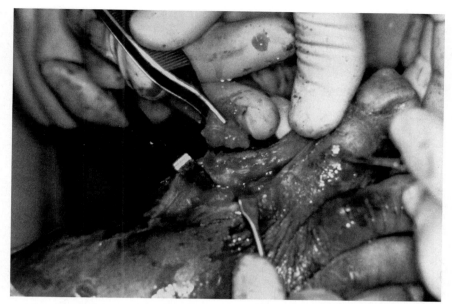

Fig. 11-18 Resected bone is sent for microbiologic and histologic examination.

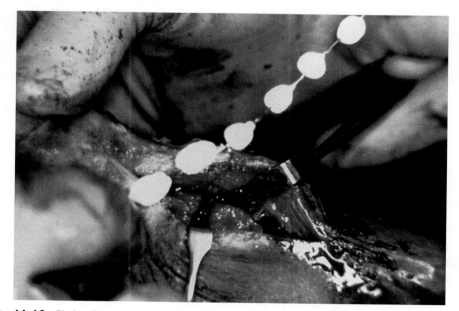

Fig. 11-19 Chain of gentamicin-impregnated PMMA beads is placed into first metatarsophalangeal joint cavity.

wound debridement and for greater success in the treatment of osteomyelitis.

Rotational flaps have very limited use in the lower extremity. As the base of the flap gets longer, the area of coverage gets smaller. Thus, random local flaps have only minimal use in the foot and ankle.[166]

The use of muscle flaps has become very popular in the treatment of osteomyelitis. In 1946, Stark recognized the effectiveness of using muscle flaps in the treatment of osteomyelitis.[167] He found that 80% of the wounds that were treated with muscle flaps remained closed, as compared to 43% of the wounds that were not covered with muscle flaps. Ger reported successful treatment of 17 consecutive patients with lower extremity osteomyelitis using debridement and muscle flap coverage.[168] Subsequently, a number of reports have appeared to support the concept of muscle-flap coverage in the treatment of osteomyelitis, using both local and free tissue transfers. Quite a few muscles are available. The arc of rotation is markedly increased by the narrowness of pedicle. The gastrocnemius and the soleus are two

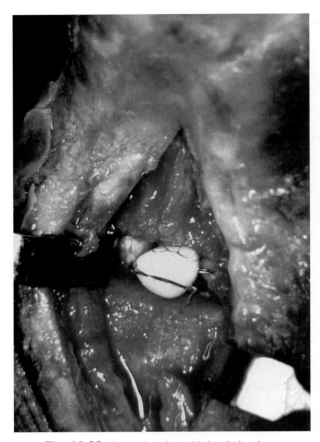

Fig. 11-20 Operative site with beads in place.

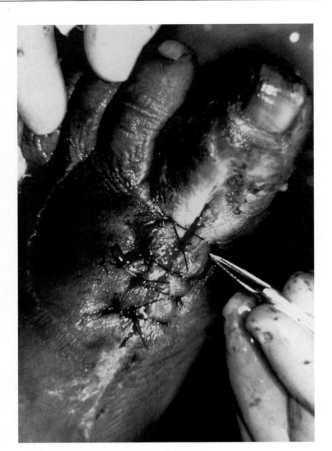

Fig. 11-21 Wound is reapproximated to allow for fluid accumulation, which is necessary for antibiotic elution.

muscles that can be utilized for rotational muscle flaps in the foot and ankle.[169,170]

The most useful and most versatile technique of skin coverage is free tissue transfer using microsvascular anastomosis. These flaps may consist of purely skin, purely muscle, skin and muscle, or skin and bone. In certain situations, composite tissues (toes, fingers, joints, growth plates, and vascularized nerves) can be transferred. Muscle can be transferred purely for the purpose of tissue coverage or, with innervation, for functioning muscle contraction.

For skin coverage, the dorsalis pedis cutaneous flap is an excellent alternative. This flap can be developed on the dorsal aspect of the foot distal to the laciniate ligament overlying the dorsalis pedis artery and first metatarsal artery.[171]

Osteocutaneous flaps can also be used to fill a defect left from extensive debridement. The free fibular graft is very popular. It is easily dissected and is based on the peroneal blood supply. It may be taken with or without skin.[172]

Free muscle flaps are also very useful. The most popular ones are the latissimus, gracilis, and rectus abdominous.[173-175]

Hyperbaric oxygen

The application of oxygen under pressure is often utilized as an adjunct to wound management in the treatment of osteomyelitis. The exact mechanism for the physiologic effects of hyperbaric oxygen (HBO) is not fully understood; however, it is felt that hyperbaric oxygen is most beneficial to patients who have a compromised oxygen delivery system.

It is believed that hyperbaric oxygen has its beneficial effects primarily through enhancement of white blood cell function and through the development of neovascularization. Hyperbaric oxygen helps to enhance the white blood cell functions of chemotaxis, phagocytosis, and oxidative destruction of bacteria, all of which are oxygen dependent.[176] Hyperbaric oxygen also provides the tissue levels of oxygen that are required for fibroblasts to produce the matrix through which neovascularization can develop.[177]

Hyperbaric oxygen may be delivered to a local body part or to the entire patient within a hyperbaric oxygen chamber. Because it is believed that hyperbaric oxygen provides most of its benefits when inspired by the patient, most hyperbaric oxygen treatment involves whole-body exposure and inspiration.[178] Hyperbaric oxygen treatment is usually delivered as intermittent, high-dose, short-term therapy. Typical treatment of osteomyelitis with hyperbaric oxygen consists of two 90-minute treatments a day for 3 weeks.

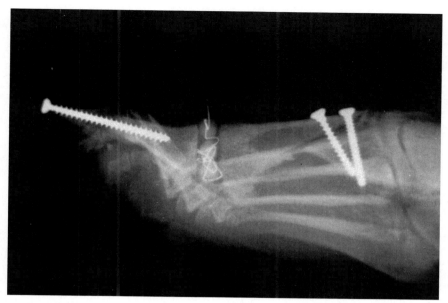

Fig. 11-22 Postoperative x-ray. Note: wire is allowed to extend dorsally from wound to facilitate removal.

CONCLUSION

The knowledge to accurately diagnose and properly treat osteomyelitis is critical to any surgeon performing elective or emergency bone surgery. Isolation of infecting organisms, adequate surgical debridement, and appropriate antibiotic therapy are essential to successful treatment.

REFERENCES

1. Nealton A: *Elements of Pathologie Chirurgicale Paris,* Paris, Baillière, 1844-1859.
2. Edwards EE: Severe candida infections: clinical perspective, immune defense mechanisms and current concepts of therapy, *Ann Intern Med* 8:91-106, 1978.
3. Chimel H, Griego MH, Zicke R: Candidal osteomyelitis: report of a case, *Am J Med Sci* 266:299-304, 1973.
4. Lefrock VL, Annangara DW: Treatment of infectious arthritis, *Clin Pharmacol Ther* 30:252-257, 1984.
5. Juttmann JW, van der Scikke W: The treatment of osteitis complicating tibial fractures, *Br J Accident Surg* 13:210-215, 1980.
6. Jacobs AM, Oloff LM: Osteomyelitis. In McGlamry ED, ed: *Comprehensive textbook of foot surgery,* Baltimore, 1987, Williams & Wilkins, pp 1041-1065.
7. Buckholz JM: The surgical management of osteomyelitis: with special reference to a surgical classification, *J Foot Surg* 26:517-524, 1987.
8. Waldvogel FA, Medoff G, Swart MN: Osteomyelitis: a review of clinical features, therapeutic considerations and unusual aspects, *N Engl J Med* 282:198-206, 1970.
9. Kelly PJ, Wilkowske CJ, Washington JA: Chronic osteomyelitis in the adult. In Adams JP, ed: *Current practice in orthopedic surgery,* St Louis, 1975, Mosby, pp 120-132.
10. Cierny G, Mader JT: Adult chronic osteomyelitis, *Orthopedics* 7:1557-1564, 1984.
11. Peterson HA: Musculoskeletal infections in children, *AAOS Instructional Course Lecture* 33:33-37, 1984.
12. Lemont H, Levy L: Osteomyelitis and the natural history of disease: a model for approaching podiatric disorders, *J Am Podiatry Assoc* 72:27-30, 1982.
13. Weinstein AJ: Osteomyelitis: microbiological and therapeutic consideration, *Prim Care* 8:557, 1981.
14. Axler DA, Terleckyi B, Abramson C: The microbiologic aspects of osteomyelitis, *J Am Podiatry Assoc* 67:691-701, 1977.
15. Aronoff SC, Scoles PV: Treatment of childhood skeletal infections, *Pediatr Clin North Am* 3:271-280, 1983.
16. Stone RA, Uhlman RA, Zeichner AM: Acute hematogenous osteomyelitis: a case report, *J Am Podiatry Assoc* 72:31-34, 1982.
17. Holzman RS, Bishko F: Osteomyelitis in heroin addicts, *Ann Intern Med* 75:693-696, 1971.
18. Adeyokuhnu A, Hendricks RG: *Salmonella* osteomyelitis in childhood: a report of 63 cases seen in Nigeria of whom 57 had sickle cell anemia, *Arch Dis Child* 55:175-184, 1980.
19. Brand RA, Black H: *Pseudomonas* osteomyelitis following puncture wounds in children, *J Bone Joint Surg* 56A:1637-1642, 1974.
20. Downey MS: Osteomyelitis in the diabetic foot. In McGlamry ED, ed: *Reconstructive surgery of the foot and leg—update '89,* Tucker, Ga, 1989, Podiatry Institute Publishing Co., pp 202-213.
21. Hill HG, Pitkow HS, Davis RH: The pathophysiology of osteomyelitis, *J Am Podiatry Assoc* 67:687-690, 1977.
22. Kehr LE, Zulli LP, McCarthy DJ: Radiographic factors in osteomyelitis, *J Am Podiatry Assoc* 67:716-732, 1977.
23. Waldvogel FA, Medoff G, Swartz MN: Osteomyelitis: a review of clinical features, therapeutic considerations and unusual aspects, *N Engl J Med* 282:260-266, 1970.
24. Waldvogel FA, Medoff G, Swartz MN: Osteomyelitis: a review of clinical features, therapeutic considerations and unusual aspects, *N Engl J Med* 282:316-322, 1970.
25. Downey MS: Osteomyelitis in the foot and ankle. In Abramson C, McCarthy DJ, Rupp M, eds: *Infectious disease of the lower extremity,* Baltimore, 1991, Williams & Wilkins.
26. Norden CW: Osteomyelitis. In Mandell GL, Douglas RG, Bennett JE, eds: *Principles and practice of infectious disease,* New York, 1979, Churchill Livingstone, pp 946-956.
27. Truet J: Studies in the development and decay of the human frame, Philadelphia, 1988, WB Saunders.
28. Light TR, McKinsey MR, Schnitze J: Bone blood flow: regional variation with skeletal maturation. In Arlet J, Ficat RP, Hugeford DS, eds: *Bone circulation,* Baltimore, 1984, Williams & Wilkins.
29. Hart UL: Acute hematogenous osteomyelitis in children, *JAMA* 41:671-680, 1937.

30. Gristina AG, Oga M, Webb LX: Adherent bacterial colonization in the pathogenesis of osteomyelitis, *Science* 228:990-993, 1985.

31. Mader JT, Calhoun JH: Long bone osteomyelitis: an overview, *J Am Podiatr Med Assoc* 78(10):476-481, 1989.

32. Giuner LB, Luddy RE, Schwartz AD: Etiology of osteomyelitis in patients with major sickle hemoglobinopathy, *J Pediatr* 99:411-413, 1981.

33. Leonard A, Comty CM, Shapiro FL: Osteomyelitis in hemodialysis patients, *Am Intern Med* 78:651-658, 1973.

34. Kelly PJ: Infected nonunion of the femur and tibia, *Orthop Clin North Am* 15(3):481-490, 1984.

35. Weiland AJ, Moore JR, Daniel RK: The efficacy of free tissue transfer in the treatment of osteomyelitis, *J Bone Joint Surg* 66A:181-193, 1984.

36. Gordon L, Chiu EJ: Treatment of infected non-union and segmental defects of the tibia with staged microvascular muscle transplantation and bone grafting, *J Bone Joint Surg* 70A:377-386, 1988.

37. Cierny G, Mader JT, Pennick JJ: A clinical staging system for adult osteomyelitis, *Contemp Orthop* 10:17-37, 1984.

38. Cierny G, Mader JT: Adult chronic osteomyelitis: an overview. In D'Ambrosia RD, Marion RL, eds: *Orthopaedic infections,* Thorofare, NJ, 1989, Slack, pp 31-47.

39. Ericson C, Lindgren L, Lindberg L: Cloxacillin in the prophylaxis of post-operative infections of the hip, *J Bone Joint Surg* 55A:808-813, 1973.

40. Lesse A, Freer C, Salata R: Oral ciprofloxacin therapy for gram negative bacillary osteomyelitis, *Am J Med* 82(suppl 4A):247-255, 1987.

41. Meyers B, Berson B, Gilbert M: Clinical patterns of osteomyelitis due to gram negative bacteria, *Arch Intern Med* 131:228-233, 1973.

42. Collins BS, Karlin JM, Silvani SH, Scurran BL: *Pseudomonas* pyarthrosis and osteomyelitis from a puncture wound of the foot, *J Am Podiatry Assoc* 75:316-320, 1985.

43. Green WE, Bruno J: *Pseudomonas* infections of the foot after puncture wounds, *South Med J* 73:146-149, 1985.

44. Norden CW: Osteomyelitis. In Mandell GL, ed: *Principal patterns of infectious diseases,* New York, 1989, Churchill Livingstone, pp 922-930.

45. Hall BB, Fitzgerald RH, Rosenblatt JE: Anaerobic osteomyelitis, *J Bone Joint Surg* 65A:30-35, 1983.

46. Raff MI, Melo JC: Anaerobic osteomyelitis, *Medicine* 57:83-103, 1978.

47. Davidson P, Horowitz I: Skeletal tuberculosis, *Am J Med* 48:77-79, 1970.

48. Marchevsky A, Damsker B, Green S: The clinicopathological spectrum of non-tuberculosis mycobacterial osteoarticular infection, *J Bone Joint Surg* 67A:925-929, 1985.

49. Kahn DS, Pritzker KH: The pathophysiology of bone infection, *Clin Orthop* 96:12-19, 1973.

50. White M, Dennison WM: Acute hematogenous osteitis in children, *J Bone Joint Surg* 34B:608, 1952.

51. Selt EB: Acute hematogenous osteomyelitis, *Pediatrics* 1:617, 1948.

52. Harris NH: Some problems in the diagnosis and treatment of acute osteomyelitis, *J Bone Joint Surg* 42B:535, 1960.

53. Riegler H, Routson G: Complications of deep puncture wounds of the foot, *J Trauma* 19:18, 1979.

54. Pinzur MS, Sage R, Stuck R, Ketner L, Osterman H: Transcutaneous oxygen as a predictor of wound healing in amputations of the foot and ankle, *Foot Ankle* 13:271, 1992.

55. Gillespie WJ, Nade S: Diagnostic and laboratory evaluation (the investigation of musculoskeletal infection). In Gillespie WJ, Nade S, eds: *Musculoskeletal infections,* Boston, 1987, Blackwell Scientific Publications, pp 141-166.

56. Braun TI, Lorber B: Chronic osteomyelitis. In Schlossberg D, ed: *Orthopaedic infection,* New York, 1988, Springer-Verlag, pp 9-20.

57. Caprioli R, Testa J, Courhoyer RW, Esposito FJ: Prompt diagnosis of suspected osteomyelitis by utilizing percutaneous bone culture, *J Foot Surg* 25:263-269, 1986.

58. Joseph WS: Osteomyelitis: antibiotic use and surgery. In Jay RM, ed: *Current therapy in podiatric surgery,* Philadelphia, 1989, BC Decker, pp 43-45.

59. Abramson C, McCarthy DT, Rupp MJ: *Infectious diseases of the lower extremity,* Baltimore, 1991, Williams & Wilkins, p 220.

60. Christman RA: The radiographic presentation of osteomyelitis in the foot, *Clin Podiatr Med Surg* 7:(3): 433, 1990.

61. Jahss MH: *Disorders of the foot and ankle,* Philadelphia, 1991, WB Saunders, pp 138-142.

62. Weissman SD: *Radiology of the foot,* Baltimore, 1989, Williams & Wilkins, pp 233-259.

63. Forrester DM, Kricum ME, Kerr R: *Imaging of the foot and ankle,* Rockville, Md, 1988, Aspen Publications, pp 164-171.

64. Kehr LE, Zulli ZP, McCarthy DJ: Radiographic factors in osteomyelitis, *J Am Podiatry Assoc* 67:10, 1977.

65. D'Ambrosia RD, Marion RL, eds: *Orthopaedic infections,* Thorofare, NJ, 1989, Slack, pp 72-73.

66. Tumeh SS, Aliabadi P, Seltzer SE: Chronic osteomyelitis: the relative roles of scintigrams, plain radiographs, and transmission computer tomography, *Clin Nucl Med* 13:1, 1988.

67. Jahss MH: *Disorders of the foot and ankle,* Philadelphia, 1991, WB Saunders, pp 1837-1840.

68. Marcinko DE, ed: *Medical and surgical therapeutics of the foot and ankle,* Baltimore, 1992, Williams & Wilkins, pp 720-722.

69. Forrester DM, Kricun ME, Kerr R: *Imaging of the foot and ankle,* Rockville, Md, 1988, Aspen Publications, pp 162-167.

70. Morrissey RT: Bone and joint sepsis in children, *AAOS Instructional Course Lectures,* 2:49-61, 1984.

71. Jahss MH, ed: *Disorders of the foot and ankle,* Philadelphia, 1991, WB Saunders, pp 2000-2001, 2516-2517.

72. D'Ambrosia RD, Marion RL, eds: *Orthopaedic infections,* Thorofare, NJ, 1989, Slack, pp 1-16.

73. Jackson MA, Nelson JD: Etiology and medical management of acute suppurative bone and joint infections in pediatric patients, *J Pediatr Orthop* 2:313-323, 1982.

74. Tachdjian MO, ed: *Pediatric orthopaedics,* Philadelphia, 1972, WB Saunders, pp 352-370.

75. Nade S: Acute hematogenous osteomyelitis in infancy and childhood, *J Bone Joint Surg* 65B:109, 1983.

76. Gristina AG, Naylor PT, Myovik QN: Mechanism of musculoskeletal infection, *Orthop Clin North Am* 22:3, 1991.

77. Marshall KC: Mechanisms of bacterial adhesion of solid water interfaces. In Souage DC, Fletcher M, eds: *Bacterial adhesion: mechanisms and physiological significance,* New York, 1985, Plenum Press, pp 133-161.

78. Schurman DJ, Smith RL: Bacterial biofilm and infected biomaterials, prosthesis, and artificial organs. In AAOS Symposium: Musculoskeletal Infection, p. 133-147, 1992.

79. Gristina AG, Costerton JW, Webb LX: Microbial adhesion, biofilms, and the pathophysiology of osteomyelitis. In D'Ambrosia RD, Marion RL, eds: *Orthopedic infections,* Thorofare, NJ, 1989, Slack.

80. Costerton JC, Geesey GF, Cheng KJ: How bacteria stick, *Sci Am* 238:86-95, 1978.

81. Costerton JW, Irvin RT, Cheng KJ: The bacterial glycocalyx in nature and disease, *Annu Rev Microbiol* 42:1093-1102, 1981.

82. Gristina AG, Habgood CD, Barth E: Biomaterial specificity, molecular mechanisms, and clinical relevance of *S. epidermides* and *S. aureus* infections in surgery. In Pulverer G, Quie PG, Peters G, eds: *Pathogenicity and clinical significance of coagulase-negative staphylococci,* Stuttgart, 1987, Gustav Fishe Verlag, pp 143-157.

83. Marrie TJ, Costerton JW: Mode of growth of bacterial pathogens in chronic polymicrobial human osteomyelitis, *J Clin Microbiol* 22: 924-933, 1985.

84. Girstina AG, Jennings RA, Naylor PT: Comparative in vitro antibiotic resistance of surface colonizing coagulase-negative staphylococci, *Antimicrob Agents Chemother* 33:813-816, 1989.

85. Naylor P, Jennings R, Myruik Q: Antibiotic sensitivity of biomaterial adherent *Staphylococcus epidermidis, Orthop Trans* 12:524-525, 1988.

86. Nichols WW, Evans JJ, Slack MPE: The penetration of antibiotics into aggregates of mucoid and non-mucoid *Pseudomonas aeruginosa, J Gen Microbiol,* 135:1291-1301, 1989.

87. Christensen GD, Buddour CM, Simpson A: Phenotypic variation of *Staphylococcus epidermidis* slime production in vitro and in vivo, *Infect Immun* 55:2870-2877, 1987.

88. Gilbert P, Brown MRW, Costerton JW: Inocula for antimicrobial sensitivity testing: a critical review, *J Antimicrob Chemother* 20:147-154, 1987.

89. Gristina AG, Rovere GD, Shoji H: An in vitro study of bacterial response to inert and reactive metals and to methylmethacryate, *J Biomed Mater Res* 10:273-281, 1976.

90. Gristina AG, Rovere GD: An in vitro study of the effects of metals used in internal fixation as bacterial growth and dissemination (abstract), *J Bone Joint Surg* 45A:1104, 1963.

91. Gristina AG, Costerton JW: Bacterial adherence and the glycocalyx and their role in musculoskeletal infection, *Orthop Clin North Am* 15:517-535, 1984.

92. Gristina AG, Costerton JW: Bacterial adherence to biomaterials and tissue: the significance of its role in clinical sepsis, *J Bone Joint Surg* 67A:264-273, 1985.

93. Ahlberg A, Carlsson AS, Lindberg L: Hematogenous infection in total joint replacement, *Clin Orthop* 137:68-75, 1978.

94. Coventry MB: Treatment of infections occurring in total hip surgery, *Orthop Clin North Am* 6:991, 1975.

95. Gillespie WJ: Infection in total joint replacement, *Infect Dis Clin North Am* 4(3):465-484, 1990.

96. Müller MS, Allgower M, Snider R, Willenegger H: Manual of internal fixation, New York, 1991, Springer Verlag.

97. Winter FE: The surgical treatment of pyogenic osteomyelitis, *Clin Orthop* 51:139-149, 1967.

98. Ditch V, Nelson J, Haltalin K: Osteomyelitis in infants and children, *Am J Dis Child* 129:1273-1278, 1975.

99. Rowling DE: The positive approach to chronic osteomyelitis, *J Bone Joint Surg* 41:681-688, 1959.

100. Cierny G, Mader J: The surgical treatment of adult osteomyelitis. In Evarts CM, ed: *Surgery of the musculoskeletal system,* New York, 1983, Churchill Livingstone.

101. Jenny G, Kempf I, Jaeger JH: The use of sulphane blue dye during surgical procedures for bone infection, *Rev Chir Orthop* 63:531-537, 1977.

102. Klemm K: Die Vitalfarbung mit Disulphine Blue ihn der Unfalchirurgie, *Schriftenr Unfallmed Tag Hauptverb Generbl Berufsgenoss* 11:177, 1970.

103. Ger R: Muscle transposition for the treatment of osteomyelitis. Instructional course lecture 204, 49th Annual Meeting of the American Academy of Orthopedic Surgeons, New Orleans, 1982.

104. Lindgren L, Torholm C: Intramedullary reaming in chronic diaphyseal osteomyelitis, *Clin Orthop* 151:215, 1980.

105. Sachs BL, Shaffer JW: Osteomyelitis of the tibia and femur: a critical evaluation of the effectiveness of the Papineau technique in a prospective study. Paper 214, 50th Annual Meeting of the American Academy of Orthopedic Surgeons, Anaheim, Calif, 1983.

106. Brodie BC: Lecture on abscess of the tibia, *Cond Med Gazette* 36:1399-1403, 1845.

107. Orr HW: The treatment of acute osteomyelitis by drainage and rest, *J Bone Joint Surg* 9:733-737, 1927.

108. Gupta RC: Treatment of chronic osteomyelitis by radical excision of bone and secondary skin grafting, *J Bone Joint Surg* 55A:371-374, 1973.

109. Kelly RP: Skin grafting in the treatment of osteomyelitic war wounds, *J Bone Joint Surg* 28:681-691, 1946.

110. Reid MR: Use of large Reverdin grafts in healing of chronic osteomyelitis, *Bull Johns Hopkins Hosp* 33:386-388, 1922.

111. Shannon JG, Woolhouse FM, Eisinger PJ: The treatment of chronic osteomyelitis by saucerization and immediate skin grafting, *Clin Orthop* 96:98-107, 1973.

112. Bicker WH, Bateman JG, Johnson WE: Treatment of chronic hematogenous osteomyelitis by means of saucerization and bone grafting, *Surg Gynecol Obstet* 96:265-274, 1953.

113. Knight MA, Wood GO: Surgical obliteration of bone cavities following traumatic osteomyelitis, *J Bone Joint Surg* 27:547-556, 1945.

114. Prigge EK: The treatment of chronic osteomyelitis by the use of muscle transplant or iliac graft, *J Bone Joint Surg* 28:576-593, 1969.

115. Starr CL: Acute hematogenous osteomyelitis, *Arch Surg* 4:567-587, 1922.

116. Buchholz HW, Engelbrecht H: Uber die Depotwirkung einiger Antibiotica bei Vermischung mit dem Kunsthartz Palacos, *Chirurg* 41:511-515, 1970.

117. Klemm K: Septopal: a new way of local antibiotic therapy. In *Local antibiotic treatment in osteomyelitis and soft tissue infections,* International Congress Series 556, Amsterdam, 1981, Excerpta Medica, pp 24-37.

118. Stabile DE, Jacobs AM: Local antibiotic treatment of soft tissue and bone infections of the foot, *J Am Podiatr Med Assoc* 80:345-353, 1990.

119. Clawson DK, Davis FJ, Hansen ST: Treatment of chronic osteomyelitis with emphasis on closed suction-irrigation technic, *Clin Orthop* 96:88-97, 1973.

120. Dombroski ET, Dunn AW: Treatment of osteomyelitis by debridement and closed wound irrigation-suction, *Clin Orthop* 43:215-231, 1965.

121. Michelinakis E: Treatment of chronic osteomyelitis with the continuous irrigation-suction method, *Acta Orthop Scand* 43:25-31, 1972.

122. Pressman M: Continuous closed suction irrigation following postoperative infection of Silastic implant, *J Am Podiatr Med Assoc* 67:746-750, 1977.

123. Jacoby RP: Closed sterile suction system, *J Am Podiatr Med Assoc* 68:834-835, 1978.

124. Schwartz NH, Marcinko DE: Suction irrigation: construction and use of a dependable closed system, *J Am Podiatr Med Assoc* 74:216-221, 1984.

125. Key AJ: Amputation for chronic osteomyelitis, *J Bone Joint Surg* 26:350-362, 1944.

126. Wardvogel FA: Treatment of osteomyelitis and septic arthritis, *Bull NY Acad Med* 58:733-749, 1982.

127. Heppenstall RB: Fracture treatment and healing, Philadelphia, 1980, WB Saunders, pp 918-920.

128. Hudspeth AS: Elimination of surgical wound infection by delayed primary wound closure, *South Med J* 66:934-938, 1973.

129. Biggs E, Ferrito JD: Delayed primary wound closure in wound healing, *J Am Podiatry Assoc* 67:56-58, 1967.

130. Dumas J, Carrel A: *Pratique de irrigation des plaies,* Paris, 1917, Maloine.

131. Smith-Petersen MN, Larsen CB, Cochran W: Local chemotherapy with primary closure of septic wounds by means of drainage and irrigation cannulae, *J Bone Joint Surg* 27:562-571, 1945.

132. Mitra RN, Grace EJ: Further studies on the treatment of chronic osteomyelitis with topical detergent antibiotic therapy, *Antibiot Ann* 4:455, 1956.

133. Goldman MA, Johnson RK, Grossberg NM: A new approach to chronic osteomyelitis, *Am J Orthop* 2:63-65, 1960.

134. McElvenny RT: The use of closed circulation and suction in the treatment of chronically infected, acutely infected and potentially infected wounds, *Am J Orthop* 3:86-87, 154-159, 1961.

135. Willenegger H, Roth W: Die antibakterielle Spüldrainage chirugischer Enfektionen, *Dtsch Med Wochenschr* 87:1485-1492, 1962.

136. Compère EL: Treatment of osteomyelitis and infected wounds by closed suction with a detergent-antibiotic solution, *Acta Orthop Scand* 32:324-333, 1962.

137. Dilmaghani A, Close JR, Rhinelander D: Drains for infections, *Acta Orthop Scand* 32:335-341, 1962.

138. Anderson LD, Horn LG: Irrigation suction technique in the treatment of acute hematogenous osteomyelitis, chronic osteomyelitis, and acute and chronic joint infections, *South Med J* 63:745-754, 1970.

139. Lawyer RB, Eyring MD: Intermittent closed suction-irrigation treatment of osteomyelitis, *Clin Orthop Rel Res* 88:80-85, 1972.

140. Iino S, Sakurai M: Intramedullary dripping and fusion with antibiotic solution for the treatment of suppurative osteomyelitis, *Orthop Surg* 20:136-141, 1979.

141. Kawashima M, Tamura H, Takao K: Closed suction irrigation. In D'Ambrosia RD, Marion RL, eds: *Orthopaedic infections,* Thorofare, NJ, 1989, Slack, pp 87-115.

142. Anthony JP, Masther SS: Update on chronic osteomyelitis, *Clin Plast Surg* 18(3):515-523, 1991.

143. Wei G, Yoshihiko K: A bioabsorbable delivery system for antibiotic treatment of osteomyelitis, *J Bone Joint Surg* 73B:246-252, 1991.

144. Sorensen ST, Sorensen AI, Merser S: Rapid release of gentamicin from collagen sponge, *Acta Orthop Scand* 61(4):353-356, 1990.

145. Klemm K: Treatment of chronic bone infections with gentamicin PMMA chains and beads, *Accid Surg* 1:20, 1976.

146. Harle A, Ritzerfeld W: The release of gentamicin into the wound secretions from polymethyl methacrylate beads, *Arch Orthop Trauma Surg* 95:65, 1978.

147. Vecsei V, Barquet A: Treatment of chronic osteomyelitis by necrectomy and gentamicin-PMMA beads, *Clin Orthop* 159:201-207, 1981.

148. Marcinko DE: Gentamicin-impregnated PMMA beads: an introduction and review, *J Foot Surg* 24:116-120, 1985.

149. Tomczak RL, Dowdy N, Storm T: Use of ceftazadine impregnated polymethyl methacrylate beads in the treatment of *Pseudomonas* osteomyelitis, *J Foot Surg* 28:542-546, 1989.

150. Calhoun JH, Mader JT: Antibiotic beads in the management of surgical infections, *Am J Surg* 157:443, 1989.

151. Adams K, Couch L, Eterny G: In vitro and in vivo evaluation of antibiotic diffusion from antibiotic impregnated polymethyl methacrylate beads, *Clin Orthop Rel Res* 278:244-252, 1992.

152. LeFrock JL, Molavi A, Prince RA: Clindamycin, *Med Clin North Am* 66:103, 1982.

153. Isaac MR, Kanat IO: Bone grafting in the management of osteomyelitis, *J Foot Surg* 25:404-406, 1986.

154. Coleman HM, Bateman JS: Cancellous bone grafts for infected bone defects: a single stage procedure, *Surg Gynecol Obstet* 83:392-398, 1946.

155. Dickson FD: Influence of infection, past or present, on the selection of cases, AAOS Lecture on Reconstruction, 1964.

156. Johnson JW, Van der Slikke W: The treatment of osteitis complicating tibial fractures, *Br J Accid Surg* 13:210-215, 1982.

157. Meyer S, Weiland AJ, Willenegger H: The treatment of infected non-union of fractures of long bones, *J Bone Joint Surg* 57A:836, 1975.

158. Smith T: Bone grafting physiology, *J Am Podiatry Assoc* 73:70, 1983.

159. Burchardt H: The biology of bone graft repair, *Clin Orthop* 174:28, 1983.

160. Hedström S, Lindgren L, Torholm C: Antibiotic containing bone cement beads in the treatment of deep muscle and skeletal infections, *Acta Orthop Scand* 51:863, 1983.

161. Reid MR: The use of large Reverdin's grafts in the healing of chronic osteomyelitis, *Bull Johns Hopkins Univ* 33:386, 1922.

162. Mowlem R: Bone and cartilage transplants: their use and behavior, *Br J Surg* 29:182, 1941.

163. Reynolds FC, Zaepfel F: Management of chronic osteomyelitis secondary to compound fractures, *J Bone Joint Surg* 30A:331, 1948.

164. Robertson IM, Barron JN: A method of treatment of chronic infective osteitis, *J Bone Joint Surg* 28:19, 1946.

165. Shannon JG, Woolhouse FM: Treatment of chronic bone infection, *J Bone Joint Surg* 36A:841, 1954.

166. McGregor IA, Jackson IT: The groin flap, *Br J Plast Surg* 25:3-16, 1972.

167. Stark WJ: The use of pedicled muscle flaps in the surgical treatment of chronic osteomyelitis resulting from compound fractures, *J Bone Joint Surg* 28:343, 1946.

168. Ger R: Muscle transposition for treatment and prevention of chronic post-traumatic osteomyelitis of the tibia, *J Bone Joint Surg* 59A:784, 1977.

169. Arnold P, Mixter R: Making the most of the gastrocnemius muscle, *Plast Reconstr Surg* 72:38, 1983.

170. Hallock G: Function preservation with the soleus muscle flap, *Orthop Rev* 14:41, 1985.

171. McGraw JB, Furlow LT: Dorsalis pedis arterialized flap: a clinical study, *Plast Reconstr Surg* 53:177-185, 1975.

172. Minami A, Masamiichi U, Toshihiko O, Manami M: Simultaneous reconstruction of bone and skin defects by free fibular graft with skin flap, *Microsurgery* 7:35-38, 1986.

173. Wood M, Cooney W, Irons G: Skeletal reconstruction by vascularized bone transfer: indications and results, *Mayo Clin Proc* 60:729-734, 1985.

174. Mathes SJ, Nahai F: *Clinical atlas of muscle and musculocutaneous flaps,* St Louis, 1979, Mosby.

175. McCraw JB, Peniix JO, Baker JW: Repair of major defects of the chest wall and spine with latissimus dorsi myocutaneous flap, *Flap Reconstr Surg* 62:1197, 1978.

176. Madur JT, Brown GL, Guckian JC, Wells CH, Reinarz SA: A mechanism for the amelioration by hyperbaric oxygen of experimental staphylococcal osteomyelitis in rabbits, *J Infect Dis* 142:1915-1922, 1980.

177. Strauss MR: Chronic refractory osteomyelitis: review and role of hyperbaric oxygen, *Hyperbaric Oxygen Rev* 231:250, 1980.

178. Strauss MB: Hyperbaric oxygen in the management of orthopaedic infections. In D'Ambrosia RD, Marion RL, eds: *Orthopaedic infections,* Thorofare, NJ, 1989, Slack, pp 117-131.

ADDITIONAL READINGS

Heard GS, Oloff LM, Wolfe DA, Little MD, Prins DD: PMMA beads versus parenteral treatment of *Staphylococcus aureus* osteomyelitis, *J Am Podiatr Med Assoc,* pp 153-164, 1997.

Kosinski MA, Smith LC: Osteoarticular tuberculosis, *Clin Podiatr Med Surg* 13:245, 1996.

Mader JT, Ortiz M, Calhoun JH: Update on the diagnosis and management of osteomyelitis, *Clin Podiatr Med Surg* 13:701-724, 1996.

Naftulin KA, Stone PA, McGarry JJ: Bilateral total calcanectomy for the treatment of chronic refractory osteomyelitis, *J Am Podiatr Med Assoc* 87:141-143, 1997.

Rogoff RS, Tinkle JD, Bartis DG: Unusual presentation of calcaneal osteomyelitis twenty-five years after inoculation, *J Am Podiatr Med Assoc* 87:125-130, 1997.

12

Major Anaerobic Infections of the Foot

David Edward Marcinko
Hope Rachel Hetico

To carry pure death in an earring, a casket, a signet, a fan-mount, a filigree basket.   Musée de Cluny

Clinical anaerobic infections of the foot are uncommon, and the fact that they are rare is indeed fortunate, since true anaerobic pathology is frequently misdiagnosed with devastating sequelae. Historically, anaerobic pedal infections have not been discussed as extensively in the literature as their counterparts in the brain, mouth, breast, pelvis, ear, liver, lungs, and intestinal tract. This may be due to the numerous confusing colloquial terms often ascribed to them. Terms such as "hospital gangrene," "gas gangrene," "acute hemolytic streptococcal gangrene," "anaerobic cellulitis," "necrotizing fasciitis," "vascular gangrene," "myofascial necrosis," "liquefaction necrosis," and the "fetid foot" are not entirely incorrect but do serve to obfuscate the correct medical definition of each specific entity.[1-5] More basically, even the term "anaerobe" may be a source of confusion. By convention, an anaerobic organism is any microbe that requires reduced oxygen tension for growth and cannot grow on a solid cultural medium, in an environment of 10% CO_2, in air (18% oxygen). Since the tolerance of anaerobic bacteria for oxygen and oxidation-reduction potentials may vary greatly, there is tremendous latitude in this definition, as many types of bacterial infections of the human body can involve anaerobes, given the proper clinical environment. For example, some anaerobes, such as *Clostridium septicum* and *Eubacterium,* are "fastidious" or "absolute"; others, such as *Escherichia coli,* are "facultative," growing in either the absence or the presence of air; others are "microaerophilic," such as *Actinomyces naeslundii* and *propionica;* and still others, such as *C. perfringens* (also known as *Bacillus aerogenes capsulatus* and *Bacillus perfringens*), are more tolerant of oxygen and possess a higher oxidation-reduction potential. Adding to bewilderment are certain other gram-positive cocci which prefer reduced oxygen tension but can still grow on solid media and which are termed "capnophilic."[6] Thus, operative definitions are an important source of clarification when the concept of anaerobic infections of the foot is discussed.

Even the taxonomy of many anaerobes is changing. For example, some *Corynebacterium* species are now classified as *Propionibacterium,* and some bacteria that have been implicated in actinomycosis (*Actinomyces propionica* and *Bifidobacterium eriksonii*) are no longer classified as *Actinomyces.* The designation *Bacteroides fragilis,* or "Frank's bacillus," even includes other species, such as *B. vulgatus, thetaiotaomicron, distasonis, ovatus,* and *uniformis.*[7,8] Therefore, the purpose of this chapter is to provide a clinical overview of anaerobic foot infections. Topics discussed will include clinical recognition, bacteriology, isolation and identification techniques, soft tissue and bone infections, specific pathologic entities, surgery, chemotherapeutic agents, and adjunctive treatment. Hopefully, armed with this information, the clinical practitioner will be imbued with an intensified awareness of this often catastrophic clinical entity.

PATHOLOGY AND PATHOPHYSIOLOGY OF CLINICAL ANAEROBIC INFECTIONS

Except for exogenously acquired infections, such as clostridia from soil, earth, or dirt, the majority of anaerobic infections are caused by organisms or toxins located within the human body and normally considered endogenous. Anaerobes are usually more plentiful than other microorganisms and outnumber aerobes 10:1 in the oral cavity and 1000:1 in the intestinal tract.[9] The skin and integumentary system house *Propionibacterium* (anaerobic diphtheroids) and anaerobic gram-positive cocci. The mouth, teeth, gums, lungs, and upper respiratory system are sources of *Bacteroides melaninogenicus* and *Fusobacterium* species. The vagina is populated with *Lactobacillus,* while the perianal and perineal skin may be populated with intestinal flora. Clostridia are found on most mucous membranes, in the ear canal and perianal skin, in the urethral meatus of both sexes, and on the skin as a transient organism. Still, all of these anaerobic organisms are beneficial in the human microbial ecosystem.[6] For example, essential physiologic roles of these organisms include intestinal vitamin K synthesis by *B. fragilis* and *E. coli,* various essential deconjugated-dedehydroxylating bile acid transformations, and fat-absorption and cholesterol-reducing metabolic processes by the enterohepatic circulation.[9] It is only when these invaders become pathologic that clinical symptoms ensue.

One major bodily defense mechanism is the normal oxidation-reduction (redox) potential (E_h) of +120 mV. A lower E_h permits anaerobic proliferation as a result of decreased vascularity, and the diminished tissue oxygenation it contributes, depending on the well-known oxygen dissociation curve.[9]

Fortunately, only a few hereditary or congenital defects exist that predispose a person to anaerobic infections, and these do not greatly affect the foot. Acatalasia, however, is a rare genetic defect, characterized by the absence of the enzyme catalase, that results in recurrent infections of the gums, mouth, and associated oral structures and may potentially seed into the lower extremities, in certain patients.[6]

Clinical scenario of infection

The clinical scenario for a patient with a pathologic anaerobic infection of the foot is both immediate and severe. It is for this reason that delayed diagnosis or misdiagnosis is not uncommon. However, the historical inquisition and inevitable subjective and objective reactions are reliable characteristics for the perspicacious practitioner.

For example, even seemingly trivial incidents, such as stepping on a nail, sustaining a small laceration, puncture, or scratch, legal or illegal drug injections, insect bites, frostbite, shock, minor foot surgery with or without epinephrine (low redox [E_h] potential), foreign body implantation, or contusion acquisition, may be important historical findings when coupled with expressions of tormenting pain, anxiety, or feelings of apprehension or impending doom.[10] Neighborhood locales or recreational areas contiguous to dairy, ranch, or farm land or other areas of fecal contamination may also be potential sites for anaerobic contamination, as well as decaying vegetable matter.[11] Even more perplexing is the fact that the time from initial contamination to clinical presentation varies from 2 to 30 days, depending on the quantity of inoculum, the virulence of the contaminating anaerobic agent(s), and the health status of the patient.[12]

Preliminary physical examination frequently demonstrates a hot, red, and swollen foot. Chills (although the actual fever may be low grade), shakes, hypotension, and the disorientation associated with the systemic signs and symptoms of any infectious process may be seen. Pain out of proportion to the eliciting event is seen in the gravely ill and spiking febrile patient. The patient may appear emotional, anxious, apprehensive, or frantic, and speak of an ill-defined feeling of death or "gloom and doom."

Patients of any race, sex, or age may be affected, including infants and the elderly. Patients with peripheral vascular disease, regardless of etiology, diabetes mellitus, obesity, herpes, lues, alcoholism, fractures, rheumatic conditions, malignancy, corticosteroid dependency, AIDS, or other disorders causing immunoincompetence may be especially affected.[13-15]

Integumentary changes are obvious and include smooth, shiny, and taunt skin. Cellulitis, myositis or myonecrosis, and gangrenous and infarcted tissue, with or without induration, may be present. Vesicles or blisters may appear, and edema is of the nonpitting variety and extends beyond the portal of entry. A bronze, azure, indigo, or dark or dusky purple ecchymotic color may be seen at the site of the injury, progressing to frank infarction and gangrene after several days. Finally, decreased cutaneous sensation or anesthesia may provide pain relief to the patient, but signals a more serious impending soft tissue slough to the astute clinician. This sloughing phenomenon is a reliable clinical stigma of the infectious process, especially in necrotizing fasciitis, and is reminiscent of a high-speed vehicular extremity degloving injury that leaves nothing but exposed skeletal bone, without the accompanying particulate foreign body implantation or fracture(s).

Other clues to the presence of clinical anaerobic foot infections may include a foul, putrid, or rotten-smelling (hydrogen sulfide) discharge; necrotic, infarcted, and gangrenous tissue with a "pseudomembrane"; black discoloration of blood containing exudates; "sulfa granule" discharges possibly indicative of actinomycosis; crepitant gas (carbon dioxide) in tissues, or discharges or on radiographs, MRIs, or CT scans; infections following animal, insect, human, or other bites; and infections related to the use of aminoglycoside antimicrobial agents, septic thrombophlebitis, or other antecedent situations predisposing to anaerobic infections, such as procedures on the gastrointestinal tract, septic abortions, or general surgery (Figs. 12-1 and 12-2).

Laboratory analysis

Laboratory evaluation may reveal acidosis and anemia as a result of erythrocyte hemolysis and a plethora of bacterial endotoxins; jaundice also may be seen as a result of anemia, with the potential for transfusion in acute cases; leukocytosis with a left shift of up to 30% and immature blast cell formations, although a lack of white blood cells may itself indicate a clostridial infection; hyperbilirubinemia; hypergammaglobulinemia with dark urine; hypocalcemia; and hypoalbuminemia.[18] In acute crises, septicemia may occur; estimates of its incidence range from 2% to 10% of all cases, predominately from the non-spore-forming gram-negative rods such as *Bacteroides*. Clinically, the picture of bacteremia consists of a sudden onset, with rigors, chills, fever, diaphoresis, and jaundice. Thrombosis and embolus formation are potential complicating factors. In addition, *Fusobacterium* produces an endotoxin that may promote septic

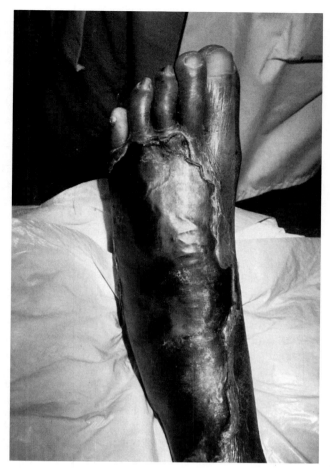

Fig. 12-1 This anaerobic infection demonstrates a dry and extensive escharotic tenacious "pseudomembranous" plaque, which is a harbinger of impending full-thickness skin slough. The dissection between soft tissue subcutaneous planes is laterally directed because of postural drainage of infected exudates. This type of infection does not predispose to localized abscess formation. *(Courtesy Dr. Keith B. Kashuk, Miami, Fla.)*

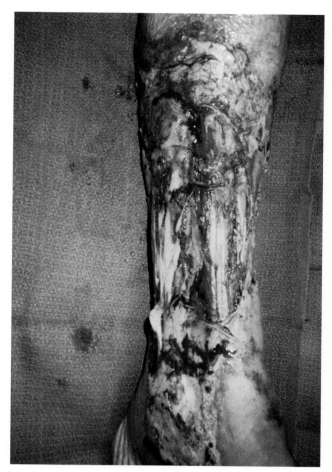

Fig. 12-2 Catastrophic deep soft tissue devitalization, reminiscent of a "degloving" injury, following a severe anaerobic infection of the leg and ankle. Fortunately, this case of necrotizing fasciitis provided near complete anesthesia as a result of damaged cutaneous nerves exiting through the contaminated superficial fascia. Plastic surgical wound coverage techniques are needed for this type of severe tissue destruction. *(Courtesy Dr. Keith B. Kashuk, Miami, Fla.)*

shock syndrome or a disseminated intravascular coagulation (DIC) phenomenon.[19-20]

SPECIMEN ACQUISITION, CULTURAL TECHNIQUES, AND BACTERIOLOGY

The continued improvement in specimen acquisition and cultural techniques will undoubtedly demonstrate the increasing prevalence of anaerobic infections in the lower extremity, particularly the diabetic foot.[21] However, since most anaerobic organisms associated with infections are benign, if not beneficial, misleading cultural data may be obtained. Therefore, special acquisition techniques, transport containers, media, and growth-processing incubators are needed for appropriate isolation and identification.

Specimen acquisition techniques

Specimen acquisition techniques include the procurement of a sufficient inoculum of material, in an expeditious manner,

to avoid the destruction of fastidious oxygen-sensitive organisms. Any abscess formation or intact instrumental layer should be decontaminated and detached, purulent material should be removed with a syringe. The most efficacious samples are taken from deep within wounds at the time of surgery, thereby avoiding secondary or cross-contamination. This method is preferred to a collection swab on a portion of exposed lesion, because saprophytic anaerobes unrelated to the infection may be obtained. In addition, since pus is made up of dead white blood cells, it is not necessary to acquire a rich purulent specimen. Two other biopsy techniques may be helpful in questionable cases. The technique described by Ulman and Kunin involves direct needle aspiration, while another technique involves a limited and local surgical procedure to evaluate the subcutaneous stroma.[22]

A frozen section for immediate diagnosis may also be attempted in selected cases. Criteria for diagnosis include (1) superficial fascial necrosis, (2) venous and arterial thrombosis with angiitis and fibrinoid necrosis, (3) dermal and fascial polymorphonuclear infiltration, (4) microorganism identification, and (5) lack of muscular involvement.[14]

After specimen procurement, a Gram stain with dark-field examination is performed for preliminary identification and comparison with cultural data.[23] Dark-field examination is helpful in demonstrating mobility, cellular morphology, and certain non–Gram staining organisms.[24]

Specimen transportation

Correct specimen transport is essential, as it represents a weak link in the chain from specimen collection to identification. Resilient anaerobes may survive while more demanding anaerobes may perish, or facultative organisms, which grow faster than anaerobes at room temperature, may outlast more absolute anaerobes, producing skewed results if appropriate precautions are not made. For example, specimens may be taken to the laboratory in a syringe and needle, if no other anaerobic transport system is available. After the specimen is collected, air is expelled from the syringe and the needle is inserted into a sterile rubber stopper. The method is not ideal, and the specimen should be delivered to the laboratory immediately and set up to culture the sample within 30 minutes.[25] Therefore, several more efficient and predictable commercially available transport systems are available for this purpose:

1. A vial transporter is an anaerobic-atmosphere glass diaphragm-stoppered bottle, which contains a solid prereduced agar mixture with E_h indicator (sodium thioglycolate or aminothiazole).
2. The anaerobic Bio-Plastic Bag Transporter may be used to transport, in its entirety, a specimen swab or syringe under sterile conditions. Upon closure of the bag, a gas generator, catalyst, and indicator are activated in an anaerobic atmosphere.
3. The cotton swab transport method utilizes a prereduced anaerobically sterilized (PRAS) cotton-tipped swab furnished in one tube and a medium column of semisolid PRAS Cary-Blair medium in another. After collection, the swab is impregnated into the medium and firmly secured.
4. A transport tube is a glass vial that is either flushed with CO_2 or placed in an anaerobic chamber for 48 hours and then sealed with a rubber diaphragm and foil cap prior to sterilization. It contains resazurin, a redox (E_h) indicator, and a bit of prereduced peptone yeast medium. Samples are collected by a syringe and introduced through the diaphragm with a needle after air is expelled from the syringe and needle lumen.
5. The Vacutainer anaerobic transporter is a double-tube, cotton swab system. After collection, the swab is placed into the inner tube, disengaging it into the central tube, simultaneously closing the puncture in the rubber stopper. The outer tube contains palladium-coated pellets that serve as a catalyst in the H_2, CO_2,

and N_2 enriched environment. The H_2 combines with the O_2 to form water and generate an anaerobic atmosphere.
6. An anaerobic (Gas-Pack) jar contains an envelope that generates hydrogen and carbon dioxide, after the addition of water, through the catalytic conversion of H_2 and O_2 to H_2O. The jar is ideal for larger specimens and may be vented for an evacuation-replacement system to be used to acquire an anaerobic milieu.

Microbial identification

Following purity testing and isolate growth, organisms are subcultured to determine whether they are obligate anaerobes, facultative anaerobes, micro-aerophiles (*Actinomyces naeslundii, Arachnia propionica,* and some positive cocci grow under reduced oxygen tension), or aerotolerant-philes (*Clostridium histolyticum* grows tenuously after initial anaerobic isolation). Tests for pathogenicity, toxin production, and spore formation (may survive boiling in alkaline solution or exposure to dry heat to 150° C, for 1 hour) are then made for the identification of certain clostridia. This is especially difficult with *C. perfringens* and *C. ramosum,* with regard to spore formation, and *C. botulinum* and *C. tetani* with regard to toxin production.[26] With few exceptions, clostridia lack the enzymes catalase, cytochrome oxidase, peroxidase, and superoxide dismutase (SOD).

The identification of non-spore-forming gram-positive bacilli is also difficult, and the current classification is based on the major acid products of glucose metabolism. For example, *Fusobacterium* species produce butyric acid, while most *Bacteroides* species do not. However, *B. splanchnicus, putredinis,* and *asaccharolyticus* produce smaller amounts of the acid but always in the isobutyric and isovaleric forms. Further species and subspecies classification is based on various idiosyncratic characteristics, such as the presence of either desoxyxholate or bile, susceptibility to certain antibiotics, or the fermentation of carbohydrates.[27]

Anaerobic gram-positive cocci are divided into to genera according to cellular morphology, while speciation is based on attributes such as indole production, carbohydrate fermentation, and nitrate reduction. Some cocci types, such as the genus *Streptococcus,* even produce lactic acid as their major metabolite. Perhaps the most common anaerobic gram-negative coccus is *Veillonella parvula,* which does not ferment hexose but converts lactate to propionate and pyruvate to acetate and propionate. Other less frequently found anaerobic gram-negative cocci are *Acidaminococcus fermentans* and *Megasphaera elsdenii.*[28] Unfortunately, a lack of positive Gram stain or cultural data is probably the rule, rather than the exception, when anaerobic infections are evaluated.

ANAEROBIC ENDOCARDITIS

In 1992, Levenson reviewed the standard medical guidelines for preoperative antibiotic prophylaxis when dealing with surgical patients considered to be at risk for aerobic endocarditis.[29] However, no mention was made of anaerobic endocarditis, as the incidence of this disorder is only slightly greater than 1% to 2% of all endocarditis cases. The population at risk includes patients over the age of 50 years, with a predilection toward older males and younger females and a tendency to spare children. Obviously, patients with rheumatic, congenital or degenerative heart disease are at increased risk.

The signs and symptoms of anaerobic endocarditis are not significantly different from those of aerobic endocarditis. Janeway lesions, for example, may occur in both forms. However, the rate of pulmonary embolism is higher, and the incidence of preexisting heart disease lower, in anaerobic-induced endocarditis than in endocarditis caused by facultative organisms. The main portal of entry (POE) is the mouth, notably from poor oral hygiene or periodontal disease, or following tooth extractions. Precipitating agents include *B. fragilis, Fusobacterium, Clostridium* (true saprophytes), and *Peptostreptococcus* (Fig. 12-3).

In an update, the American Heart Association published its guidelines for the prevention of bacterial endocarditis. Recommendations for dental procedures and those involving the respiratory tract were put forth when *Streptococcus viridans* was the most common enterococcal pathogen. However, the overall effectiveness of prophylaxis remains undetermined.

In recent studies, the potential for transient bacteremia resulting from foot surgery was evaluated in 42 non-cardiac-risk patients. In no instance did bacteremia or septicemia result.[30] However, despite these results, most authorities concluded that sampling of a larger population would be required before the discontinuance of prophylactic antibiotics should be considered.

Currently, all patients considered at risk for developing aerobic or anaerobic endocarditis should receive antibiotics to prevent the onset or recurrence of endocarditis postop-

eratively. The antimicrobial agent is preferably administered prior to the procedure to provide optimal coverage and prevent development of resistant strains of organisms. The agents are bactericidal rather than bacteriostatic, with the particular exception in penicillin allergies, which would require the administration of erythromycin. One such anaerobic antimicrobial agent is metronidazole (Flagyl), which shows consistently good bactericidal activity in vivo and in vitro.[31]

SPECIFIC PATHOLOGIC ENTITIES OF THE FOOT

To avoid confusion and promote disciplined order, the following specific conditions are cited in a progressive fashion according to increasing severity and clinical morbidity.[32]

Anaerobic crepitant cellulitis

MacLennon has defined anaerobic cellulitis as a localized soft tissue anaerobic infection that does not involve muscle mass.[33] Although the condition may be characterized by a malodorous discharge and gas in the tissues, it does not induce great pain or edema, and any discharge may be minimal with a small potential for systemic toxicity. Any gas-producing non-spore-forming or facultative anaerobes may produce the condition, but an infection that involves clostridial contamination will be most severe. Anaerobic crepitant cellulitis is common in diabetic patients and is treated with debridement and antibiotics, as described by Greenberg and Greenberg in 1989.[34] Concomitant vascular compromise may necessitate radical resection or amputation. Prompt treatment prior to muscle involvement may lower the mortality rate by 20%.

Chronic undermining anaerobic ulceration of Meleney

Meleney's ulceration (MU) is an atypical soft tissue excoriation that is progressive and deep and that spreads diffusely, producing multiple sinus tracts and necrotic foci from subcutaneous planes to the skin.[35] Aerophilic streptococci are the usual offenders. Treatment, with debridement and antibiosis, is infuriatingly slow.

Progressive bacterial synergistic gangrene

Progressive bacterial synergistic gangrene (PBSG) is an unusual form of anaerobic infection. Common bacterial miscreants include *Peptostreptococcus* species and *S. aureus,* working in synergy to produce ulcerative necrosis of both skin and subcutaneous and fascial tissue planes.[36]

Anaerobic infected vascular gangrene

Anaerobic infected "dry" vascular gangrene (AIVG) is typically caused by anaerobic organisms in the face of an ischemic limb resulting from either generalized peripheral vascular disease or other local arterial flow compromise.[37] In

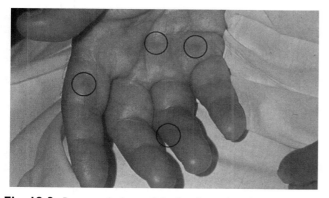

Fig. 12-3 Janeway lesions of the hand, produced by anaerobic-induced endocarditis. The major portal of entry is the mouth. Precipitating agents include *B. fragilis, Fusobacterium, Clostridium,* and *Peptostreptococcus. (From Feingold FM, Sutter VL: Anaerobic infections,* Kalamazoo, Mich, 1983, Scope-Upjohn Publications.)

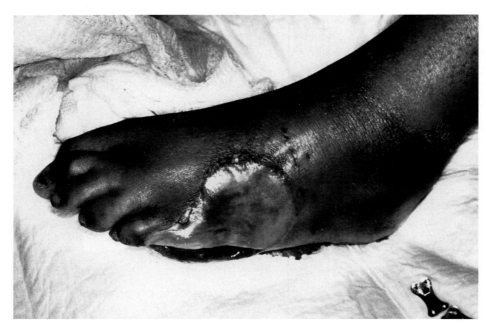

Fig. 12-4 Case of a 19-year-old black female with insulin-dependent diabetes mellitus and a 5-day history of a swollen and red lateral left foot. She had no history of trauma but did have a long-standing lesion underneath the fifth metatarsophalangeal joint. Demonstrates initial incision and drainage of the plantar lateral aspect of the left foot. *(Courtesy Dr. Charles Gudas, Hinsdale, Ill.)*

contradistinction to anaerobic cellulitis, there is usually a great degree of edema with gas formation, but again there is only slight systemic bacteriemia capability. Facultative organisms such as *B. fragilis* or *perfringens* are common causative agents, not uncommonly from fecal fallout.

Necrotizing fasciitis

Necrotizing fasciitis (NF) is a serious limb- and life-threatening infection that is noted for its rapid progression among soft tissue fascial planes. It was extensively investigated during the Civil War and became known as "hospital gangrene," "acute hemolytic streptococcal gangrene," or "necrotizing erysipelas."[38] The classical description of NF was produced by Meleney, in 1924.[39] Regardless of designation, the depiction of a dark-gray or ashen subcutaneous fascia remains a stigma of a process that continues to possess high morbidity and mortality because of major end-organ collapse, acute septic shock, pulmonary embolism, or disseminated intravascular coagulation.

A list of differential diagnoses for NF includes erysipelas, streptococcal myositis, and the previously mentioned pathologic anaerobic entities.[40] According to Mahan, in 1991, the diagnostic criteria for NF include (1) extensive necrosis of superficial fascia, with the undermining of surrounding soft tissue structures, (2) moderate to severe systemic toxicity with mental disorientation, (3) absence of clostridia as the predominant pervading pathogen, (4) absence of muscle destruction and major vascular occlusion, and (5) an intense leukocytic infiltrate on pathologic examination of involved necrotic structures.[41] Consequently, the difficulty in establishing the diagnosis is based on the triad of nonexistent or

trivial trauma, confusing integumentary changes, and rapid progression of the disease process.

Implicated microorganisms include hemolytic streptococci, staphylococci, and *B. fragilis,* although one study of 16 patients, by Pessa and Howard, in 1985 identified 75 species of both aerobic and anaerobic bacteria in such wounds, while others have grouped NF into two types based on cultural data.[42] The first, type I, contains both absolute and facultative anaerobes, while the second, type II, possesses group A streptococci alone or in combination with staphylococci and in the absence of aerobes. In addition, the use of oral nonsteroidal antiinflammatory agents has been associated with NF by Rimailho, Riou, Richard, and Auzepy, in 1987.[43]

Treatment of NF includes medical stabilization of the patient through electrolyte and transfusion supplementation, appropriate parenteral antibiosis, aggressive surgical incision and drainage with debridement, surgical reexploration within 24 to 48 hours, nutritional support, and wound coverage by secondary or tertiary means. The use of intravenous fluorescein dye may assist in the determination of viable versus infarcted and necrotic tissue[44] (Figs. 12-4 to 12-7).

Myofascial clostridial necrosis (gas gangrene)

Myofascial clostridial necrosis (MCN), or "gas gangrene," is one of the most anxiety-producing lower extremity infections for both patient and physician. Clostridial wound contamination is more common than realized and may approach 10% to 30% of all wounds in patients with diabetes or neoplastic disease. Typical clinical features include a

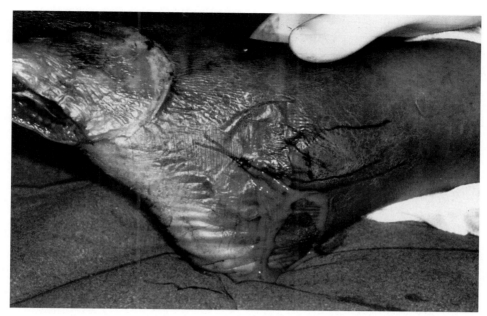

Fig. 12-5 Shows incision and drainage of lateral ankle with purulence noted from the incision. Subsequent culture revealed an anaerobic streptococcus and *Peptostreptococcus* infection. *(Courtesy Dr. Charles Gudas, Hinsdale, Ill.)*

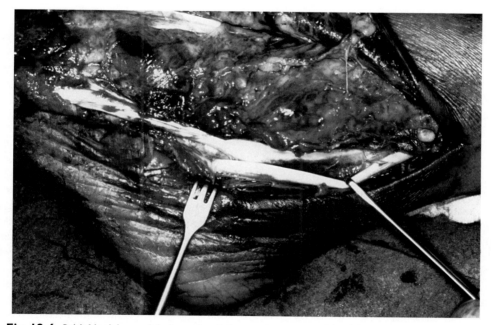

Fig. 12-6 Initial incision and drainage involving septic tenosynovitis of the peroneal muscle-tendon complex. *(Courtesy Dr. Charles Gudas, Hinsdale, Ill.)*

painfully tense and pale edema, turquoise-tinted ecchymosis, bullae formation, protracted necrosis, crepitant gas in 80% of soft tissue structures, and eventual toxemia. Differential diagnoses include synergistic nonclostridial anaerobic myonecrosis (SNCAM) (also known as cutaneous necrotizing myositis or synergistic necrotizing cellulitis) and anaerobic streptococcal myositis (ASM).[45] SNCAM is a virulent soft tissue infection not involving bone. Extensive "liquefaction" necrosis may occur, producing "dishwater pus."

Bacteroides sp. (gram-positive rods, spore formers or non–spore formers), anaerobic streptococci, and facultative gram-negative bacilli are inculpated in this disease. ASM is characterized by pain, toxemia, and seropurulent exudate with edema. Debridement, antibiotics, and anti–gas gangrene antitoxin are often needed for successful treatment.[46]

Human or animal fecal fallout and farmland contamination are archetypal environmental sources of gas gangrene contamination, and blowflies may play a role in

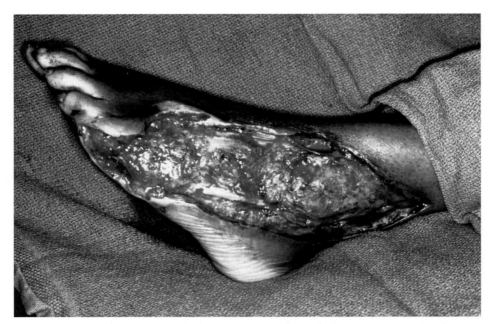

Fig. 12-7 Operative stage II, 3 days after incision and drainage with debridement of necrotic skin and soft tissue. The patient underwent a split-thickness skin graft 10 days later, with complete healing and infection resolution. *(Courtesy Dr. Charles Gudas, Hinsdale, Ill.)*

its transmission as a vector to humans. Etiologic agents include *C. perfringens* (aromatic gas producer with alpha toxin production), *C. septicum* (rapid symptom producer, especially in patients with cecal carcinoma), *C. novyi*, *C. histolyticum*, *C. tertium*, *C. paraputrificum*, *C. sardiensis*, *C. butyricum*, *C. fallox*, *C. beiferinckii*, *C. ramosum*, *C. sporogens*, *C. capitovale*, *C. bifermentans*, and *C. sartagoformum*.[47] Nonclostridial aerobic culprits, which may also produce gas in tissue planes, include: *K. pneumoniae*, *E. coli*, *Enterobacter*, and *Proteus* (gram-negative rods), *S. pyogenes*, and *S. aureus* (gram-positive cocci).

The presumptive diagnosis of *C. perfringens*, type A, may be made by the presence of colonies on human, rabbit, or sheep blood agar plates. It is characterized by nonmotile subterminal, oval spores, which can ferment sucrose with exceptional gas production known as "stormy fermentation," producing nitrates and sulfides. *C. perfringens* is also known to produce eight minor toxins (theta [cardiotoxic], kappa [collagenase], mu [hyaluronidase], nu [deoxyribonuclease], fibrinolysin [protease], neuraminidase [splits tertiary sialic acid], hemagglutinin [neutralizes blood group factor A], and circulating factor [inhibits phagocytosis]) and several enterotoxins. The species can be subdivided into five types (A to E), on the basis of the four major toxins, known as alpha or lecithinase, beta, epsilon, and iota. The development of a "double zone" of hemolysis, when *C. perfringens* is grown on enriched agar, known as the Nagler reaction, is pathognomonic.[6] This occurs when the clostridial enzyme lecithinase, or phospholipase C, attacks the egg yolk in the media and produces a clear opaque-like area around bacterial growth, by splitting lecithin into

diglyceride and phosphorylcholine. Typically, the inner zone is completely hemolyzed while the outer zone is usually incomplete. *C. paraperfringens* may also produce this reaction but is not often encountered in clinical practice.

Tetanus (lockjaw)

Tetanus (trismus or "lockjaw") is a noncommunicable infectious disease, caused by the pervasive, anaerobic, gram-positive, spore-forming resident agent of dirt and the bowel, *C. tetani*. The organism itself is not invasive, grows slowly to the size of 0.5 μm × 2.5 μm, and is harmless except for the production of a plasmid-mediated neurotoxin (consisting of tetanolysin, which is oxygen sensitive, and tetanospasmin, which is intracellular), which acts on the CNS to reduce inhibitory motor activity. Circulating blood levels of neurotoxin less than 0.01 IU/ml at the time of onset are indicative of diagnosis. The common route of transmission is a break in the skin (needle sticks, nail punctures, lacerations, animal bites, scratches, insect bites, bullet wounds) in an outdoor setting.

Common conditions associated with tetanus include gangrene, frostbite, ulcerations, osteomyelitis, and dental abscesses and procedures. Up to 40% of human intestines are colonized with *C. tetani*.

The clinical characteristic of tetanus were first described by Hippocrates and then in 1884, by Carle, when the etiologic agent was first identified. Early clinical features of localized tetanus, within 3 days to 3 weeks of inoculation, include pains and spasm confined to the injured area. Generalized tetanic signs and symptoms include headaches,

TABLE 12-1 Tetanus prophylaxis protocol

Immunization Data	Course of Action
Complete immunization with last booster with 1 year.	None needed
Complete immunization within last 10 years but no booster follow-up.	Administer 0.5 cc tetanus and diphtheria adult toxoid (Td)
Complete immunization and subsequent booster within last decade.	Administer 0.5 cc Td
Complete immunization but no booster within last decade. Clean minor wound promptly treated.	Administer 0.5 cc Td
Complete immunization more than a decade ago with no booster within past 5 years.	Administer 0.5 cc Td and 250 units human tetanus immune globulin
Wound other than minor and/or not treated promptly.	(TIGH), at separate sites with separate syringes. Give 500 units if wound is clostridia prone.
No record of immunization with clean minor wound treated promptly.	Start immunization with 0.5 cc Td and schedule further immunization.
No record of immunization with other than clean wound and/or treated promptly.	Administer 250 units TIGH and begin immunization with 0.5 cc Td. Give 500 units TIGH if wound is clostridia prone. Use separate syringes at separate sites.

TABLE 12-2 Expanded tetanus immunization recommendation for women of childbearing age

Dose one: Early in pregnancy or first contact
Dose two: Four weeks later
Dose three: Subsequent pregnancy or 6 to 12 months later
Dose four: Subsequent pregnancy or 1 to 5 years after dose three
Dose five: Subsequent pregnancy or 1 to 10 years after dose four

Modified from Issues in neonatal infection control, EPI/GAG/87/WP. 11, World Health Organization, 1987.

constipation, sweating, tachycardia, dysphagia, trismus with neck stiffness, risus sardonicus, local and fascial cramps, ipsilateral hyperreflexia, and anxiety.[50] Cephalic tetanus occurs with lesions of the head and face and present with atonic nerve palsies of cranial nerves III, IV, IX, X, and XII. It is more common in males. Aggressive respiratory and supportive care, with sedation, is needed, as death is due to respiratory collapse. Moreover, tetanus antitoxin and toxoid should be administered, at different sites, along with wound debridement and penicillin antibiosis. Descombey, in 1924, prepared a toxoid, chemically changed toxin, which induced neutralizing antibodies without inducing the illness, and began the wholesale process of tetanus prophylaxis.

Recently, Gumann reiterated the protocol of Karlin, regarding tetanus prophylaxis in open wound fractures[51,52] (Table 12-1). Once the three-dose primary immunization series has been completed, along with at least one booster dose every 10 to 15 years thereafter, routine supplementary boosters at the time of additional injury are not needed. In fact, too frequent booster administration may increase the likelihood of hypersensitivity reactions to immunization.

Tetanus toxoid is safe and immunogenic and protects through neutralizing antibodies (Table 12-2). Nearly all primary recipients are protected. Interestingly, the underadministration of tetanus prophylaxis in the United States appears to be the exception rather than the rule of care.

Recent studies suggest that 1% to 6% of patients receive less than the recommended prophylactic amounts of Td (adsorbed tetanus toxoid), with or without TIG (tetanus immune globulin), indicated by their clinical wound statuses and historical reviews. On the other hand, 12% to 17% receive more than the recommended dose.

Wound botulism

The concept of wound botulism was first noted in the early 1940s. Most affected patients were young males, and wounds were often deep and avascular with associated osseous pathology. More recently, an increased incidence of wound botulism has been associated with intravenous drug use or the chronic use of nasalar cocaine. Signs and symptoms include the usual gastrointestinal and CNS stigmata of botulism. The diagnosis is confirmed with the isolation of *C. botulinum* from the infected wound or the presence of botulinal toxin in the serum. The fatality rate is about 16%, but the prognosis improves with the availability of respiratory support. Local wound treatment includes surgical debridement, drainage, and penicillin antibiosis.[48-49]

SURGICAL TREATMENT OF ANAEROBIC INFECTIONS

Appropriate surgical intervention is the initial therapeutic treatment in most infections, and anaerobic defilement is no exception. It is the *sine qua non* of therapy. In the initial acute condition, the simplest approach to wound care is extensive debridement of infective bone and soft tissue, under general anesthesia. A temperate finger-probing technique may be used to ascertain the extent of necrosis, as infected soft tissue structures may disintegrate under slight pressure. Aggressive and extensive "netoyage" and resection of infected osseous tissue structures is essential, even if it approaches a radical intensity. Segments of necrotic skin, subcutaneous tissues, ligaments, muscles, or tendons, as well as plantar fascia, may even have to be removed to expose the depths of the infection or to permit adequate drainage of tendon sheaths, tissue planes, or the plantar vault. Fractures must be stabilized, and if large muscle mass loss occurs, or if limb function is seriously compromised, consideration must be given to amputation. Therefore, a knowledge of the plantar arch architecture is vital, since anaerobic organisms and necrosis may lurk in its associated spaces.[53]

The plantar vault consists of three fundamentally segregated compartments: medial (abductor hallucis muscle), lateral (abductor and flexor digiti minimi muscles), and central. The central compartment is further divided into medial (flexor hallucis longus, flexor hallucis brevis, and adductor hallucis), superficial (flexor digitorum brevis, flexor digitorum longus, quadratus plantae, and lumbricales), and deep chambers (interossei). The central compartment is still further subdivided into four laminated potential spaces, known as M1 to M4, interspersed between the four definitive muscle layers of the foot. Therefore, as delineated by Bauer, this anatomic composition must be fully appreciated when the infectious process within the plantar vault is tracked and explored.[54]

Later, vascular reconstruction may be needed, although the infection management protocol usually comes first in a life-threatening situation.[55] Of course, resected stumps, rays, and feet will heal in time, if adequately perfused, but the prime objective of the surgery is to remove necrotic tissue and bone as well as drain infection fluids.[56]

Once the foot has been surgically decompressed, the next step in recovery involves daily debridement, and even a return to the operating room within 24 to 48 hours of the initial surgery. Liberal wound irrigation is also a helpful but often neglected portion of the debridement regimen. Various solutions may be used, such as sterile normal saline, hydrogen peroxide, or povidone-iodine in a concentration of 1%.

If the wound or cavity is significant in size, open wound packing with sterile gauze impregnated with iodophor, or some other antiseptic that is not irritating to delicate granulation tissue, is indicated. However, aerobic infections are more prone to leave large cavities after debridement, while anaerobes are predisposed to destroy a more extensive but shallow surface area.

The encouragement of fluid removal is beneficial, as well as daily wound debridement and the avoidance of desiccation through the use of wet-to-dry dressings. Once granulation tissue begins to flourish, periodic Gram stains and cultures are needed to evaluate wound progress in anticipation of healing. Delayed primary closure is usually not indicated in anaerobic corruption.[58] These wounds must usually be packed open.

Once the clinical setting and wound cultures do not demonstrate overt infection, temperature normalizes, and granulation tissue growth commences, the final stage of local wound management may begin, by second intention, skin grafts, or flaps.[59-64]

CHEMOTHERAPEUTIC AGENTS FOR ANAEROBIC INFECTIONS

Although surgical decompression is the treatment foundation for many infections, antimicrobial agents are also extremely important to reduce the likelihood of recurrent disease. Many infections in which anaerobes are established also involve facultative and aerobic organisms, which will influence the choice of antimicrobial agents. Ecumenically, antimicrobial therapy for anaerobic infections will require high doses and prolonged administration because of tissue necrosis and regression potential, and any agent may result in the superinfection overgrowth of nonsusceptible organisms, including fungi. Therefore, the following is a list of common agents, as proposed by Dickinson and Lipkin in 1992, used to treat anaerobic infections regardless of anatomic location.[65]

Penicillin G (natural penicillin) is active against many anaerobic infections, including anaerobic streptococci, clostridia, *Actinomyces,* and *Fusobacterium,* but penicillin alone is not recommended for seriously ill patients and is not effective against *B. fragilis.* The usual dose is 1.2 to 24 million units per day. High doses of piperacillin, carbenicillin, amoxicillin and clavulanate (Augmentin) and ticarcillin and clavulanate (Timentin) may be useful in some cases.[66]

Most cephalosporins are less active against anaerobes than penicillin G. Cefoxitin (Mefoxin) and cefotetan (Cefotan) are active against most isolates of *B. fragilis,* but no cephalosporin should be used to treat serious clostridial infections. Some third-generation agents such as ceftizoxime (Cefizox) are moderately active against many anaerobes but offer no advantage over other agents for anaerobic infections.[67]

The lincosamide clindamycin (Cleocin) inhibits bacterial protein synthesis by binding to the 50S ribosomal unit. It should not be used concurrently with other antibiotics that act in a similar manner, such as erythromycin and chloramphenicol. Plasmid-mediated resistance has been reported in *B. fragilis.* Clindamycin is active against *B. fragilis* and other anaerobic microorganisms and gram-positive cocci but not enterococci or methicillin-resistant staphylococci. Essentially, all aerobic gram-negative bacilli are resistant. It is useful against *B. fragilis, C. perfringens, Fusobacterium,* and anaerobic streptococci and as an alternative to penicillin in allergic patients. It is also more effective than lincomycin in terms of activity and oral absorption.[68]

Metronidazole (Flagyl) is a nitroimidazole compound that is metabolized by bacterial anaerobic nitroreductase with production of short-lived, cytotoxic intermediates that disrupt bacterial DNA. It is bactericidal and also affects certain parasitic organisms. Therapeutic uses include infections caused by anaerobic gram-negative rods such as *Bacteroides* and *Fusobacterium,* including septicemia, osteomyelitis, and septic arthritis. Some gram-positive obligative anaerobes and microaerophiles are resistant, along with most aerobic organisms.

Chloramphenicol (Chloromycetin) inhibits bacterial protein synthesis by binding to the 50S ribosomal unit. Binding is competitively inhibited by clindamycin and erythromycin. Plasmid-mediated resistance resulting from production of acetyltransferase enzyme has been recorded. It may also code for resistance to tetracyclines and ampicillin. Chloramphenicol demonstrates a broad spectrum of activity, with variable antimicrobial affects against a wide range of gram-positive and gram-negative bacteria, chlamydia, rickettsiae, and *B. fragilis.*[70]

Finally, the tetracyclines inhibit bacterial protein synthesis by binding to the 30S ribosomal subunit but are generally not used in the treatment of anaerobic infections because of plasmid-mediated resistant strains. Some clostridia, *F. varium,* aerobic cocci (microaerophilic cocci), and the *Eubacterium* are also resistant.[65]

The aminoglycosides are considered inactive against the majority of anaerobic infections, and their activity against enterococci is inadequate when used as monotherapy. It is important to note that penicillins may inactivate aminoglycosides in vitro and therefore should not be in the same solution or administered through the same IV line; dosing times should be altered as well.

Vancomycin (Vancocin) is a complex glycopeptide derived from the actinomycete *Streptomyces orientalis* and functions through cell wall inhibition. It is useful against certain anaerobic species and antibiotic-associated enterocolitis caused by *C. difficile.*

The anaerobic activity of the 4-quinolone ciprofloxacin (Cipro) is poor.

Gas gangrene antitoxin

Gas gangrene antitoxin was produced from hyperimmunized horse plasma, which often produced a sensitivity reaction. Then, a globulin-modified polyvalent *(C. perfringens, C. histolyticum, C. sordelli, C. novyi)* antitoxin was available, for a brief period of time. Both are no longer in vogue, and the latter is unavailable for general use.[71,72]

ADJUNCTIVE THERAPY

Although the use of hyperbaric oxygen (HBO), a toxic gas, in the treatment of anaerobic infections is controversial, its use was articulated by Malay in 1991.[73] Essentially, it involves placing the entire patient ("complete immersion") into an oxygen chamber with increased barometric pressure. Under this situation, the body acts as a liquid container, and the physical gas laws of Henry, Boyle, and Dalton exert their influence. This is to distinguish it from older, more local modalities, which encompassed only the affected body part, and have since proven much less effective. The toxic effects of oxygen, on the lungs and the CNS, are also mitigated in this fashion, but pulmonary fibrosis (Lorrain-Smith effect) and eardrum rupture may still occur and myringotomy may be needed, in the unconscious patient, to equilibrate pressure changes.

Typically, the patient receives 20 to 25 treatments of 60 to 90 minutes, three times per week, at 90 psi of pressure (1 atmospheric pressure = 14.7 psi). The mechanism of action was thought to be directly related to the bactericidal activity of oxygen. Critics cite increased oxygen-radical formation, which may actually induce cellular injury.[74] However, slight hyperoxia from oxygen radicals may antagonize rather than potentiate lipid peroxidation.

A more recent hypothesis suggests an indirect mechanism of action: increased neovascularization through white blood cell chemotaxis and phagocytosis with increased osteoclastic activity. Regardless of which hypothesis is correct, HBO remains an adjunctive modality, useful more for the residual effects of the anaerobic infectious process than for actual curative treatment.[75]

CONCLUSION

Anaerobic infections of the foot may cause significant morbidity and mortality. Acceptable treatment must include prompt diagnosis, appropriate surgery, and therapeutic antibiotics. Long-term follow-up care may also entail additional reconstructive surgical techniques to ameliorate the ravages of the pestilence. The clinician must possess impressive protean skills in order to render adequate care to cope with this severe disease process.

ACKNOWLEDGEMENTS

Production of this chapter was supported by The Upjohn Company and Don A. Madren, R.Ph. Portions were modified and reprinted, with permission, from Finegold SM and Sutter VL: *Anaerobic infections,* Kalamazoo, Mich, 1983, Scope-Upjohn Publications.

REFERENCES

1. Finlay GH, Hazelhurst JA, Franz RC: Gangrenous erysipelas and necrotizing fasciitis, *SA Medical J* 62:125, 1982.
2. Sudarsky LA., Lashinger JC, Coppa CF, et al: Improved results from a standardized approach treating patients with necrotizing fasciitis, *Ann Surg* 206:661, 1987.
3. Nekata MN, Lewis RP: Anaerobic bacteria in bone and joint infections, *Rev Infect Dis* 65:165-170, 1984.
4. Meleney F: Clinical aspects and treatment of surgical infections, Philadelphia, 1949, WB Saunders.
5. Cline KA, Turnbull TL: Clostridial myonecrosis, *Ann Emerg Med* 14:459, 1985.
6. Finegold SM, Sutter VL: *Anaerobic infections,* Kalamazoo, Mich, 1983, Scope-Upjohn Publications.
7. Barron S: *Medical microbiology,* Menlo Park, Calif, 1986, Addison-Wesley Publishing Co.
8. Berkow R: *The Merck manual,* ed 13, Rathway, N.J., 1977, Merck & Co.
9. Sim FH: Anaerobic infections, *Orthop Clin North Am* 6:1049, 1975.
10. Foster W, Lobe TE, Bortros N: Gangrenous soft tissue infections, *Inf Surg* 5:837, 1985.
11. Rea WJ, Wyrick WJ: Necrotizing fascitis, *Am Surg* 172:957, 1970.
12. Green D, Walter J, Heden R, Menacker L: The effects of local anesthetics containing epinephrine on digital blood perfusion, *J Am Podiatry Assoc* 69:397, 1979.

13. VanHook R, Vandervelde AG: Gas gangrene after intramuscular injection of epinephrine: report of a fatal case, *Ann Intern Med* 83:669, 1975.

14. Goldberg GN, Hansen RC, Lynch PJ: Necrotizing fascitis in infancy: report of three cases and review of the literature, *Pediatr Dermatol* 2:55, 1984.

15. Defore WW, Mattox KL, Dang MH, et al: Necrotizing fascitis: a persistent surgical problem, *J Am Coll Emerg Physicians* 6:62, 1977.

16. Harris EJ: Diagnostic imaging of infections. In Abramson C, McCarthy DJ, Rupp MJ, eds: *Infectious diseases of the lower extremities,* Baltimore, 1991, Williams & Wilkins.

17. Schlefman BS: Radiographic modalities and interpretation. In Marcinko DE, ed: *Medical and surgical therapeutics of the foot and ankle,* Baltimore, 1992, Williams & Wilkins.

18. Rupp MJ: The clinical laboratory as a diagnostic tool. In Abramson C, McCarthy DJ, Rupp MJ, eds: *Infectious diseases of the lower extremities,* Baltimore, 1991, Williams & Wilkins.

19. Joseph WS: Clinical and laboratory diagnosis of lower extremity infections, *J Am Podiatr Med Assoc* 79:505, 1989.

20. Dennis KJ: Diagnostic laboratory analysis. In Marcinko DE, ed: *Medical and surgical therapeutics of the foot and ankle,* Baltimore, 1992, Williams & Wilkins.

21. Finegold S: Anaerobic bacteria: their role in infections and their management, *Postgrad Med* 81:141, 1987.

22. Ulman SJ, Kunin CM: Needle aspiration in the diagnosis of soft tissue infections, *Arch Intern Med* 135:959, 1975.

23. Svensson LF, Brookstone AJ, Wellsted M: Necrotizing fascitis in a contused area, *J Trauma* 25:260, 1985.

24. Finegold SM, Sutter VL: *Anaerobic infections,* Kalamazoo, Mich., 1979, Scope-Upjohn Publications.

25. Bauer JD: *Clinical laboratory methods,* ed 8, St. Louis, 1974, Mosby.

26. Axler DA: Microbiology of diabetic foot infections, *J Foot Surg* 26:93, 1987.

27. Marcinko DE: Osteomyelitis. In McGlamry ED, ed: *Comprehensive textbook of foot surgery,* Baltimore, 1992, Williams & Wilkins.

28. Drugs for anaerobic infections, *Med Lett Drugs Ther* 26:87, 1984.

29. Levenson M: Infective endocarditis and the foot specialist. In Marcinko DE, ed: *Medical and surgical therapeutics of the foot and ankle,* Baltimore, 1992, Williams & Wilkins.

30. Trepal MJ, Burnetti V, Hodge, WR: Intra-operative bacteremia during foot surgery, *J Foot Surg* 27:47, 1988.

31. Kaye D: *Infective endocarditis,* Baltimore, 1976, University Park Press.

32. Abramowicz M: Drugs for anaerobic infections, *Med Lett Drugs Ther* 26:87, 1984.

33. MacLennon JD: The histotoxic clostridial infections of man, *Bact Tev* 26:177, 1962.

34. Greenberg PM, Greenberg H: Crepitant cellulitis: polymicrobic infection of the diabetic lower extremity, *J Am Podiatry Assoc* 79:197, 1989.

35. Meleney F: Bacterial synergism in disease processes with confirmation of the synergistic bacterial etiology of a certain type of progressive gangrene of the abdominal wall, *Ann Surg* 94:961, 1931.

36. Stone HH, Martin D: Synergistic necrotizing cellulitis, *Surg Gynecol Obstet* 161:357, 1985.

37. Kidawa AS: The vascular system and related disorders: diagnosis and treatment. In Marcinko DE, ed: *Medical and surgical therapeutics of the foot and ankle,* Baltimore, 1992, Williams & Wilkins.

38. Hart GB, Lamb RC, Strauss MB: Gas gangrene: a collective review, *J Trauma* 23:9891, 1983.

39. Jones J: Investigations upon the nature, causes and treatment of hospital gangrene and its prevalence in the Confederate armies, 1861-1865. US Sanitary Commission. Surgical memoirs of the war of rebellion, 1871. In Meleney: Treatise on surgical infections, New York, 1948, Oxford University Press.

40. Joseph WS: Infections following lower extremity trauma. In Scurran BL, ed: *Foot and ankle trauma,* New York, 1989, Churchill Livingstone.

41. Mahan KT: Necrotizing fasciitis. In Abramson C, McCarthy DJ, Rupp MJ, eds: *Infectious diseases of the lower extremities.* Baltimore, 1991, Williams & Wilkins.

42. Pessa M, Howard R: Necrotizing fasciitis, *Surg Gynecol Obstet* 161:357, 1985.

43. Rimaihlo A, Riox B, Richard C, Auzepy P: Fulminating necrotizing fasciitis and nonsteroidal anti-inflammatory agents, *J Infect Dis* 155:143, 1987.

44. Bartolomei FJ: Subcutaneous infections. In Abramson C, McCarthy DJ, Rupp MJ, eds: *Infectious diseases of the lower extremities,* Baltimore, 1991, Williams & Wilkins.

45. Moehring HD: Postoperative clostridial infection: a case report, *Clin Orthop* 228:265, 1988.

46. Jamison JP, Ivey FM: Non-traumatic clostridial myonecrosis: a case report, *Orthop Rev* 15:65, 1986.

47. Bessman AN, Wagner N: Nonclostridial gas gangrene: a report of 48 cases and review of literature, *JAMA* 233:448, 1975.

48. Werry DG, Meek RN: *J Trauma* 26:280, 1986.

49. Sanders LJ, Murray-Leisure KA: Infections of the diabetic foot. In Abramson C, McCarthy DJ, Rupp, MJ, eds: *Infectious diseases of the lower extremities,* Baltimore, 1991, Williams & Wilkins.

50. Brill LR, Harris GM, Kinberg P: Nosocomical postoperative tetanus infection, *J Foot Surg* 23:235, 1984.

51. Gumann GS: Lower extremity traumatology. In Marcinko, DE, ed: *Medical and surgical therapeutics of the foot and ankle,* Baltimore, 1992, Williams & Wilkins.

52. Karlin JM: Management of open fractures, *Clin Podiatry* 2:217, 1985.

53. Marcinko DE: *Protocol manual for pedal infections,* Brentwood, Tenn, 1989, PICA Publications.

54. Bauer GR: Plantar space infections: anatomic and surgical considerations. In Abramson C, McCarthy DJ, Rupp MJ, eds: *Infectious diseases of the lower extremities,* Baltimore, 1991, Williams & Wilkins.

55. Marcinko DE, Carlson R: Psychological considerations of the surgical patient: an emerging issue, *J Am Podiatry Assoc* 74:441, 1984.

56. Harris W, Alpert W, Marcinko DE: Nitrous oxide and valium use for production of conscious sedation, *J Am Podiatry Assoc* 72:505-509, 1982.

57. Marcinko DE: Materials used in foot surgery. In McGlamry ED, ed: *Comprehensive textbook of foot surgery,* Baltimore, 1989, Williams & Wilkins.

58. Miller SJ: Edema, hematoma and infection. In McGlamry ED, ed: *Comprehensive textbook of foot surgery,* Baltimore, 1992, Williams & Wilkins.

59. Marcinko DE: Plastic surgery in podiatry (simplified illustrated techniques), *J Foot Surg* 27:103, 1988.

60. Marcinko DE: Lower extremity limb salvage, *J Foot Surg* 27:145, 1988.

61. Turek D: Skin grafts of the lower extremity, *J Am Podiatry Assoc* 67:28, 1977.

62. Julien P, Marcinko DE, Gordon S: Reconstruction of soft tissue defects about the great toe, *J Foot Surg* 27:116, 1988.

63. Dockery GL: Skin grafting techniques. In Jay RM, ed: *Current therapy in podiatric surgery,* Philadelphia, 1989, BC Decker.

64. Saponora GC, Warren AM: Pinch grafts: application in podiatric wound closure, *J Foot Surg* 27:111, 1988.

65. Dickinson B, Lipkin L: Antimicrobial agents of choice. In Marcinko DE, ed: *Medical and surgical therapeutics of the foot and ankle,* Baltimore, 1992, Williams & Wilkins.

66. Abramowicz M: Antimicrobial drugs of choice: In *Handbook of antimicrobial therapy,* New Rochelle, N.Y., 1982, The Medical Letter, Inc.

67. Abramowicz M: Antimicrobial drugs of choice, *Med Lett Drugs Ther* 30:33, 1988.

68. Moellering RC: Use and abuse of antibiotic combinations, *RI Med J* 55:341, 1972.

69. Steigbiegel N: Erythromycin, lincomycin, and clindamycin. In *Principles and practice of infectious diseases,* ed. 2, New York, 1985, Wiley.

70. Corey SV: Antimicrobial selection. In Abramson C, McCarthy DJ, Rupp MJ, eds: *Infectious diseases of the lower extremities,* Baltimore, 1991, Williams & Wilkins.

71. Rosenblatt JE: Laboratory tests used to guide antimicrobial therapy, *Mayo Clin Proc* 58:14, 1983.

72. Tilton RC: MCI's and MBC's, *Infections in Medicine,* May/June, 1986, pp 218-225.

73. Malay SD: Muscle infections. In Abramson C, McCarthy DJ, Rupp MJ, eds: *Infectious diseases of the lower extremities,* Baltimore, 1991, Williams & Wilkins.

74. Hirn M, Ninikoski J: Hyperbaric oxygen in the treatment of clostridial gas gangrene, *Ann Gynaecol* 77:37, 1988.

75. Peacock EE, Van Winkle W Jr: *Wound repair,* Philadelphia, 1977, WB Saunders.

ADDITIONAL READINGS

Castellano B: Emergency surgery in the septic diabetic patient. In *Comprehensive Clinic of Foot Surgery,* Tucker, Ga, 1997, Podiatry Institute Publications.

Phillips, AJ: Pedal amputation in the diabetic foot. In *Comprehensive Clinic of Foot Surgery,* Tucker, Ga, 1977, Podiatry Institute Publications.

Sheffield PJ, Brakora MJ: Hyperbaric oxygen therapy for diabetic wounds, *Clin Podiatr Med Surg* 12(1):105-117, 1995.

Taylor RP: Wound care concepts (principles and products). In *Comprehensive Clinic in Foot Surgery,* Tucker, Ga, 1997, Podiatry Institute Publications.

Section Four

Medical and Surgical Treatment of Foot Infections

13

Antimicrobial Agents

Alvario Lopez
David Edward Marcinko

I drank of poppy and cold mandrake juice, and being asleep, belike they thought me dead.   Marlowe

THE PENICILLINS

Penicillin was discovered by Sir Alexander Fleming, in 1928, but it was Florey and Chain who isolated its structure, described its properties, and produced a true antimicrobial agent. The first patient was treated in 1941. By the end of the 1940s, penicillin G was widely available in the United States.[1]

Members of the penicillin family share a common structure that consists of three components: a five-membered thiazolidine ring, a beta-lactam ring, and a side chain. It is the side chain that determines the antibacterial spectrum and pharmacologic properties of a particular penicillin. The cephalosporins and carbapenems have generally similar structures, as do to a lesser degree the monobactams.

The penicillins differ among themselves in their resistance to beta-lactamase because of penicillin-binding proteins (PBPs), their penetration characteristics through gram-negative cell walls, and their susceptibility to gastric acid.

The advantages of penicillins include the fact that they are bactericidal, have good tissue distribution and penetration, are excreted by the kidneys, and are relatively safe.

Penicillin disadvantages include a short serum half-life (approximately 30 minutes for natural penicillins to 60 minutes for the extended-spectrum penicillins), instability produced by gastric acids, and inactivity against methicillin (oxacillin) resistant *Staphylococcus* (MRSA, MRSE) and, most recently, *Enterococcus* species.

Penicillin's adverse reactions include anaphylaxis, allergic skin reactions, gastrointestinal distress, and neurologic, hematologic, and other electrolyte disturbances. The penicillins can be reviewed in the following logical manner.[2]

Natural penicillins

The natural penicillins are used for non-penicillinase-producing staphylococci, streptococci, gram-negative cocci, some gram-positive or gram-negative rods, spirochetes, and actinomycetes. More specifically, they are effective against streptococcus groups A, C, G, and viridans, most enterococci, non-penicillinase *Neisseria gonorrhoeae, Pseudomonas multocida,* and most anaerobes other than the *Bacteroides* species. Examples are included in Table 13-1.

Penicillinase-resistant (antistaphylococcal) penicillins

The penicillinase-resistant (antistaphylococcal) penicillins are less active than the natural penicillins against organisms sensitive to the latter. Their use should be reserved for infections known to be caused by staphylococci that produce beta-lactamase. Interestingly, their antibacterial activity is sufficiently high to eradicate most streptococci (except enterococci). These agents include methicillin, nafcillin, the isoxazolyl penicillins (cloxacillin, dicloxacillin, oxacillin), and flucloxacillin.

Aminopenicillins

The aminopenicillins are similar to penicillin G, with coverage extending to some gram-negative rods. They are less active than penicillin G but more active against enterococci. Examples include ampicillin, hetacillin, pivampicillin, bacampicillin, epicillin, cyclacillin, and amoxicillin. The aminopenicillins are generally indicated for treatment of *Streptococcus* species (equivalent activity to natural penicillins) and *Enterococcus* species (increased activity compared to natural penicillins). Aminopenicillins have poor activity against most *Staphylococcus* species and activity against some gram-negative organisms, including *Escherichia coli, Proteus mirabilis, Shigella, Salmonella,* and *Haemophilus influenzae.*

Carboxypenicillins

Ticarcillin and carbenicillin were the first penicillins to be used in the treatment of *Pseudomonas* infections. They are less active than penicillin G against gram-negative cocci but

TABLE 13-1 Natural penicillins

Penicillin G	Various
Penicillin V	V-Cillin, Pen-Vee K
Procaine penicillin G	Wycillin
Benzathine penicillin G	Bicillin-LA, Permapen

cover certain gram-positive rods. Examples include carbenicillin, ticarcillin, temocillin, indanylcarbenicillin, and carfecillin. Carboxypenicillins are inactive against most *Staphylococcus* species and *Streptococcus* species and have increased gram-negative activity with coverage against most Enterobacteriaceae and *Pseudomonas aeruginosa* (usually in combination with aminoglycoside) strains. Combination therapy with an aminoglycoside is often recommended in this scenario.

Ureido-piperazine penicillins

These broad-spectrum agents possess enhanced coverage for gram-negative rods. Examples of the ureidopenicillins include azlocillin, mezlocillin, and piperacillin. They are similar to the carboxypenicillins but have greater activity for the Enterobacteriaceae than ticarcillin and carbenicillin. They can also be used for *Pseudomonas* infections.

THE PENICILLINS AND BETA-LACTAM INHIBITORS

Penicillins can be combined with the three beta-lactamase inhibitors (clavulanic acid, sulbactam, and tazobactam), which are potent inhibitors of many plasmid-mediated and some chromosomal beta-lactamases. Each inhibitor is available only as a fixed-combination preparation that includes an active beta-lactamase antibiotic as the companion agent; minor clinical differences in potency occur. These agents include amoxicillin plus clavulanate, ticarcillin plus clavulanate, ampicillin plus sulbactam, and piperacillin/tazobactam. Only amoxicillin/clavulanate is available orally; the others must be given parenterally.[3]

The spectrum of activity includes methicillin (oxacillin)-sensitive *Staphylococcus* species (particularly the ampicillin and amoxacillin combinations), streptococci, enterococci, aerobic gram-negative rods, *Pseudomonas aeruginosa* (except the ampicillin and amoxacillin combinations), and anaerobes. They are particularly useful for postoperative, diabetic, and integumentary foot infections caused by *S. aureus, B. fragilis,* and Enterobacteriaceae. *Serratia* spp., *C. freundii, Enterobacter* spp., *P. aeruginosa,* and some Enterobacteriaceae may produce chromosomally mediated beta-lactamases that are resistant to these drugs.[4]

Clavulanate

The beta-lactamase inhibitor clavulanate was found in cultures of *S. clavuligerus.* Initially, it demonstrated only a low level of antibacterial action, but when combined with penicillin G, inhibition of *Klebsiella,* normally resistant to penicillin, was noted. Potassium clavulanate has subsequently been shown to inhibit certain types of beta-lactamases from a number of clinically important gram-positive and gram-negative organisms, such as *E. coli, Neisseria, Staphylococcus,* and *H. influenzae.*[5]

Clavulanate in combination with amoxicillin (Augmentin) has proven useful to treat bite wounds and skin structure infections due to streptococci and staphylococci, anaerobes, and aerobic gram-negative bacteria. Fortunately, few side effects have been reported with clavulanate combination use, although diarrhea may follow its use, especially when a patient is dosed orally in a thrice-daily schedule.[6]

Parenteral ticarcillin-clavulanate (Timentin) has been used to treat skin and osseous tissue infections. To treat neutropenic patients, a combination with an aminoglycoside may be necessary.

Sulbactam

Sulbactam is a broader-spectrum beta-lactamase inhibitor than clavulanic acid, but it is also less potent. Sulbactam is used in combination with ampicillin in a ratio of 0.5 g of sulbactam per 1 g of ampicillin, as a parenteral formulation for IV administration (Unasyn). Reported side effects have been minimal.[7]

Tazobactam

Tazobactam is a penicillanic acid sulfone beta-lactamase inhibitor with a structure not unlike sulbactam. Its spectrum is similar to that of sulbactam, but its potency is more similar to that of clavulanic acid. It is commercially available for parenteral administration in combination with piperacillin (Zosyn) in a ratio of 8:1 by weight. This drug has the most activity against enterococci and *Pseudomonas aeruginosa,* compared to other members of its class. The adult dose is 12 to 16 g/day of piperacillin, with 1.5 to 2 g/day tazobactam, administered in divided doses every 6 to 8 hours for creatinine clearance greater than 40 ml/min. Few adverse reactions have been reported.[8]

Table 13-2 lists examples of the penicillinase-resistant antimicrobials.

THE CEPHALOSPORINS

The cephalosporins are probably the most widely used antibiotics in the world. The fungus was discovered in the sewers of Sardinia, by Professor Giuseppe Brotzu from the University of Cagliari, in the mid-1940s. Subsequently, Abraham and co-workers identified the active antibacterial factors from which the antibiotics were eventually derived.[9]

Cephalosporins have a beta-lactam structure. However, the thiazolidine ring typical of penicillins is replaced by a six-member dihydrothiazine ring. These agents appear to inhibit bacterial cell wall synthesis in a manner similar to that of penicillins. The cephalosporins and derivatives

TABLE 13-2　Penicillinase-resistant antimicrobials

Cloxacillin	Tegopen
Dicloxacillin	Dynapen
Nafcillin	Unipen
Oxacillin	Prostaphlin
Methicillin	Staphcillin
Carboxypenicillins	
Carbenicillin	Geopen
Ticarcillin	Ticar
Ureidopenicillins	
Azlocillin	Azlin
Mezlocillin	Mezin
Piperacillin	Pipracil
Combinations with Beta-Lactamase Inhibitors	
Ampicillin/sulbactam	Unasyn
Amoxicillin/clavulanate	Augmentin
Ticarcillin/clavulanate	Timentin
Piperacillin/tazobactam	Zosyn

demonstrate variable resistance to degradation by bacterial beta-lactamases. Cephalosporins are ineffective against methicillin-resistant staphylococci (altered PBPs) and enterococci. Organisms resistant to most cephalosporins include methicillin (oxacillin)-resistant *Staphylococcus* species, *Enterococcus* species, *Xanthomonas maltophilia*, *Acinetobacter,* and *Clostridium difficile.* First-generation agents are often used in preoperative surgical prophylaxis.

The main advantages of cephalosporin therapy include their bactericidal nature, good half-life, good tissue distribution and penetration, oral activity, and relative safety. Disadvantages include inactivity against certain organisms and the fact that parenteral use is limited mainly to the intravenous route.

Adverse reactions include hypersensitivity or allergic reactions, minimal nephrotoxicity (do not potentiate toxicity of aminoglycosides), diarrhea with or without *C. difficile* colitis, impaired aggregation of platelets, interference with vitamin K metabolism, disulfiram reaction with alcohol, neutropenia, and potential thrombophlebitis. Agents of cautious use include cefamandole, cefmetazole, cefoperazone, cefotetan, and moxalactam. The last drug is no longer available in the United States.[10]

Classification of cephalosporins

The cephalosporins are usually classified by "generations." This classification is based on the general features of antibacterial activity. In addition, first-generation agents most closely resemble the penicillins in their chemical structure and should not be used in patients with known hypersensitivity to penicillins. The overall risk of developing allergic reactions to cephalosporins is about 10% for patients with any history of reaction to penicillins. Although all the cephalosporins are considered broad-spectrum agents, none has adequate activity against enterococci, methicillin-

resistant *Staphylococcus,* penicillin-resistant *Streptococcus pneumoniae,* and *Listeria.*[11]

The first-generation compounds have a narrow spectrum of activity focused primarily on the gram-positive cocci. First-generation indications include methicillin (oxacillin)-sensitive *Staphylococcus* species (penicillinase- and non-penicillinase-producing organisms); *Streptococcus* species (no *Enterococcus* species); gram-negative organisms, including *E. coli, P. mirabilis,* and *Klebsiella* species; and anaerobic organisms (no *Bacteroides* species).

Examples include Cefazolin (Ancef, Kefzol), cephalothin (Keflin, Seffin), cephapirin (Cefadyl), cephalexin (Keflex), cefadroxil (Duricef), and cephradine (Anspor, Velasef).

The second-generation compounds have variable activity against gram-positive cocci but have increased activity against gram-negative bacteria. Second-generation indications include methicillin (oxacillin)-sensitive *Staphylococcus* species (typically less active than first-generation agents, with exceptions), *Streptococcus* species, increased activity against elective gram-negative bacilli, including *H. influenzae, Klebsiella* species, and indole-negative *Proteus,* specific agents with activity against *Enterobacter, Serratia,* indole-positive *Proteus* and *Neisseria* species, and anaerobic organisms (including *Bacteroides*). There is no activity against *Pseudomonas* species.

Examples include cefamandole (Mandol), cefoxitin (Mefoxin), cefuroxime (Zinacef, Kefurox), cefotetan (Cefotan), cefonocid (Monocid), cefaclor (Ceclor), and ceforanide (Precef). In addition, cefuroxime axetil (Ceftin), is an oral agent in this class.

The third-generation compounds may be divided into two subgroups based on their activity against *Pseudomonas aeruginosa.* Drugs such as cefotaxime (Claforan), ceftizoxime (Cefizox), ceftriaxone (Rocephin), and cefixime (Suprax) are poorly active against *Pseudomonas* but retain broad activity against gram-positive cocci and gram-negative rods. In contrast, ceftazidime (Fortaz and Tazidime) and cefoperazone (Cefobid) are active against *Pseudomonas* and gram-positive rods but are less active against gram-negative cocci. None of the agents within this group is active against methicillin-resistant staphylococci, enterococci, or *Listeria.* The anaerobic activity of drugs in this class is comparable to cefoxitin.

The fourth generation of cephalosporins represents agents with unique combinations of antistaphylococcal and antipseudomonal activity. These agents have activity against gram-positive cocci and a broad spectrum of gram-negative bacteria, including *P. aeruginosa,* and the Enterobacteriaceae with inducible chromosomal beta-lactamases.

Examples include cefepime (Maxipime), which has superior activity against *S. pyogenes, S. aureus, S. pneumoniae,* and the Enterobacteriaceae. Cefpirome (investigational), a parenterally administered cephalosporin, has superior activity against streptococci, *S. aureus, Neisseria, H. influenzae,* and Enterobacteriaceae. Finally, cefpiramide (investigational) is less active than other third-generation cephalosporins against Enterobacteriaceae.

Routes of cephalosporin administration and dosage

A. First Generation
1. Cefazolin; IM, IV; 1-2 g q8h
2. Cephalothin; IV; 1-2 g q4-6h
3. Cephalexin; PO; 0.5-1 g q6h
4. Cefadroxil; PO; 500 mg q12h
5. Cephradine; PO; 500 mg q6h
B. Second Generation
1. Cefamandole; IM, IV; 1-2 g q6h
2. Cefoxitin; IM, IV; 2 g q6-8h
3. Cefuroxime; IM, IV; 0.75-1.5 g q8h
4. Cefuroxime; PO; 250-500 mg q12h
5. Cefotetan; IM, IV; 1-3 g q12h
6. Cefonocid; IM, IV; 1-2 g q24h
7. Ceforanide; IM, IV (investigational)
8. Cefaclor; PO; 250-500 mg q8h
C. Third Generation
1. Cefotaxime; IM, IV; 1-2 g q8h
2. Ceftizoxime; IM, IV; 1-2 g q8-12h
3. Ceftriaxone; IM, IV; 2 g q24h
4. Ceftazidime; IM, IV; 1-2 g q8-12h
5. Cefoperazone; IM, IV; 2 g q8-12h
6. Cefixime; PO; 400 mg q24h
7. Cefpodoxime; PO; 200-400 mg bid
8. Ceftibuten; PO (investigational)
D. Fourth Generation
1. Cefepime; IM, IV; 0.5-2 g q12h
2. Cefpiramide (investigational)
3. Cefpirome (investigational)

RELATED BETA-LACTAM ANTIBIOTICS

Carbapenems

Carbapenems are more closely related to the penicillins in their chemical structure than the cephalosporins. Carbapenems are derivatives of thienamycin, a compound produced by *Streptomyces cattleya*. There are two members of the class: imipenem-cilastatin (Primaxin) and meropenem (Merrem), which has recently entered the U.S. market. The former drug is composed of the active portion (imipenem) compounded with cilastatin, a molecule that prevents the destruction of imipenem in urine but has no antibacterial activity of its own.

The mechanism of action if imipenem includes its high affinity for PBPs of both gram-positive and gram-negative bacteria, subsequently producing cellular lysis. On the other hand, carbapenems show a postantibiotic effect (PAE), which is in contrast to penicillins and cephalosporins, and analogous to aminoglycosides and fluoroquinolones.

The spectrum of activity of carbapenems include aerobic gram-positive cocci, including methicillin-sensitive staphylococci as well as the streptococci and enterococci. They are not typically active against methicillin-resistant staphylococci, *Corynebacterium*, and some *Bacillus* species. Resistant species of enterococci have also been described. Activity against anaerobes is generally excellent, with the exception of *Clostridium difficile*. The carbapenems have excellent activity against aerobic gram-negative bacilli, including Enterobacteriaceae and *Pseudomonas*, including those species resistant to cephalosporins.

Carbapenems are resistant to most beta-lactams and have excellent tissue penetration. Their metabolism is primarily renal. They have little cross-resistance to other beta-lactams. Disadvantages of imipenem include cost, potential seizures in those with seizure history, potential GI upset (*C. difficile* colitis), and possible resistance when used as single therapy for *Pseudomonas* infection. Carbapenem may have a lower incidence of seizures than imipenem. Neither drug should be used in patients with known hypersensitivity to penicillin.[12]

Our recommendation is that these drugs should be reserved for severely ill patients or for those whose bacterial isolates are resistant to other available drugs. Appropriate indications include life- or limb-threatening infections, nosocomial infections, or polymicrobic infections that would otherwise require multiple other antibiotics. For patients with severe *Pseudomonas* infections, addition of an aminoglycoside for synergy should be considered. The recommended dose of imipenem is 0.5-1 g IV q6-8h for most patients with normal renal function. Dose adjustments are required for diminished renal function. The usual dose of meropenem is 1.0 g IV q8h, with adjustments for creatinine clearance below 50 ml/min.

Aztreonam (Azactam)

Aztreonam is a monocyclic beta-lactam with no appreciable antibacterial activity against gram-positive or anaerobic bacteria; its coverage is limited to gram-negative bacilli. It inhibits most Enterobacteriaceae and acts synergistically with aminoglycosides against *P. aeruginosa*. Indications include urinary tract infections (UTIs) lower respiratory tract infections, infections of the skin and soft tissue (including postoperative wounds, ulcerations, and burns), intraabdominal infections, and gynecologic infections. Since there is no cross-reactivity with other beta-lactam antibiotics, aztreonam can be safely used in patients with severe allergies to penicillin and cephalosporins. The usual dose is 1 to 2 g, q6-8h, IV or IM. The drug is not yet approved for pediatric use, but few significant adverse reactions have been reported.

THE QUINOLONES

The first of the quinolone antibiotics, an analogue of nalidixic acid, was a 1,8-naphthyridine structure identified by Lesher in 1962,[13] a synthetic compound not derived from fungi or molds. It took the combination of fluorine- and piperazine-substituted derivatives to renew interest in the compound.

TABLE 13-3 Quinolone tissue levels

Greater than Serum Levels

Urine
Kidney
Prostate
Feces
Bile
Lung
Neutrophils
Macrophages

Lower than Serum Levels

Saliva
Prostate fluid
Osseous
CSF

All quinolone derivatives in clinical use have a dual ring structure, with a nitrogen located at position 1, a carbonyl group at position 4, and a carboxyl group attached to the carbon atom at the third position of the first ring.[14]

Today, a broad spectrum of activity, good oral absorption, bactericidal nature, and good bone distribution with reliable GI tolerance have resulted in extensive clinical use of the fluoroquinolones. These agents work by inhibiting bacterial DNA gyrase (gyr A and gyr B), a topoisomerase that nicks and seals DNA in the process of transcription. Resistance may be caused by mutation, although plasmid resistance may be possible, though rare.[15]

Ciprofloxacin (Cipro) demonstrates a broad spectrum of activity against many gram-positive and gram-negative pathogens, Enterobacteriaceae, *Neisseria, H. influenzae,* and some *mycobacteria*. Although active against *Staphylococcus aureus* (both methicillin-sensitive and methicillin-resistant), it is not recommended for serious infections caused by this pathogen. Although some streptococci may demonstrate in vitro sensitivity to ciprofloxacin, penicillin remains the drug of choice. Anaerobic activity is also weak. Oxfloxacin may be better than ciprofloxacin against gram-positive cocci but slightly weaker against *Pseudomonas*.[16,17]

Clinical uses of fluoroquinolones include urinary tract infections, respiratory tract infections, GI infections, skin and soft tissue infections, osteomyelitis, and sexually transmitted diseases (Table 13-3). Several trials have demonstrated their successful use as prophylactic agents in granulocytopenic patients. These drugs should not be used for infections of the CNS. Because of their popular use, resistance is increasing, and many authorities recommend avoiding their routine use when other agents may be substituted.[18]

Use in pediatric or obstetric patients is precluded because of osteochondrosis. CNS toxicity, including convulsions, may occur in some patients, particularly the elderly when given high doses. The most frequent complaint is GI distress. Interference may also occur with hepatic metabolism of oral anticoagulants.[19] Recent reports of heel cord rupture with ciprofloxacin may be anecdotal and are not yet clinically proven.

Adverse drug interactions include: (1) theophylline, by inhibiting metabolism and clearance and increasing blood levels of theophylline; therefore, blood levels must be monitored and adjusted to avoid theophylline-related adverse reactions; (2) caffeine, by inhibiting caffeine clearance, increasing blood levels of caffeine; (3) antacids, iron supplements, and zinc supplements, which chelate with the quinolones and lower their absorption and serum levels; these drugs should not be taken 2 hours before or 2 hours after quinolone administration.[20]

The following quinolones are in clinical use or under developmental investigation, and may be classified in the following manner:

A. 4-Quinolones
   1. Norfloxacin
   2. Ofloxacin (Floxin)
   3. Lomefloxacin (Maxaquin)
   4. Sparfloxacin
B. Nalidixic acid
   1. Pefloxacin
   2. Ciprofloxacin (Cipro)
   3. Fleroxacin
   4. Tosufloxacin
C. Oxolinic acid
   1. Amifloxacin
   2. Enoxacin
   3. Clinifloxacin

Dosage and administration are as follows: ciprofloxacin: 250-750 mg q12h, not to exceed 1500 mg/day; ofloxacin: 400 mg bid (i.e., 400 mg every 12 hours).

VANCOMYCIN, TEICOPLANIN, AND RIFAMPIN

Vancomycin

Vancomycin (Vancocin) is a complex glycopeptide, with a weight of 1450 daltons, elaborated from the actinomycete *Streptomyces orientalis.* It inhibits bacterial cell wall synthesis. When the drug was first commercially introduced, one third of its impurities contributed to most adverse reactions. More currently, with better processing techniques, side effects have diminished greatly. Now there is no cross-resistance between vancomycin with other antibiotics, and resistance is rare.[21]

The vancomycin spectrum of activity consists of aerobic and anaerobic gram-positive organisms. It is bactericidal against most strains of staphylococci and nonenterococcal streptococci. It is bacteriostatic against most strains of enterococci. Vancomycin is effective against gram-positive organisms, including aerobic and anaerobic species. It is indicated in the treatment of infections due to methicillin-resistant *S. aureus* (MRSA) or *S. epidermidis* (MRSE). It is used in infections caused by staphylococci or streptococci in patients who are allergic to beta-lactams, antibiotic-associated enterocolitis caused by *C. difficile,* and infections, including those involving prosthetic devices or implants, caused by gram-positive organisms with multiple antibiotic resistance. It is also used in foot surgical prophylaxis if the patient is allergic to beta-lactam antibiotics or if surgery is performed at a center where MRSA and/or MRSE are problem pathogens. Vancomycin is 75% to 90% excreted by glomerular filtration, possess a long half-life, minimal toxicity, and good tissue penetration, and has rare allergic potential.

The disadvantages of vancomycin include slow parenteral administration (60 to 90 minutes). The drug is not readily absorbed orally, and oral administration is used only for treatment of *C. difficile* colitis. A unique adverse reaction is the "red man syndrome/reaction," which is characterized by an erythematous face, neck, and upper torso. A flush hot feeling with pruritus may occur, with hypotension. It is related to the speed of administration and is not a true allergy. Symptoms are relieved with antihistamines.

Other problems include pain and spasm and ototoxicity (auditory nerve, high-pitch hearing loss, irreversible deafness) and associated risks, which are increased with concomitant use of an aminoglycoside or other ototoxic drug. Nephrotoxicity, neutropenia, and chemical thrombophlebitis are possible (occurs in 13% of patients with peripheral venous cannulas).[22]

In the past, peak and trough serum levels were recommended to monitor vancomycin serum concentrations after a steady state had been achieved. Currently, the routine need for this sort of testing has been challenged, although no absolute recommendations can be made at this time.

Teicoplanin

Teicoplanin is a glycopeptide antibiotic derived from the fermentation process of *Actinoplanes teichomyceticus.* Typically used in gram-positive infections, teicoplanin is approved for investigational use in the United States. It has a longer half-life than vancomycin, is more lipophilic, and has few inactive metabolites. Toxicity, while similar to that of vancomycin, is less profound in all respects. Teicoplanin is potentially an effective alternative to vancomycin and may be useful for patients who have a vancomycin allergy. It has also been combined with PMMA beads and used for local implantation.

Administered once daily (400 mg IM or IV) in the treatment of MRSA infections, teicoplanin is thought comparable to vancomycin in efficacy. In combination with an aminoglycoside, teicoplanin may be a suitable alternative to ampicillin or penicillin G for the treatment of enterococcal infections.

The safe and effective daily use of teicoplanin makes it a potentially useful adjunct in the antimicrobial armamentarium if future clinical studies warrant.[23]

The rifamycins

Rifampin is a semisynthetic derivative of rifamycin B, a macrolide antibiotic produced by the mold *Streptomyces mediterranei* and first isolated in 1957. Rifampin is a zwitterion and exerts a bactericidal effect by inhibiting DNA-dependent RNA polymerase at the beta subunit. This mechanism of action prevents chain initiation but not elongation.

Rifampin possesses good activity against staphylococci and streptococci and all mycobacteria, and some gram-negative activity against *Neisseria* and *Haemophilus.* It is also useful in the treatment of brucellosis, *Legionella,* and rickettsiae. It has been used for infections due to resistant *Pseudomonas aeruginosa* and may be active against the fungi *H. capsulatum* and *Aspergillus.*

Rifampin penetrates abscess fluids better than most other antibiotics with similar antimicrobial activity. It is indicated in combination therapy with vancomycin, ciprofloxacin, or trimethoprim/sulfamethoxazole for treatment of MRSE or MRSA infections. It can also be used in treatment with other antistaphylococcal antibiotics (nafcillin, vancomycin, or azithromycin) against tolerant staphylococci. A recent uncontrolled study of rifampin combined with ciprofloxacin for the treatment of staphylococcal and streptococcal prosthetic implant infections was encouraging. The combination therapy leads to improved serum bactericidal levels against tolerant staphylococcal species. It may be used with other antistaphylococcal and antibiotics for treatment of chronic staphylococcal osteomyelitis, septic arthritis, endocarditis, vascular graft infections, and CNS shunts. Rifampin is also the drug of choice for prophylaxis of meningitis resulting from *Neisseria meningiditis* and *H. influenzae.*

Disadvantages of rifampin include a rapidly developing drug resistance, enhanced hepatic metabolism, and decreased half-life and effectiveness of medications that are detoxified by the liver (i.e., warfarin, digoxin, and oral birth control pills).

Rifampin is readily absorbed from the GI tract following oral administration. It distributes readily into tissues, including cerebrospinal fluid. Elimination is by hepatic cytochrome P-450 and therefore may increase the hepatic clearance of other drugs. No dose adjustment is required in renal failure.

Adverse reactions include an orange-red discoloration of body fluids and contact lenses and flu-like symptoms with a high maculopapular rash and transient elevation of transaminase. Severe hepatotoxicity occurs in about 0.6% of patients taking the drug. The dose schedule of rifampin is 600 mg PO q24h for adults and 10 to 20 mg/kg/day q12-14h for children.

Interestingly, rifampin has been used to treat a number of noninfectious conditions, such as biliary pruritus, rheumatoid arthritis and ankylosing spondilytis, Crohn's disease, and acute myelogenous leukemia. Newer synthetic rifamycins include Rifabutin (Mycobutin), an agent principally used in the prevention and treatment of *M. avium-intracellulare* infection in AIDS patients. Other agents include rifapentine, rifaximin, and the various benzoxazinorifamycins.[24]

TABLE 13-4 Recommended serum concentrations of selected aminoglycosides

	Daily Dosage		Serum Concentration	
	Loading Dose (mg/kg)	Total (mg/kg)	Divided into (doses given)	Peak/Trough (μg/ml)
Amikacin	5.0-7.5	15	q8h	20-30; 5-10
Gentamicin	1.5-2.0	3-5	q8h	4-6; 1-2
Netilmicin	1.5-2.0	3-5	q8h	4-6; 1-2
Tobramycin	1.5-2.0	3-5	q8h	4-6; 1-2

THE AMINOGLYCOSIDES

The aminoglycosides have been used to treat bacterial infections since the 1940s. Streptomycin was the first agent produced from *Streptomyces* sp., while neomycin, kanamycin, and gentamicin are natural fermentation products. Amikacin, netilmicin, dibekacin, and isepamicin are semisynthetic derivatives of the natural products. Nine aminoglycosides are currently available for commercial use in the United States. Some, such as paromomycin, have been used to treat protozoan pathogens, while others, such as spectinomycin, may be used to treat *N. gonorrhoeae*. Although all share the common potential adverse effects of nephrotoxicity, ototoxicity, and neuromuscular blockade, the prevalence of aminoglycoside resistance has remained low, and plasmid-mediated enzymatic modification is the most common mechanism of drug resistance. Although newer beta-lactam and fluoroquinolone antibiotics may share the same antibacterial spectrum, the efficacy and cost-effectiveness of the aminoglycosides, and the resistance problems encountered with newer agents, indicate a continued clinical need for them.[25]

Aminoglycosides are organic bases that are water soluble, existing as polycations at body pH and possessing molecular weights in the range of 445 to 600 daltons. Their polarity is an important determinant of their pharmacokinetics and toxicity. They are thermostabile, have a half-life of about 2 hours, possess satisfactory tissue distribution and penetration, and are excreted by the kidneys. All have an essential six-membered ring with the amino group substitute aminocyclitol. The moniker aminoglycoside results from the glycosidic bonds between the aminocyclitol and two or more non-amino-containing sugars.

Common characteristics of the aminoglycosides include poor absorption from the GI tract and limited binding to plasma proteins, with distribution primarily within extracellular fluid. The aminoglycosides exert bactericidal effects by inhibiting bacterial protein synthesis at the 30S ribosomal subunit. To reach the ribosomes, the aminoglycosides must penetrate the cell wall and bacterial cytoplasmic membrane. Their transport is significantly impaired in inflamed, anaerobic, or necrotic (hyperosmolar) environments. Uptake may be facilitated by beta-lactam antibiotics or vancomycin, and antimicrobial effects may be synergistic with antipseudomonal penicillins or third-generation cephalosporins. This combination provides augmented activity against a number of pathogens; however, penicillins may inactivate aminoglycosides in vitro and should not be mixed in the same solution or given through the same IV line. Dosing times should also be alternated.[26]

The aminoglycosides have a fairly broad spectrum, including some gram-negative cocci and, most importantly, enteric gram-negative bacilli. They are ineffective against anaerobic organisms, and their activity against enterococci is inadequate for single-drug therapy. Common indications for aminoglycosides include *Pseudomonas aeruginosa,* severe enterococcal infections, initial or definitive therapy for suspected or proven gram-negative rod infections with multiple organisms, mixed surgical infections, and use with antibiotic-impregnated PMMA beads.[27]

Because of their narrow therapeutic index, the serum concentrations of aminoglycosides generally must be monitored during therapy. Therapeutic drug monitoring ensures adequate antibiotic levels and lessens the chance of renal toxicity and ototoxicity.

The most commonly used aminoglycosides are listed below:

1. Gentamicin (Garamycin)
2. Streptomycin
3. Kanamycin (Kantrex, Klebcil)
4. Netilmicin (Netromycin)
5. Neomycin D (Mycifradin)
6. Tobramycin (Nebcin)
7. Amikacin (Amikin)
8. Sisomicin

Serum concentrations and dose

Aminoglycosides are distributed primarily within the extracellular fluid (ECF) compartment and eliminated almost entirely by glomerular filtration. Subsequently, various nomograms or formulas have been developed as a guide for the dosing of the aminoglycosides. Essential to most of these approaches is the assumption that aminoglycoside clearances are similar and can be estimated from creatinine clearances as a measure of renal function. Dosing strategies ultimately must provide peak and trough levels in the proper range. In general, the size of the dose is varied in order to adjust the peak level, and the dosing interval is varied in order to adjust the trough level. (See Table 13-4.)

Initially, the standard loading dose is based on the patient's ideal body weight. More precisely, the dose required to establish a desired serum level (C_{max}) can be estimated from the following formula: Dose = $C_{max} \times$ Vd (where Vd is an estimate of ECF fluid volume, which normally equals 25% of body weight).

Peak serum levels are obtained 30 minutes after IV administration. Therapeutic response is most likely if the peak/MIC ratio is at least 4, while trough serum levels are obtained within 30 minutes before the next dose.

Gentamicin and tobramycin peak values are 6 to 10 µg/ml, and trough values are less than 2 µg/ml. Amikacin has a peak value of 18 to 30 µg/ml, while its trough value is less than 10 µg/ml.

The maintenance dose can then be estimated by using three different but standardized methods.[28]

1. Since aminoglycoside clearance is dependent on glomerular filtration rate (GFR), one can assume that GFR equals creatinine clearance, according to the Cockcroft-Gault equation:

$$GFR\ (creatinine\ Cl) = \frac{(140 - age)(wt\ kg)}{72 \times serum\ creatinine\ (mg/dl)}$$

Then, daily dose = normal dose × creatinine Cl/100. For females, the creatinine clearance is multiplied by a factor of 0.85.

2. According to the nomogram of Sarrubi, the maintenance dose (as a percentage of the loading dose) may be determined on the basis of the patient's corrected creatinine clearance, C(c)cr(ml/min), where: C(c)cr male = 140 − age/serum creatinine; and C(c)cr female = 0.85 C(c)cr male; and the percentage of the loading dose required is based on the dosage interval. The nomogram predicts serum t½ based on a corrected creatinine clearance and translates this information to maintenance doses required to maintain desired peak serum levels.

3. Finally, the half-life of the aminoglycoside can be estimated from the creatinine clearance according to the following equation:

$$t\frac{1}{2} = \frac{0.69\ (Vd)}{Creatinine\ Cl}$$

The normal daily dose is then administered every three half-lives.

Unfortunately, pitfalls of nomogram reliance include varying pharmacokinetics, varying changes in Vd, and poor correlation between age-adjusted renal function and creatinine clearance (half-lives tend to be shorter in younger patients than older ones).[29]

Adverse effects

All aminoglycosides have the potential to produce nephrotoxicity and ototoxicity. In addition, they may potentiate neuromuscular blocking drugs or worsen symptoms in patients with neuromuscular disease.

Factors predisposing patients to nephrotoxicity include advanced age, preexisting renal disease, previous administration of aminoglycosides, prolonged administration, low blood volume, septicemia, concurrent nephrotoxic drug usage, concurrent loop diuretics, and concurrent high-dose cephalosporins, and a high trough value is more important than a high peak value for therapeutic efficacy. In this regard, gentamicin is probably more nephrotoxic than tobramycin and amikacin probably less than so than gentamicin or tobramycin.

Creatinine and blood urea nitrogen (BUN) may be monitored as a guide to renal impairment. Typically, serum creatinine is ordered before therapy, then roughly every other day, and a 0.4 mg/dl change indicates likely renal impairment. Serum blood urea nitrogen is a secondary test and is less specific for renal function than creatinine.

Factors predisposing patients to ototoxicity (cranial nerve VIII destruction is permanent, affects higher frequencies, and is derived from destruction of vestibular or cochlear cells) include advanced age, preexisting hearing loss, previous administration of aminoglycosides, prolonged administration of aminoglycosides, preexisting renal impairment, concurrent ototoxic drug usage, and renal dialysis. High trough value is more important than high peak value for monitoring, although ototoxicity is less dependent on serum concentration than nephrotoxicity.

Factors predisposing patients to neuromuscular blockade include general anesthesia with tubocurarine, succinylcholine, or similar agents. The blockade results from the presynaptic and postsynaptic release of acetylcholine. The blockade is rapidly reversed by using IV calcium gluconate, although the use of neostigmine is variable.[32]

Alternative dosing schedule

An alternative approach to aminoglycoside dosing involves its administration in large, single daily doses. This is designed to maximize the peak level, minimizing trough level and taking advantage of the drug's "postantibiotic" effect. This approach is particularly useful for patients requiring long-term therapy. Clinical studies have so far demonstrated clinical efficacy comparable with traditional multidose regimens, with less toxicity.

THE MACROLIDE AND LINCOSAMIDE ANTIBIOTICS

The macrolide antibiotics (erythromycin, azithromycin, clarithyromycin, and others) and the lincosamide antibiotics (clindamycin, lincomycin, and others) are not chemically related but possess similar biologic properties. Erythromycin is the most important macrolide but has few primary indications and is usually used as an alternative to penicillin G. Azithromycin and clarithromycin possess advantages over erythromycin in antimicrobial effects, pharmacokinetics, and the potential for use in certain AIDS-related infections. Clindamycin is important in the treatment of anaerobic infections, while lincomycin is mainly of historical interest.

Erythromycin

Erythromycin is the most important of the macrolide "large-ring" antibiotics. It was derived, in 1952, from a strain of *Streptomyces erythreus* obtained from soil in the Philippines. It consists of a 14-member macrocyclic lactone ring, attached to two sugar moieties (desosamine and cladinose).

Erythromycin is poorly soluble in water, has a pK of 8.8, and is rapidly degraded by gastric acid. Its serum half-life is 1.4 hours, and it is concentrated in the liver and excreted in the bile and feces.

Erythromycin inhibits bacterial RNA protein synthesis by binding reversibly to the 50S ribosomal subunit. The binding site is competitive with that of chloramphenicol and clindamycin, suggesting common binding sites for these agents.

Erythromycin is active against gram-positive cocci (except enterococci or methicillin-resistant staphylococci). Moderate activity is directed toward some gram-positive bacilli. Erythromycin is largely inactive against most aerobic gram-negative rods. It exerts primarily bacteriostatic effects and should not be used for serious infections, which generally should be treated with bactericidal agents.

Erythromycin is indicated for the treatment of skin and soft tissue infections due to streptococci and for minor staphylococcal infection of the cutaneous variety. It is the drug of choice for several dermatologic infections: erysipelas *(Streptococcus),* erythrasma *(Corynebacterium),* bullous impetigo *(Staphylococcus/Streptococcus),* and erysipelothrix *(Erysipelothrix insidiosa).* It is a poor alternative choice to penicillin in soft tissue infections. However, it is an alternative antibiotic for subacute bacterial endocarditis, as prophylaxis, and for recurrence of acute rheumatic fever. It is an excellent alternative oral antibiotic to amoxicillin for endocarditis prophylaxis and is also effective against *Clostridium tetanii* and *Bacteroides.* Lastly, it is the drug of choice against *Legionella* and is active against *Chlamydia* species.

Adverse effects include a rapid resistance developed by staphylococcal organisms during treatment, and the drug can elevate SGOT. It also may cause GI irritation and allergic reactions (fever, eosinophilia, skin eruptions), and the estolate formulation can cause cholestatic hepatitis. Pseudomembranous colitis has been occasionally reported with erythromycin use. Incompatibility during administration with other drugs has also been noted. These include vitamins B and C, colistin, cephalothin, tetracycline, heparin, metaraminol, chloramphenicol, midazolam, carbamazepine, theophylline, triazolam, and phenytoin.

Several preparations are available for oral use:

1. Erythromycin base (Ilotycin, Robimycin, Kessomycin, E-Mycin, Erytab, Eryc)
2. Erythromycin stearate (Bristamycin, Ethril, Pfizer-E, Erypar)
3. Erythromycin ethylsuccinate (Pediamycin, Erythrocin)
4. Erythromycin estolate (Ilosone)

Enteric-coated (E-Mycin) and timed-release (Eryc) preparations cause the least GI irritation. Food should be avoided for 1 hour before or after taking erythromycin base. Food is acceptable for salt and ester forms. The drug is not usually given intramuscularly because of pain on injection. However, erythrocin lactobionate is helpful in this regard, if administered slowly (30 to 60 minutes).

The usual dose of erythromycin is 250 to 500 mg q6h. As endocarditis prophylaxis, the usual dose is 1 g, 2 hours before the anticipated surgical procedure, and 500 mg q6h thereafter. It should not be used alone for the treatment of deep staphylococcal infections because of the potential for drug resistance. The drug should also not be given simultaneously with penicillin because of antagonism.

Dirithromycin (Dynabac)

This is a recently approved long-acting macrolide. It is approved only for patients older than 12 years with mild to moderate infections, such as acute exacerbations of chronic bronchitis, community-acquired pneumonia, upper respiratory infections, and uncomplicated skin and skin structure infections. It is given once daily with food at a dose of 250 mg per day. Its side effect profile, mechanism of action, and spectrum of activity are essentially identical to those of erythromycin.

Azithromycin (Zithromax)

In recent years, USPG Pfizer has spearheaded the search for a new macrolide antibiotic that has better oral absorption, a longer half-life, a greater spectrum of activity, and less GI distress than traditional erythromycin. Azithromycin (CP-62993) (Zithromax) seems to have some of these attributes. The agent is derived from erythromycin, having a methyl-substituted nitrogen in its 15-member lactone ring. Like the other macrolides, the agent is bacteriostatic and almost all MRSA or MRSE contaminants are resistant.[33]

Zithromax is indicated for uncomplicated skin and skin structure infections caused by gram-positive aerobes, such as *S. aureus, S. pyogenes,* and *S. agalactiae.* It is also used to treat gram-negative aerobic respiratory infections, such as *H. influenzae, M. catarrhalis,* and *C. trachomatis.* It should be given at least 1 hour before, or 2 hours after, a meal.

The mechanism of action of Zithromax is its unique intracellular concentration in phagocytes and fibroblasts. The ratio of intracellular to extracellular concentration is greater than 30 after a 1-hour incubation period.

Adverse reactions include mild cardiovascular palpitations, GI irritability, vertigo, and allergic photosensitivity with angioedema.

The recommended dosage of Zithromax, for patients greater than 16 years of age, is a single oral loading dose of 500 mg on the first day, followed by 250-mg doses on days 2 through 5, for a total of 1.5 g.[34]

Clarithromycin (Biaxin)

Another derivative of erythromycin is clarithromycin, which like azithromycin has improved oral absorption compared to the parent compound. Its mechanism of action is similar to that of the other macrolides, causing inhibition of RNA-dependent protein synthesis. Its spectrum of activity is similar to that of azithromycin, although it has less activity against *Mycobacterium avium-intracellulare,* unlike erythromycin. Bacteria resistant to erythromycin will also be resistant to azithromycin and clarithromycin.

The side effect profile of clarithromycin is similar to that of azithromycin. An increased number of drug interactions have been noted for clarithromycin compared to azithromycin. In particular, increased levels of carbamazepine and theophylline have been noted. Neither drug should be used with antihistamines, because of the risk of development of lethal cardiac arrhythmias.

Clarithromycin is indicated for the treatment of upper and lower respiratory infections caused by susceptible pathogens. It is also approved for uncomplicated skin and skin structure infections and for the treatment and prophylaxis of *Mycobacterium avium-intracellulare* infections. Its usual dose is 250 to 500 mg PO given twice daily.

Clindamycin (Cleocin)

Lincomycin was isolated, in 1962, from the organism *Streptomyces lincolnensis,* found in soil from Lincoln, Nebraska. Although lincomycin is now essentially abandoned, the related drug clindamycin (Cleocin) is prepared as the hydrochloride salt of its base and as a palmitate ester. Clindamycin inhibits bacterial protein synthesis by binding to the 50S ribosomal unit. Protein synthesis is thus inhibited in early chain elongation by transpeptidation interference.

Clindamycin possesses a good half-life (2.4 hours), has excellent tissue distribution and penetration (except CSF), and is available through IM, IV, oral, or topical administration. It is metabolized by the liver and voided through renal and biliary excretion. It can be combined and mixed with aminoglycosides in the same solution. Clindamycin should not be used concurrently with other antibiotics that act in a similar manner, such as erythromycin and chloramphenicol. Plasmid-mediated resistance has been reported in *B. fragilis* (5% to 25%).

Clindamycin has some limited activity against *B. fragilis* and other anaerobic microorganisms and gram-negative cocci, but not enterococci or methicillin-resistant staphylococci. It is used for soft tissue, decubitus ulcers and anaerobic bacteremia caused by *Clostridium perfringens, Fusobacterium,* or anaerobic (viridans) streptococci (alternative to penicillins in allergic patients). It may also be used in infections due to *S. aureus,* including osteomyelitis, as an alternative to beta-lactams. Essentially, all aerobic gram-negative bacilli are resistant. It is not used for MRSA, MRSE, or enterococcus infections. It has no activity against gram-negative aerobic bacteria or *Clostridium difficile.*

Adverse effects of clindamycin include *Clostridium difficile* toxin-mediated pseudomembranous colitis (1:2500). Interestingly, most cases are associated with penicillins (ampicillin) and cephalosporins rather than clindamycin. With clindamycin, the condition has a variable incidence and is diagnosed by stool cultures (high sensitivity: variable rate of false positives), although cytotoxin assay is highly specific but of moderate sensitivity. The demonstration of plaques on proctoscopy or sigmoidoscopy is diagnostic. Treatment is by discontinuing the precipitating agent, administering oral vancomycin (125 to 500 mg q6h for 7 to 10 days) or metronidazole (250 mg q6h for 10 days), and providing supportive therapy (fluids and electrolytes).[35] Cholestyramine (Questran) may be used to bind the toxin. Agents that inhibit peristalsis worsen the problem. Other side effects include GI distress, such as nausea, anorexia, vomiting, and diarrhea; hematologic changes; allergic reactions; and neuromuscular blockade.

Dosage and administration of clindamycin are as follows: oral, 150-450 mg q6-12h; IM, 150-900 mg q8h; IV, 600-2700 mg/day in 3 or 4 divided doses. Hepatic or renal disease requires cutting the dose by 50%.

Recently, clindamycin and primaquine have been used to treat AIDS-related *Pneumocystis carinii* pneumonia.

Metronidazole (Flagyl)

Metronidazole was developed in 1959 for the treatment of *Trichomonas vaginalis* infections. It is a nitroimidazole agent with the chemical formula 1-(2-hydroxyethyl)-2-methyl-5-nitroimidazole. It has a low molecular weight of 171.

Metronidazole is metabolized by bacterial nitroreductase (anaerobic), with production of short-lived, cytotoxic intermediates that disrupt bacterial DNA. It is bactericidal and also affects certain parasitic organisms. It has an excellent half-life (8 hours), possesses good tissue distribution and penetration, and is available for parenteral or oral administration.

Metronidazole is used to treat anaerobic infections due to gram-positive bacteria, such as *Peptococcus* (limited activity), *Peptostreptococcus* (limited activity), *Clostridium perfringens,* and *Clostridium difficile.* It is used to treat infections due to anaerobic gram-negative rods, such as *Bacteroides* and *Fusobacterium,* including septicemia, osteomyelitis, and septic arthritis. It is also used for other parasitic infections, such as giardiasis and amebiasis. It has limited activity against some anaerobic gram-positive cocci, and is inactive against aerobic gram-positive and gram-negative organisms.[36]

Metronidazole should be used cautiously in patients with hepatic disease; the dose may have to be reduced by 50%. In addition, the agent may produce a metallic taste, nausea, vomiting, diarrhea, headaches, paresthesias, reversible neutropenia, cutaneous eruptions, and convulsive seizures with peripheral neuropathy (rare).

A disulfiram-like reaction will occur, and therefore alcohol must be avoided. Metronidazole inhibits warfarin and interferes with certain chemical analyses for SGOT, with falsely low or negative values. Antacids, barbiturates, and cholestyramine decrease serum concentrations of the drug. In addition, *Clostridium difficile*–associated pseudomembranous colitis may occur rarely.[37]

Dosage and administration of metronidazole are as follows:

Oral: 1-2 g/day in 2-4 divided doses
Parenteral: loading dose, 15 mg/kg; subsequent doses, 7.5 mg/kg q6h

Resistance to metronidazole is plasmid and chromosomally mediated, but rare. Marginally resistant isolates include *P. bivia, P. malaninogenicus, B. ureolyticus,* and some *B. fragilis.* Several cases of metronidazole-resistant *T. vaginalis* have also been reported.

THE TETRACYCLINES AND CHLORAMPHENICOL

Tetracyclines

Chlortetracycline was discovered by Professor Benjamin M. Duggar, a meticulous mycologist, more than 50 years ago. He designated the organism *S. aerofaciens,* and named the first product Aureomycin.

The tetracyclines are sparsely indicated for bone and soft tissue extremity infections, but as broad-spectrum agents, they have in vitro efficacy against gram-positive and gram-negative organisms, some anaerobes, *Chlamydia, Mycoplasma,* and *Rickettsia.* The tetracyclines are effective orally, with variable absorption rates from the GI tract, in the following percentages: chlortetracycline (30%), oxytetracycline and tetracycline (60% to 80%), doxycycline (95%), minocycline (100%). All the tetracyclines inhibit bacterial protein synthesis by binding to the 30S ribosome subunit.[38]

In general, tetracyclines are not indicated for extremity infections except as an alternative in the treatment of clostridial infections in patients unable to tolerate penicillin G, or for actinomycosis in patients allergic to penicillin G. Additionally, these agents should not be used to treat staphylococcal, group A beta-hemolytic streptococcal, or *S. pneumoniae* infections, because of the occurrence of resistant strains. Resistance is plasmid mediated through coding for proteins that interfere with bacterial transport of the drug.

Today, there are three tetracycline analogs, based on differences in their pharmacology.

A. Short-acting agents
1. Chlortetracycline (Aureomycin): dose, 250 mg q6h; range, 1-2 g
2. Oxytetracycline (Terramycin): dose, 250 mg q6h; range, 1-2 g
3. Tetracycline (Achromycin, Tetracyn): dose, 250 mg q6h; range, 1-2 g
B. Intermediate-acting agents

1. Demethylchlortetracycline (Declomycin): dose, 150-300 mg q6-12h; range, 0.3-1.2 g
2. Methacycline (Rondomycin): dose, 150-300 mg q6-12h; range, 600 mg
C. Long-acting agents
1. Doxycycline (Vibramycin): dose, 50-100 mg q12h; range, 200 mg day no. 1, then 100 mg/day
2. Minocycline (Minocin, Vectrin): dose, 50-100 mg q12h; range, 200-mg loading dose, then 100 mg q12h.

There are few serious adverse reactions with the tetracyclines. Absorption is impaired by dairy products, aluminum hydroxide gels, and calcium and magnesium salts through the process of chelation. Tetracyclines are not indicated in children under 7 or 8 years and in pregnant women, because deposition in calcified tissue such as teeth and bone is possible. Hypoplasia of enamel and retardation of bone growth in human fetuses and children may occur. Adverse effects include gastrointestinal irritation, hepatic damage that may manifest as acute liver necrosis, phototoxic dermatitis, vestibular symptoms, and renal toxicity and azotemia. Cross-sensitization among the tetracyclines is universal. Minocycline can cause vestibular toxicity.

The tetracyclines are excreted in urine and feces. The half-life for tetracycline is 6 to 9 hours, except for doxycycline and minocycline, which have half-lives of 17 to 20 hours.

Chloramphenicol (Chloromycetin)

Like the early tetracyclines, chloramphenicol was discovered by screening organisms for their antimicrobial activity. Isolated by Burkholder from a mulched field near Caracas, Venezuela, the organism produced the active compound *Streptomyces venezuelae.* Chloramphenicol was introduced in 1949 and was one of the first agents whose chemical synthesis was economically feasible. Unfortunately, reports soon linked this highly effective agent with aplastic anemia, and it quickly fell into disfavor. Thiamphenicol, a related compound not producing aplastic anemia, is not available in the United States.

Chloramphenicol inhibits bacterial protein synthesis by binding to the 50S subunit, of the 70S ribosomal locus, which retards attachment of the aminoacyl-tRNA binding region unit. Binding is competitively inhibited by clindamycin and erythromycin. Plasmid-mediated resistance due to production of acetyltransferase enzyme has been reported. Plasmids may also code for resistance to tetracyclines and ampicillin. Chloramphenicol is a bacteriostatic agent, with a variable half-life (1.6 to 4.1 hours) and good oral absorption leading to wide distribution, with exceptional ability to penetrate lipid barriers, including the blood-brain barrier.

Chloramphenicol demonstrates a broad spectrum of activity, with relatively strong antimicrobial effects against a wide range of gram-positive (except MRSA, MRSE) and gram-negative bacteria, *B. fragilis,* chlamydiae, and rickettsiae. It has variable effectiveness against *Enterococcus.* Gram-negative bacterial exceptions include *Klebsiella, Enterobacter, Serratia, Acinetobacter,* and *P. aeruginosa.*[39]

Elimination of chloramphenicol is primarily hepatic via glucuronide conjugation. Neonates may develop "gray baby syndrome" as a result of low levels of glucuronyl transferase. This condition, which occurs in premature infants and newborns, is rare but potentially fatal; it is characterized by abdominal distention, cyanosis, and vasomotor collapse.

The "idiosyncratic" bone marrow aplasia (aplastic anemia [1 in 25,000 to 50,000]) associated with chloramphenicol is typically unpredictable; it occurs weeks to months after completion of the antibiotic, and the resulting pancytopenia is irreversible and typically fatal. There may be an associated reversible bone marrow depression, which is dose related (>4 g/day of 25 mg/ml serum levels) and may present as anemia, leukopenia, or thrombocytopenia. Furthermore, optic neuritis (3% to 5%) may occur in children, along with drug interactions based on inhibition of hepatic cytochrome P-450, causing a decrease in the hepatic clearance of oral hypoglycemics, rifampin, warfarin, or phenytoin.

The dosage in adults is 50 to 100 mg/kg/day in 3 or 4 divided doses (IV). The dosage in children and neonates is specialized. The serum concentration should be monitored closely in patients with hepatic dysfunction (10 to 30 g/ml is recommended).

Chloramphenicol is rarely indicated in bone or soft tissue extremity infections. Its use is restricted to seriously ill patients in clearly defined situations.

THE SULFONAMIDES AND TRIMETHOPRIM

The modern era of antibacterial therapy began in 1932 with the recognition of the protective properties of prontosil (sulfachrysodine) by Gerhard Domagk, a chemist in the German dye industry. During the next several decades, the basic sulfanilamide compound was altered to remove unwanted side effects. Further modifications resulted in compounds of more specific utility, such as 2,4-diaminopyrimidine (trimethoprim–not a sulfonamide), a structural analogue of para-aminobenzoic acid (PABA), which inhibits folic acid synthesis in bacteria. Antimicrobial effects are ultimately mediated by an inhibition of DNA and nucleic acid synthesis, as diagrammed below.[40]

$$\text{(Sulfa)} \qquad\qquad \text{(Trimethoprim)}$$
$$\text{PABA} \xrightarrow{\;-/\!/\;} \text{Dihydrofolic acid} \xrightarrow{\;-/\!/\;} \text{Folic acid}$$
$$\downarrow$$
$$\text{(Precursors)} \longrightarrow \text{Purines} \longrightarrow \text{DNA}$$

In the decade of the 1970s, the combination of trimethoprim-sulfamethoxazole (TMP-SMX) was made available in fixed combinations, demonstrating action against a wide variety of organisms. Resistance to sulfa is widespread and increasingly common in both community and nosocomial strains of bacteria, as well as *Actinomyces, Chlamydia, Plasmodia,* and *Toxoplasma.* Resistance typically may occur through mutated enzymes or elevated levels of bacterial PABA synthesis.

Topical sulfa agents are bacteriostatic and are used to slowly minimize the microcolinization of sensitive bacteria on wounds or burns, or after nail avulsions or chemical matrixectomy. Burns, rashes, or topical allergic reactions may occur. Topical agents include the following:
1. Sulfacetamide (Isopto, Cetamide)
2. Mafenide acetate (Sulfamylon)
3. Silver sulfadiazine (Silvadene)

The main indications for systemic sulfa drugs include soft tissue infections requiring broad-spectrum coverage when there is an allergy to other appropriate agents or when sensitivity studies find the infecting organism susceptible to TMP-SMX. Sensitive microorganisms include gram-positive and gram-negative cocci, many gram-negative bacilli, actinomycetes, and *Pneumocystis carinii.* However, these drugs demonstrate virtually no activity against anaerobes. Systemic (oral/parenteral) agents include the following:
1. Sulfisoxazole (Gantrisin, SK-Soxazole)
2. Sulfamethoxazole (Gantanol)
3. Sulfacytine (Renoquid)
4. Sulfamethizole (Thiosulfil)
5. Phthalylsulfathiazole (Sulfathalidine)
6. Sulfasalazine (Azulfidine)
7. Sulfadiazine

More specifically, trimethoprim-sulfamethoxazole (Septra, Bactrim) is primarily indicated as an alternative antibiotic in the treatment of infections due to staphylococci, including methicillin-resistant staphylococci (MRSA or MRSE); infections due to *Neisseria* and susceptible strains of *H. influenzae* and *S. pneumoniae;* and infections due to Enterobacteriaceae (as alternatives to beta-lactams or aminoglycosides). TMP-SMX may also be used in the neutropenic or immunosuppressed patient, as a prophylactic agent.

The mean half-life of these agents is 10 to 12 hours (normal renal function) with an optimal synergistic ratio is 1:5 to 1:4 (TMP/SMX). Sulfonamides are excreted in the urine.[41]

Dosage and administration are as follows:
A. Tablets
   1. 80 mg TMP/400 mg SMX
   2. 160 mg TMP/800 mg SMX (DS)
B. Oral suspension: 40 mg TMP/200 mg SMX per 5 ml
C. Dosage must be reduced in patients with renal insufficiency.
D. Usual adult dose: Septra DS or Bactrim DS, 160 TMP/800 SMX q12h, for 10-14 days

Adverse reactions of the sulfa drugs include skin and mucous membrane hypersensitivity, drug fever, serum sickness, and hepatitis. Although rare, severe dermatologic reactions, including Stevens-Johnson syndrome, Lyell's syndrome, and exfoliative dermatitis, may occur. Hematologic reactions include hemolytic or megaloblastic anemia. Sulfa drugs are contraindicated in patients with sickle-cell disease (trait), glucose-6-PD deficiency, or folic acid deficiency. They should not be used in infants less than 2 months old. Drug interactions are based on protein binding in agents such as warfarin, Coumadin, and oral hypoglycemics.

Resistance to trimethroprim is common, especially in the Enterobacteriaceae and *Shigella* and *Salmonella* spp.[42]

SYSTEMIC AND CUTANEOUS ANTIFUNGAL AGENTS

Griseofulvin

The systemic treatment of chronic noninflammatory ringworm conditions of the skin, hands, soles, feet, toenails, and hair is often preferred to topical treatment. Traditionally, griseofulvin has been the usual treatment because of its efficacy and low cost. Griseofulvin binds to fungal microtubules and is active against the various species of dermatophytes, such as *Microsporum, Epidermophyton,* and *Trichophyton.* The drug is deposited in keratinocytes, making these cells resistant to fungal invasion. In the skin, griseofulvin is delivered to the stratum corneum by sweat glands. Ketoconazole or itraconazole can be used for griseofulvin-resistant conditions, although candidiasis of the nails or skin is not responsive. For toenails, at least 6 months of therapy with one of the following is required:

1. Grifulvin V (250-500 mg bid)
2. Fulvicin P/G (165-330 mg bid)
3. Grisactin-Ultra (125-250-330 mg bid)

Monthly blood counts are recommended during prolonged therapy. Griseofulvin is contraindicated in patients with porphyria or hepatic dysfunction. It may also produce headaches or dizziness and may produce allergy photosensitivity with penicillin in allergic patients.

Ketoconazole

Ketoconazole (Nizoral) is a member of the imidazole group of antifungal agents, and oral absorption varies among individuals. Its antimycotic affects involve multiple sites, including inhibition of the synthesis or function of fungal cell membranes and intracellular accumulation of hydrogen peroxide. Although the drug is active in other systemic fungal infections, the most important use of ketoconazole is in the treatment of chronic mucocutaneous candidiasis. It is also approved for use in dermatophyte infections, fungal infections of the toenails, and cutaneous sporotrichosis. The usual dose is 200 to 400 mg/day, especially in patients allergic to iodide, although itraconazole may be a more effective agent in nonallergic patients. Adverse effects include hepatotoxicity and possible testosterone and cortisol suppression.

Itraconazole

Itraconazole may be used to treat ringworm, onychomycosis, candidiasis, and tinea versicolor. Available as Sporanox, in 100-mg capsules, a parenteral form is currently unavailable, but an oral suspension, Cyclodextrin, is under clinical investigation. The bioavailability of itraconazole is enhanced with food; rifampin and phenytoin decrease absorption, while Claritin and Seldane increase blood levels. Side effects include rash, pruritis, and decreased sexual function in males. Itraconazole should be avoided in pregnancy and used cautiously in patients taking the following drugs: amphotericin B, astemizole, calcium channel blockers, carbamazepine, cyclosporin, digoxin, isoniazid, midazolam or its derivatives, phenobarbital, phenytoin, quinine, rifampin, and warfarin.

Terbinafine

Terbinafine (C21 H26 CIN), slightly soluble in water and marketed as Lamisil, is indicated for the treatment of onychomycosis due to dermatophytes (*T. rubrum* and *T. mentagrophytes*). One 250-mg tablet daily is used for 6 weeks to treat fingernail infections and up to 12 weeks for toenail infections. Adverse reactions include GI, dermatologic, taste, visual, and liver alterations. Hepatic function studies are suggested in prolonged (>6 weeks) toenail conditions. Cautious use is suggested in patients taking cimetidine, phenobarbital, or rifampin.

Fluconazole

Fluconazole is well absorbed from the GI tract and, as Diflucan, is available in doses that range from 50 to 200 mg/day. Cutaneous sporotrichosis may respond to fluconazole, but data on ringworm or tinea versicolor are sparse. Side effects include diarrhea, rashes, and, in extreme cases, hepatic necrosis and Stevens-Johnson syndrome. Cautious use is suggested in patients taking astemizole, coumadin, oral contraceptives, rifampin, sulfonylureas, or theophylline.

INVESTIGATIONAL SYSTEMIC ANTIFUNGAL AGENTS

According to Hay, saperconazole and SCH 39304 are new triazole agents being tested for use in systemic fungal infections. Both combine good blood absorption with a broad spectrum of activity. Cilofungin, on the other hand, is a cell wall biosynthesis inhibitor active against a more narrow range of fungal agents, while nikkomycin which blocks chitin synthesis, is active against several different fungi, including *C. albicans.*[43]

TOPICAL ANTIFUNGAL AGENTS

One of the newest agents for the topical treatment of cutaneous superficial noninflammatory fungal infections of the pedal skin is butenafine HCl 1% cream (Mentax). Indicated for the treatment of tinea pedis caused by *E. floccosum, T. mentagrophytes, T. rubrum* and *T. tonsurans,* butenafine HCl cream has not been studied in immunocompromised patients. Reported side effects are minimal but may include erythema, irritation and itching in less than 2% of patients studied. It is not known if butenafine HCl is excreted in human milk, and its safety and efficacy in patients below the age of twelve have not been determined.

REFERENCES

1. Chambers HF, Neu HC: Penicillins. In Mandell GL, Bennett JE, Dolan R, eds: *Mandell, Douglas, and Bennett's principles and practice of infectious disease,* New York, 1995, Churchill Livingstone.
2. Corey SV: Penicillins. In Ruch JA, ed: *Reconstructive surgery of the foot and leg,* Atlanta, 1992, Podiatry Institute.
3. Chambers HF, Neu HC: Other beta-lactam antibiotics. In Mandell GL, Bennett JE, Dolan R, eds: *Mandell, Douglas and Bennett's principles and practice of infectious disease,* New York, 1995, Churchill, Livingstone.
4. Neu HC: Oral beta-lactam antibiotics (1960-1993), *Infect Dis Clin Pract* 6:394, 1993.
5. Weiss ME, Adkinson NF: Beta lactam allergy. In Mandell GL, Bennett JE, Dolan R, eds: Beta lactam allergy: In *Mandell, Douglas, and Bennett's principles and practice of infectious disease,* New York, 1995, Churchill, Livingstone.
6. Hopkins JM, Towner KJ: Enhanced resistance to cefotaxime and imipenem in *E. aerogenes, J Antimicrob Chemother* 25:49, 1990.
7. Martin DE: Imipenem-cilastatin and aztreonam. In Ruch JA, ed: *Reconstructive surgery of the foot and leg,* Atlanta, 1992, Podiatry Institute.
8. Ross CD: Imipenem/cilastatin: its use in the treatment of foot infection in the compromised host, *J Am Podiatr Med Assoc.* 78(7):361, 1988.
9. Gustaferro CA, Steckelberg JM: Cephalosporin antimicrobial agents and related compounds, *Mayo Clin Proc* 66:1064, 1991.
10. Karchmer AW: Cephalosporins. In Mandell GL, Bennett JE, Dolan R, eds: *Mandell, Douglas and Bennett's principles and practice of infectious disease,* New York, 1995, Churchill, Livingstone.
11. von Aksen U, Noller HF: Footprinting the sites of interaction in antibiotics, *Science* 260:1500, 1993.
12. Amin NM: New antibiotics: carbapenems, monobactams-quinolones, *Am Fam Physician* 38(3):125, 1988.
13. Asahina Y, Ishizaki KT: Recent advances in structure related relationships in new quinolones, *Prog Drug Res* 38:57, 1992.
14. Downey MS: Quinolones. In Ruch JA, ed: *Reconstructive surgery of the foot and leg,* Atlanta, 1992, Podiatry Institute.
15. Reese RJ, Maxwell A: DNA gyrase (structure and function), *Crit Rev Biochem Mol Biology* 26:335, 1991.
16. Dworkin R, Modin G, Kuntz S: Comparative efficacies of ciprofloxacin, perfloxacin and vancomycin in combination with refampin in a rat model of MRSA in osteomyelitis, *Antimicrob Agents Chemother* 34:1014, 1990.
17. Gotfried MH, Ellison WT: Safety and efficacy of lomefloxacin versus cefaclor in the treatment of acute exacerbations of chronic bronchitis, *Am J Med* 92(S-4A) 108-113, 1992.
18. LeFrock JL: Use of ciprofloxacin in podiatric medicine, *J Am Podiatr Med Assoc* 79:497, 1989.
19. Mouton Y, Leroy O: Efficacy of intravenous ofloxacin, *J Antimicrob Chemother* 26(S):115-121, 1990.
20. Ulmer W: Fleroxacin versus amoxicillin in the treatment of chronic bronchitis, *Am J Med* 94(S):136-141, 1993.
21. Lam S, Singer C, Tucci V: The challenge of vancomycin-resistant enterococci, *Am J Infect Control* 23:170, 1995.
22. Taylor C: Vancomycin and rifampin. In Ruch JA, ed: *Reconstructive surgery of the foot and leg,* Atlanta, 1992, Podiatry Institute.
23. Greenwood D: Microbiological properties of teicoplanin, *J Antimicrob Chemother* 21(A):1-3, 1988.
24. Tan JS, File TM: Diagnosis and treatment of staphylococcal disease, *J Am Podiatr Med Assoc* 79:492, 1989.
25. Downey MS: Aminoglycosides. In Ruch JA, ed: *Reconstructive surgery of the foot and leg,* Atlanta, 1992, Podiatry Institute.
26. Gilbert DN: Aminoglycosides. In Mandell GL, Bennett JE, Dolan R, eds: *Mandell, Douglas and Bennett's principles and practice of infectious disease,* New York, 1995, Churchill, Livingstone.
27. Marcinko DE: Gentamicin impregnated PMMA beads, *J Foot Surg* 24:116, 1985.
28. Dickinson BD: Antimicrobial agents of choice. In Marcinko DE, ed: *Medical and surgical therapeutics of the foot and ankle,* Baltimore, 1992, Williams & Wilkins.
29. Dickinson BD, Lipkin L: Pharmacology and anesthetics for the foot specialist. In Marcinko DE, ed: *Medical and surgical therapeutics of the foot and ankle,* Baltimore, 1992, Williams & Wilkins.
30. Joseph WS: Clinical and laboratory diagnosis of lower extremity infections, *J Am Podiatr Med Assoc* 79:505, 1989.
31. Corey SV: Antimicrobial selection. In Abramson C, McCarthy DJ, Rupp MJ, eds: *Infectious diseases of the lower extremities,* Baltimore, 1991, Williams & Wilkins.
32. Snow DA: Medical management. In Abramson C, McCarthy DJ, Rupp MJ, eds: *Infectious diseases of the lower extremities,* Baltimore, 1991, Williams & Wilkins.
33. Perronne C, Gikas A: Activities of sparfloxacin, azithromycin, temafloxacin and rifapentine compared with that of clarithromycin against multiplication of *M. avium, Antimicrob Chemother* 35:1356, 1991.
34. Clarithromycin and azithromycin, *Med Lett Drugs Ther* 34:45, 1992.
35. Yu GV: Clindamycin, metronidazole and chloramphenicol. In Ruch JA, ed: *Reconstructive surgery of the foot and leg,* Atlanta, 1992, Podiatry Institute.
36. Bartlett JG: Anti-anaerobic antibacterial agents, *Lancet* 2:478, 1992.
37. Oloff L: Clinical scenario of the fetid foot. In Marcinko DE, ed: *Medical and surgical therapeutics of the foot and ankle,* Baltimore, 1992, Williams & Wilkins.
38. Nikaido H: Outer membrane barrier as a mechanism of antimicrobial resistance, *J Infect Dis* 33:1831, 1989.
39. Dretler RH, Castellano BD: Antibiotic therapy in diabetic patients. In McGlamry ED, ed: *Reconstructive surgery of the foot and leg,* Tucker, Ga, 1988, Podiatry Institute.
40. Bartles RH, van der Spek JA: Acute pancreatitis due to TMP/SMX, *South Med J* 85:1006, 1992.
41. Ray A, Newton V: Use of chromatography to monitor stability of tetracyclines and chlortetracycline in susceptibility determination, *Antimicrob Agents Chemother* 35:1264, 1993.
42. Miller SJ: Sulfonamides. In Ruch JA, ed: *Reconstructive surgery of the foot and leg,* Atlanta, 1992, Podiatry Institute.
43. Hay RJ: Antifungal drugs on the horizon, *J Am Acad Dermatol* 31(5): 82-86, 1994.

ADDITIONAL READINGS

Chiritescu MM, St Chiritescu ME, Scher RK: Newer systemic antifungal drugs for the treatment of onychomycosis, *Clin Podiatr Med Surg* 13(4):741-758, 1996.

Edin ML, Miclav T, Lester GE: Effects of cephazolin in osteoblasts, in vitro, *Clin Orthop Rel Res* 333(12):245-251, 1996.

Friedman C: A brave new world of information and communication for infection control professionals, *Am J Infect Control* 24(6):417-420, 1996.

Isiklar ZU, Darouiche RO, Landon GC: Efficacy of antibiotics alone for orthopedic device related infections, *Clin Orthop Rel Res* 332(11): 184-189, 1996.

Joseph WS, Kosinski MA: Prophylaxis in lower extremity infectious diseases, *Clin Podiatr Med Surg* 13(4):647-660, 1996.

Joseph WS, LeFrock J: The use of oral antibiotics in lower extremity infections, *Clin Podiatr Med Surg* 13(4):683-700, 1996.

Kushwaha VP, Shaw BA, Gerardi JA: Musculoskeletal coccidioidomycosis: a review of 25 cases, *Clin Orthop Rel Res* 332(11):190-199, 1996.

Midgley G, Moore MK, Cook JC: Mycology of nail disorders, *J Am Acad Dermatol* 315:68-74, 1994.

Moussa FW, Gainor BJ, Angelen J: Disinfecting agents for removing adherent bacteria from orthopedic hardware, *Clin Orthop Rel Res* 329 (8):255-262, 1996.

Recommendations for preventing the spread of vancomycin resistance: recommendations of the Hospital Infection Control Practices Advisory Committee (HICPAC), *Am J Infect Control* 23:87, 1995.

Reyes C, Barnauskas S, Hetherington V: Retrospective assessment of antibiotic and tourniquet use in ambulatory foot surgery, *J Foot Surg* 36(1):55-62, 1997.

Simeds ST, Goertzen D, Ivarsson D: Influence of temperature on mixing bone cement properties, *Clin Orthop Rel Res* 334(1):326-334, 1997.

Tan JS, File TM: Management of staphylococcal and streptococcal infections, *Clin Podiatr Med Surg* 3:4, 793-810, 1996.

Thakor K, Glatt AE: Vancomycin resistant enterococci, *Clin Podiatr Med Surg* 13(4):661-670, 1996.

14

Wound Healing, Surgical Decompression, and Soft Tissue Coverage in the Infected Foot

David Edward Marcinko
Rachel Pentin-Maki

I look back upon my medical studies as the school which taught me, in a more penetrating and convincing way than any other, the eternal principles of scientific work, principles so simple yet continually forgotten, so clear and yet so ever shrouded by a deceptive veil. Helmholtz

The basic rules for treating most foot infections are (1) appropriate clinical recognition, (2) correct laboratory and radiographic analysis, (3) accurate cultural data, and (4) judicious surgical debridement, drainage, and wound closure. This chapter will describe the surgical drainage, debridement, and wound closure techniques that are useful in treatment of the infected foot.

THE INFECTED FOOT: ACUTE PHASE

In the acute phase of any well-perfused foot infection, especially with a known or suspected abscess formation, the simplest approach to surgical treatment is debridement. Without proper incision and drainage of abscesses or infected spaces, all other adjuncts to care may be to no avail. Decompression may involve the removal of sutures or the release of purulence from the wound. It also may entail the deep removal of any implant device, fixation hardware, or other possible foreign body or focus of infection. Prosthetic implant infection is classified into three types: (1) An "acute infection" (occurring within the first 4 to 6 weeks of surgery) presents with the cardinal signs of inflammation. Radiographs are normal, but the erythrocyte sedimentation rate (ESR) or C-reactive protein (CRP) may be elevated. A differential diagnosis is hematoma, but conformational diagnosis is through aspiration and cultural data. (2) A "delayed acute-onset" infection (signs occur after a year of normalcy) presents with an acute attack of first metatarsophalangeal joint pain, with normal radiographs but an elevated white blood cell (WBC) count. Again, joint aspiration confirms the diagnosis. (3) Finally, a "chronic infection" (present longer than 4 to 6 weeks without acute

signs and symptoms) presents with a history of inflammatory changes for many weeks. ESR and WBC changes may be seen, along with an open or draining sinus tract. Radiographs may or may not be normal, and bone scans may be positive in many cases.

Generally, the suspicious fixation or implant device is left intact if deemed clinically stable, and removed if unstable. This is performed in order to allow unhindered drainage of infected exudates in the foot and reduce the likelihood of occult infection. However, since the excision of an infected implant prosthesis may prove problematic, its fate may be subject to the algorithm shown in Table 14-1 for consideration.

It cannot be overstressed that adequate and extensive drainage and debridement of necrotic tissue are essential. This usually means a trip to the operating room to have the procedure performed under sterile conditions. General or local anesthesia (generally without epinephrine) is most commonly used, with the infiltrative block administered well away from the site of active infection. Tourniquets are not typically used.

The incision should be linear and sloped to form a trough for ease of postural drainage. The often ill-conceived notion of foot elevation counters this concept and may involve the patient resting in a prone position to encourage gravity drainage. It makes no sense to elevate a foot to allow infected exudates to travel through tissue planes proximally, and possibly infect uncontaminated rearfoot, ankle, or lower leg tissue planes. Normal post-inflammatory edema will subside naturally with proper decompression, antibiosis, and debridement. Typical incision placement sites following routine foot surgical procedures may extend from the first or

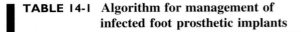

TABLE 14-1   Algorithm for management of infected foot prosthetic implants

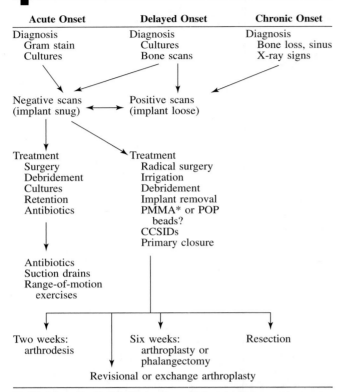

Modified from Gustilo RB: Management of infected total knee replacement. In Gustillo RB, ed: *Orthopedic infection: diagnosis and treatment,* Philadelphia, 1989, WB Saunders.
PPMA, Polymethyl methacrylate; *POP,* plaster of Paris; *CCSID,* continuous closed suction-irrigation drain.

lesser metatarsophalangeal joints, to the interdigital toe web spaces, over the dorsum of the foot to the arch area or around the heel, anterior ankle, or posterior leg. Segments of necrotic extensor or flexor tendons, as well as plantar fascia or muscles, may even have to be removed to expose the depths of the infection or to permit adequate drainage of tendon sheaths or tissue planes.[1-4]

Soft tissue, fascial, and tendon debridement is the prime prerequisite to eventual wound healing and recovery after the infectious process has occurred. These tissue are not vital, because of their poor vascular status, and can usually be removed without serious adverse effects. A pulsatile irrigation system enhances debridement of infected tissues. The criteria for infected muscle debridement are based on four parameters: consistency, contractility, perfusion, and color. Osseous structures are very dependent upon an intact blood supply, which entails both the macrocirculation and the microcirculation. Therefore, bone as well as any other tissue that does not bleed when incised is necrotic, and should be removed. Saucerization or exteriorization is performed to bevel bone edge surfaces, to promote tissue coverage at a later date.

Stabilization of osseous fragments is done with external fixation devices, placed proximal and distal to the affected bone margins, well away from the site of infection. Rigid fixation provides favorable conditions for infected fractures, because of the potential for primary bone healing, minimal sequestration, and less bone resorption. Osteosynthesis (AO/ASIF) material is used with caution.

Avascular bone, cartilage, and joints tolerate infection poorly, and ultimately the infected bone in the digits or feet may have to be resected. Until the ultimate decision is made by the attending clinician or consultant as to salvage or amputation, the aim and first priority is to provide proper dependent drainage to the affected part(s).

At times, a necrotic toe or ray may be associated with an abscess around its metatarsophalangeal joint and be the cause of cellulitis or lymphangitis as it streaks up the leg. This usually occurs on the medial aspect of the foot or ankle and involves the medial saphenous vascular and lymphatic tree. However, when cellulitis exists at some site proximal to the focus of infection, one must resist the urge to incise and drain the area. Injudicious surgery in the face of cellulitis is contraindicated and can do more harm than good by spreading the infection and prolonging recovery from iatrogenically induced open wounds. In the event of cellulitis without abscess formation, it is acceptable to infiltrate a small amount of sterile saline subcutaneously, and then evacuate the specimen for cultural examination. Of course, prior to complete localization and "pointing" of an abscess, warm Turkish towels, dependency, and bed rest are ideal aids to hasten the localization process.

At other times, when a gangrenous digit is associated with a mummified dry black toe or a weeping cyanotic wet toe, the patient is best served by resecting the digit itself with its associated bones and joints. Such removal of a toe or ray must properly be considered radical debridement, for it is not an amputation in the true sense that the wound is expected to heal by first intention. Of course, such stumps and rays will heal in time, but the prime objective of the surgery is to remove necrotic tissue and bone as well as drain infection fluids.

It is obvious that most foot infections do not require the extensive salvage surgery described here. However, the basic principles must always be remembered. Once the foot has been surgically decompressed, and if delayed primary or tertiary healing is not anticipated, the next step in recovery involves daily debridement in the office or hospital setting. If pain is a deterrent to this therapy, then proximal wound blocks, nitrous oxide sedation, ketamine, or intravenous agents such as diazepam may be used. Periodically, the patient may even be returned to the operating room for additional debridement, for as many times as needed. Chemicals, enzymatic agents, and whirlpool baths also aid in the cultivation of granulation tissue. Care must be taken when using whirlpools to prevent additional waterborne contaminants such as gram-negative infections.

Liberal wound irrigation is also a helpful but often neglected portion of the daily debridement regimen. Various solutions may be used, such as normal sterile saline, hydrogen peroxide, or povidone-iodine in a concentration of 1%. When *Pseudomonas* is involved, weak acetic acid (vinegar) solution will inhibit the growth of organisms via changes in pH. If the wound cavity is significant in size with a large "dead space," open wound packing with sterile gauze impregnated with iodophor or some other antiseptic that is not irritating to delicate granulation tissue is indicated.

The encouragement of fluid removal through the use of various wicks, drains, or gauze strips is also beneficial. Of course, daily wound debridement is done by the attending surgeon, rather than the nursing staff, and strict sterile conditions must be maintained. The wound must never be exposed to the contaminated air for more than a brief period, and desiccation must be avoided at all costs. This can be accomplished through the use of wet-to-dry dressings, applied two or three times daily.

Once granulation tissue begins to flourish, periodic Gram stains and cultures are needed to evaluate wound progress in anticipation of healing by second intention, delayed primary closure, or skin grafting techniques.[4]

Finally, philosophical considerations of the foot specialist inherently seem to favor the above limb salvage techniques rather than amputation. Although these techniques are more risky, painful, time intensive, and cost intensive, most specialists and patients opt for an attempt to save the limb rather than remove it. Whether such heroic measures are appropriate in all cases is a societal question (Fig. 14-1).

THE INFECTED FOOT: CHRONIC PHASE

Once wound cultures prove less serious, temperature and laboratory parameters normalize, granulation tissue growth commences, and the patient clinically improves, the final stage of local wound management may begin. Essentially, this involves three healing possibilities: (1) second intention, (2) delayed primary closure, and (3) skin grafting techniques.

Healing by second intention

Healing by second intention is the most predictable method in the terminal phase of wound healing. It is also the most damaging, frustrating, time consuming, economically devastating, and traditional method of postinfection wound repair. As we have seen, in this method the wound is simply allowed to granulate in until closed, providing adequate blood supply is available. It produces fibrous adhesions to directly involved, as well as indirectly involved, vital other structures. In many cases, dense scarified tissues may laminate or glue together vital structures, rendering the body part functionless or disfigured. Unfortunately, however, it still seems to be the most medicolegally sound course of action to pursue following infected cases, since it is known that the risk of acute infection is decreased with a packed wound, although chronicity is another matter. On the other

hand, a primarily closed wound does gain resistance to infection, from subsequent colonization, faster than one that is left open. It is especially feasible in the case of a small wound, such as one that follows digital or lesser metatarsal surgery. Frequently, follow-up care can be nicely rendered in the outpatient, office, or home setting.[5]

Delayed primary wound closure

Again, delayed primary closure refers to the suturing of a previously infected wound. Usually this means a wound rendered clean but not necessarily sterile, with no overt bone contamination. The procedure may involve several weeks of hospitalization and parenteral antibiotics in preparation for the closure. It may also involve the "freshening" and undermining of wound margins in order to mobilize adjacent soft tissue structures. Negative serial cultures are not required prior to closure, since such a wound might rightly be considered culturally contaminated but not clinically infected.

The wound is usually closed *per primam* with nonbraided and nonabsorbable suture materials, preferably with simple or horizontal mattress sutures and with absolutely no wound tension on fragile edges. Infectious disease consultation is highly desirable when one is contemplating the delayed primary closure of a wound, since timing is of critical importance.[4,5]

SKIN GRAFTING AND PLASTIC SURGICAL TECHNIQUES

The history of skin grafting dates back to the early 1880s. A skin graft is properly defined as transplanted tissue that has been detached from a donor site and moved to a recipient bed. Skin graft nomenclature includes the following types: (1) autograft (tissue transplanted from one site to another on the same individual); (2) isograft (tissue transplanted between genetically identical individuals); (3) allograft or homograft (graft between two individuals of the same species); and (4) xenograft or heterograft (graft between two different species).

Skin for grafting purposes is available from several body sites, including the top of the foot, the lateral malleolus, the popliteal fossa, and the inguinal ligament region. The elasticity, color, thickness, and durability of the skin vary with site, age, and sex. The dermal skin layer comprises most of the actual skin thickness and contains various skin appendages, such as hair follicles and sebaceous and sweat glands.

Skin grafting of a previously infected wound is performed when an extensive amount of soft tissue has been lost and the wound is not considered to be colonized by pathogenic bacteria. The acquisition of a uniform and regular bed of granulation tissue is of utmost importance, since it is the single most important factor for graft survival or "take." Characteristics of an ideal bed include well-vascularized granulation tissue and maintenance of intimate contact with

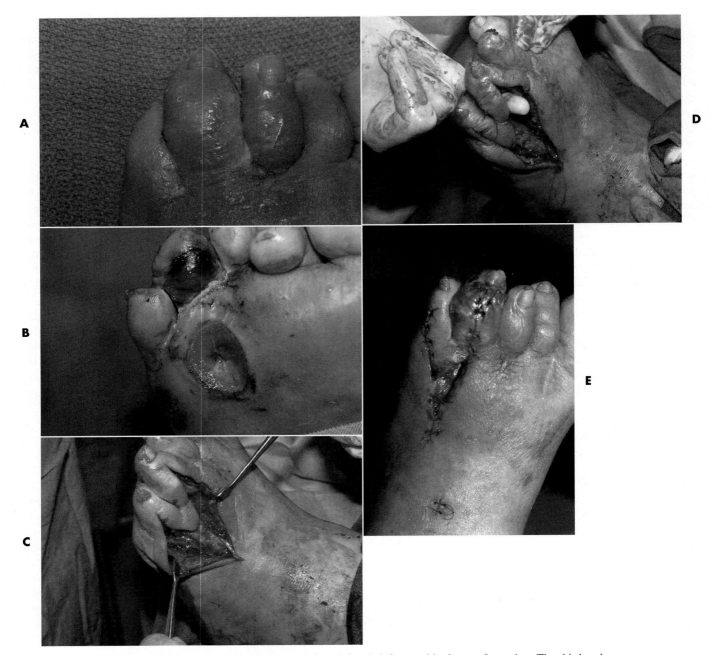

Fig. 14-1 A, Dorsal view of acute infected fourth left toe with abscess formation. The third and fifth toes and the entire forefoot are red, warm, and swollen. **B,** Plantar view of fourth toe pulp abscess and vascular compromise due to increased compartmental space pressure. Full-thickness ulceration, tracking to bone, connects to the web space wound. Purulent drainage is noted. **C,** The forefoot and respective fourth and fifth rays are surgically explored. **D,** "Finger probe" technique demonstrates through-and-through nature of irrigation and drainage. **E,** Fourth and fifth toes are sutured closed. The proximal incision was packed and left open to drain. Wounds subsequently healed without incident.

the graft until mature. A skin graft cannot be applied directly to bare bone or tendinous tissue because a delicate interface is needed for vascularization. Once cultivated, however, virtually any tissue type with a vascular and granulating stroma may be an acceptable bed for a skin graft. The wound is grafted with a split- or full-thickness skin graft, harvested

from the contralateral anterior thigh and applied dermal side down on the recipient bed. It can be sutured in place or can be affixed with adhesive plastic strips or a Vaseline-impregnated gauze dressing.

The process of graft survival are divided into three phases: (1) fibrin adhesion immediately after placement on the recipient bed, (2) plasmatic absorption for initial graft nourishment, and (3) inosculation that reestablishes new circulation within the graft, after 48 to 72 hours. Factors adverse to graft survival include the following:

1. Movement: disrupts vascular attachments; however, a bridging phenomenon may occur over a small area less than 0.5 cm in diameter.
2. Hematoma or seroma: fluid under the graft may lead to necrosis as well as movement. If a hematoma or seroma is identified early, "rolling" or aspiration may be performed to evacuate the contents and prevent the graft from floating away.
3. Infection: skin grafts are particularly prone to water-loving *Pseudomonas* sp. and cellulitis-producing streptococcal organisms. Ironically, grafting over an open or granulating wound may actually reduce bacterial counts and serve to prevent an infection by acting as a biologic barrier.

Split-thickness skin grafts

A split-thickness skin graft (STSG) consists of the epidermis and variable portions of the dermis. Depending on the amount of dermis present, the STSG can be classified as thin (0.008 to 0.0012 inch), medium (0.012 to 0.016 inch), or thick (0.016 to 0.020 inch). A full-thickness skin graft (FTSG) contains the epidermis and entire dermal layer. An STSG is more likely to survive than an FTSG but may leave an unsightly scar and is less durable than its full-thickness counterparts. STSGs are usually harvested with a pneumatic or electric dermatome from the anterior thigh, fenestrated, and applied dermal side down on the wound, after perforation. Small portions of skin may be taken freehand with a straight razor or Humby knife.

The technique used with a power dermatome first lubricates and tenses the skin with sterile mineral oil. The blade is then advanced slowly, with uniform pressure and speed. As the cut skin is peeled away, an assistant grasps it to prevent folding in front of the dermatome blade and shredding of the freshly harvested graft. Local anesthesia is used for donor site acquisition, and the specimen is perforated for drainage. It may also be stored for future use, under moist refrigeration at 0° to 5° C. The donor site is covered with a nonstatic dressing and typically is more painful to the patient than the recipient bed. A vascularized donor site may be ready for reharvesting in about 3 weeks.[6] If a larger area must be grafted, the graft can be "piecrusted" or "crosshatched" with a mesher to increase its surface area and allow fluid seepage. Once the graft site is healed, a molded shoe can be fabricated to prevent irritation and protect the friable site. The technique is economically advantageous and psychologically palatable and fosters a more rapid period of rehabilitation. Skin graft cosmetic results are superior to healing by second intention but generally less pleasing than a delayed primary wound closure. Obviously, the technique is available only to the experienced foot surgeon.[8]

Full-thickness skin grafts

As noted, full-thickness skin grafts differ from split-thickness skin grafts in that the latter are more likely to survive and the former are more cosmetically acceptable. Furthermore, a full-thickness graft is more likely to contract but also provides a more durable surface. Typical donor sites include the dorsum of the foot, the malleoli, and the inguinal fold. Anatomically, the graft is composed of both the dermis and the epidermis, which contains the protein elastin, which increases durability.[7]

When the graft is harvested, a surgical template is used to mark the necessary pattern, although a bit more skin is usually taken than needed; as the elastin produces a degree of contractility to the graft and some shrinkage occurs. The specimen is denuded of its fat and placed dermal side down over the wound. Because the graft is full thickness, the blood vessels available for ingrowth are relatively large and few in number. It is then dressed with a stent bandage, and examined within 72 hours.

Skin flaps

A skin flap is a segment of subcutaneous tissue that is transferred to restore a soft tissue defect, but remains permanently or temporarily attached to the donor site for blood supply. The base of the flap, which contains the blood supply, is called the pedicle. There are three basic types of skin flaps:

1. A "random" flap is vascularized from the random intradermal and subdermal plexus. Because of perfusion limitations, a random flap can supply only a fixed length of tissue regardless of its base, with approximately a 1:1 length-to-width ratio. It therefore has limited use.
2. An "axial" flap consists of an artery and a vein that are incorporated into the pedicle. This increases perfusion and may be useful in digital or metatarsophalangeal joint infections. Essentially, the appropriate toe is filleted and used for wound coverage.
3. An "island" flap is similar to an axial flap, except that the soft tissue and vascular elements have been removed to increase mobility, as it may be rotated through an arc of 180 degrees or more.

Muscle flaps

Local muscle flaps, for the secondary closure of chronic wounds, have been used since the 1920s. Most treatment areas are in the axial skeleton, or in the femur or tibia. The gastrocnemius or soleus muscles are most commonly used.

Specialized skin flaps

Three additional flap techniques may be used in the foot, following certain infection and wound defect types.

1. The "neurovascular island" flap contains a nerve located within the vascular plexus. This flap maintains tactile sensation and is being increasingly used in foot surgery.

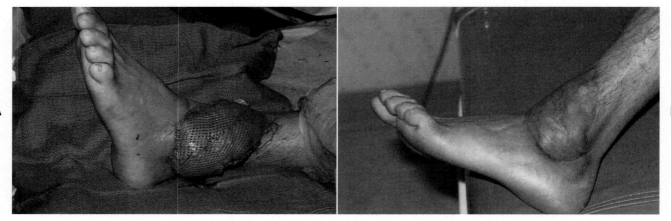

Fig. 14-2 **A,** Muscle free flap from latissimus dorsi covered with split-thickness skin graft. **B,** Same patient healed, with typical bulky contour. *(Courtesy Dr. Thomas J. Merrill, Barry University School of Podiatric Medicine, Miami Shores, Fla.)*

2. The "myocutaneous" (musculocutaneous) flap is a special anatomic variation that permits the transfer of a portion of the muscle underlying the skin on a single neurovascular pedicle. The tissue may be used as an axial or island flap, or it can be detached and transferred as a free flap to cover a peripheral defect in a single procedure. As example of this flap type is a "cross-leg flap" (Fig. 14-2).

3. The "tree" flap is an axial flap in which the blood supply has been severed and the flap transferred to its recipient site. Circulation is reestablished by microvascular anastomosis of its respective artery and vein. There is generally a 20% risk of flap loss with this type of transfer, and many wound defects can be adequately managed with the other types of techniques.

Viability of skin flaps

Unlike the situation with skin grafts, the usual cause of flap failure is vascular embarrassment, produced by mechanical tension, excessive edema, restrictive bandages, or tight sutures. Flap viability may be evaluated through clinical appearance, Doppler ultrasound, fluorescein dye, and digital plethysmography. Treatment is symptomatic but usually fails if vascular embarrassment is not recognized early.

Miscellaneous skin graft techniques

Small full-thickness "postage stamp" grafts are used to "pepper" a wound defect and allow epithelialization to fill in remaining spots. Larger, rotational pedicle and bilobed skin flaps are used for localized defects left by the infectious process.

A dermal (reverse) overlay graft is used when circulation will not support an STSG. First, the STSG is harvested and the dermis removed. The STSG is placed over the donor site, and the remaining dermal graft is reversed and placed over the recipient bed with its superficial layer facing down. Five to seven days later, another STSG is placed over it and allowed to heal. This procedure is only occasionally used in foot surgery.

Finally, the concept of soft tissue expansion, through the use of soft tissue expanders (stretchers), is increasingly being used to cover soft tissue defects. In this technique, deflated plastic silicone balloons are inserted under the subcutaneous tissue layer, but above the fascial plane. The bladders are then slowly expanded, to allow the overlying tissue to adapt and respond to the challenge. Upon removal of the bladder, the redundant tissue is harvested for immediate or later use. The surgical site is then primarily closed.

INFECTED SURGICAL OR TRAUMATIC NONUNIONS

The case of an iatrogenic or traumatic nonunion of the foot is indeed a complex one. Much has been published in the medical literature about various treatment regimens. According to Gustillo, they can be distilled into the following general principles[9]:

1. Radical debridement of infected and necrotic bone and surrounding soft tissue structures
2. Achievement of fracture stability, especially with external hardware fixation devices placed proximal and distal to the break
3. Promotion of granulation tissue and abundant cancellous bone grafting to fill large skeletal defects
4. Frequent dressing changes for proper wound toilet
5. Skin and soft tissue coverage, through the techniques just described
6. Avoidance of weight bearing until the fracture has healed
7. Appropriate antimicrobial therapy, through any of the vehicles described in the next chapter

CONCLUSION

The surgical treatment of the infected foot entails many different surgical, medical, mechanical, and physiologic processes. These often begin with the normal or abnormal stages of wound healing, progress to the acute and/or chronically infected phases, and usually terminate with different types of plastic or reconstructive surgical techniques. The purpose of this chapter has been to review some of these techniques, in order to appreciate the multifaceted challenge the infected foot presents to the informed clinician.

REFERENCES

1. Fenton CF, Marcinko DE: Wound healing. In Marcinko DE, ed: *Medical and surgical therapeutics of the foot and ankle*, Baltimore, 1992, Williams & Wilkins.
2. Marcinko DE: Radiotherapeutic treatment of a plantar keloid scar, *Podiatry Tracts* 1:49, 1988.
3. Marcinko DE, Tursi F: Pedal burn contractures, *J Am Podiatry Assoc* 78:396, 1988.
4. Marcinko DE: *Protocol for the diagnosis and treatment of pedal infections*, Brentwood, Tenn, 1987, PICA.
5. Marcinko DE: *Advanced protocol for the diagnosis and treatment of pedal infections*, revised edition, Brentwood, Tenn, 1987, PICA.
6. Rothstein AS: Skin grafting techniques, *J Am Podiatry Assoc* 73:79, 1983.
7. Marcinko DE: Plastic surgery in podiatry (simplified illustrated techniques), *J Foot Surg* 27:103, 1988.
8. Bryant WM: Wound healing, *Clin Symp* 29:1, 1981.
9. Gustilo RB: Management of infected non-union. In Gustilo RB, ed: *Orthopedic infection: diagnosis and treatment*, Philadelphia, 1989, WB Saunders.
10. Marcinko DE, Carlson R: Psychological considerations of the surgical patient: an emerging issue, *J Am Podiatry Assoc* 74:441, 1984.

ADDITIONAL READINGS

Albreski DA, Huey C, Spadone SJ: *Aeromonas hydrophila:* a fresh water pathogen and its pedal manifestations, *J Am Podiatr Med Assoc* 86:135-138, 1996.

Drennan JC: *The child's foot and ankle,* New York, 1992, Raven Press.

Hanna JR, Giacopelli JA: A review of wound healing and wound dressing products, *JFAS* 36:2-14, 1997.

Mann RA, Coughlin MJ: *Surgery of the foot and ankle,* St Louis, 1993, Mosby.

Rose EH: Management of skin loss. In Scurran BL, ed: *Foot and ankle trauma,* New York, 1995, Churchill Livingstone.

Rudolph R: Current concepts in wound healing. In Scurran BL, ed: *Foot and ankle trauma,* New York, 1995, Churchill Livingstone.

Servatjoo P: Deep vein thrombosis, *J Am Podiatr Med Assoc* 5:224-232, 1997.

15

New Treatment Modalities for the Infected Foot

David Edward Marcinko
Hope Rachel Hetico

The medical errors of one century constitute the popular faith of the next. Alonzo Clark

Several newly developed antibiotic delivery systems are useful in treatment of the infected foot. These include plaster of Paris pellets, implantable antibiotic delivery pumps, and chemotherapeutic phagocytic delivery vehicles.[1]

ANTIBIOTIC-IMPREGNATED PLASTER OF PARIS PELLETS

The use of antibiotic-impregnated polymethyl methacrylate (PMMA) beads, for the local elution of antimicrobial agents into a wound environment, is well known.[2-15] However, the use of plaster of Paris (POP) pellets, for the same purpose, is less well known.[16-28] According to the historical literature, plaster of Paris pellets have been used to fill dead spaces in bone, left by the ravages of tumors, cysts, and osteomyelitis, since the end of the nineteenth century, when it was proposed that an antibiotic called Rivanol be added to POP shaped pellets. Kovacevic then proposed the use of penicillin and sulfonamides, in 1953.[29] Therefore, the two functions of POP, to fill voids and deliver antibiotics to the infected site, were established. Further animal and human studies revealed good tissue tolerance to POP without significant foreign body macrophage reaction, an absence of bone growth, and fracture inhibition, without osteogenetic stimulation.

In addition, POP beads were found to be absorbed after implantation and did not demonstrate the temporary hypercalcemia seen by Norden in animal models.[30] More recent human trials have produced similar encouraging results in the treatment of chronic osteomyelitis. For example, Bouillet et al used POP beads impregnated with fucidic acid or amoxicillin, with good results, in 1989.[31] Since an increasing percentage of osseous infections are caused by *Staphylococcus aureus* and *S. epidermidis,* and the increasing resistance of these microorganisms to antibiotics has been noted, Dacquet and colleagues used the new agent teicoplanin as the active agent in POP pellets.[32] This drug, a recently discovered antibiotic complex obtained from the fermenta-

tion product of *Actinoplanes teicomyceticus,* is structurally related to the vancomycin-ristocetin group of antibiotics. It is a mixture of six closely related glycopeptide components identified in high-performance liquid chromatography. It possesses potent bactericidal activity against a wide variety of aerobic and anaerobic gram-positive bacteria and is not effective against anaerobes. Teicoplanin possesses major joint osteoarticular antistaphylococcal activity, with weak staphylococcal resistance. The minimum inhibitory concentration (MIC) of teicoplanin for most strains of *S. aureus* is 0.5 to 1 µg/ml., regardless of its resistance to methicillin or penicillin.

Plaster of Paris pellets are fashioned according to a dehydration technique described by Mackey and Varlet, in 1982.[33] The powdered antibiotic teicoplanin and sterile saline are added while the pellets are hand fabricated from the resulting admixture under aseptic conditions. Usual concentrations are 500 to 1000 mg teicoplanin per 10 g plaster of Paris. Pellet size is $6 \times 4 \times 3$ mm. Forty pellets may be double packed in polyethylene sacs and sterilized by gamma irradiation.

Dacquet et al then determined, through in vitro studies, that teicoplanin was initially released in a rapid massive manner, followed by a slower diminished release lasting about 30 days.[32] Additionally, it was seen that the higher the initial antibiotic dose, the longer the sustained release of active ingredient. An analysis of release properties demonstrated that antibiotic levels over the MIC 90 can be achieved for up to 9 days and maintained in the therapeutic range for up to 21 days in experimental conditions. It is logical to assume, then, that higher in vivo concentrations can be maintained for a longer period with the daily addition of additional antibiotic eluted from the antibiotic pellets already at the infected site.

Therefore, the delivery of an antibiotic directly to the site of infection, by means of an absorbable, space-filling compound, represents a dramatically new and viable alternative in the treatment of osteomyelitis, especially in cases in which local vascularity may be compromised.[33-50]

IMPLANTABLE ANTIBIOTIC FLUID DELIVERY PUMPS

Implantable antibiotic fluid delivery pumps (IADFPs) are a new modality for the administration of antimicrobial agents in the treatment of severe bone and soft tissue infections. A typical pump (Shiley Infusaid, Norwood, Mass.), consists of two chambers. One chamber is filled with the active ingredient and the other with medical grade Freon. The chambers are separated by collapsible metal bellows. As the Freon changes from a liquid to a gaseous state, it expands and compresses the chamber that contains the drug, which is then driven out the egress tube of the pump and into the egress catheters. The pump is refilled percutaneously at weekly intervals. When the drug chamber is reexpanded, it compresses the chamber filled with Freon back into its liquid state and recharging the pump. The antibiotic delivered by the pump is usually an aminoglycoside at an initial concentration of 50 mg/ml. The pump delivers between 4 and 7 ml of drug per day; therefore 200 to 350 mg of drug is administered per day. The pump is surgically implanted subcutaneously in the ipsilateral lower abdominal quadrant for lower extremity infections. After implantation, the egress catheters are tunneled subcutaneously, brought through the skin, coiled, and held in place with adhesive tape. Parenteral prophylactic antibiotics are given for five doses to prevent pump site infection and to treat the cellulitis frequently associated with severe skeletal infections. Serum creatinine and aminoglycoside levels are monitored at weekly intervals along with appropriate audiograms. Clinical and radiographic response to treatment is monitored in the usual fashion.

In 1992, Perry and colleagues reported their study of 12 patients with acutely infected hip arthroplasties that were treated with debridement and amikacin delivered through an implantable pump.[51] The infection was suppressed in 10 cases. Intracellular levels of amikacin were measured in eight cases. These levels ranged from greater than 150 μg/ml to 1688 μg/ml. The systemic level of amikacin remained below 10 μg/ml in all but one case. Duration of hospitalization averaged 19 days, and there were no significant toxic side effects to the drug.

In another study by the same author, an implantable pump was used in seven patients treated for active osteomyelitis, with positive wound cultures and draining sinus tracts, who were followed for more than 1 year. S. aureus was the pathogen in four cases, and pump treatment was with amikacin, with serum drug level kept above 2.5 μg/ml. Drainage stopped during pump treatment in all seven patients, but recurred in two after pump excision. Tissue biopsy was positive at pump removal in one patient.

Later critical review revealed that amikacin should probably not have been used in many cases. The primary pathogen, and the lack of ototoxicity and nephrotoxicity, should have made the penicillinase-resistant penicillins or the cephalosporins, the preferred drugs for long-term treatment. Also, agents such as ceftriaxone or cefonicid might have allowed for outpatient intramuscular therapy. In addition, the current concept of medical cost containment might have precluded the use of amikacin in this situation.

CHEMOTHERAPEUTIC PHAGOCYTIC DELIVERY VEHICLES (CPDVs)

In 1990, Glaude and Snider demonstrated that fibroblasts are capable of concentrating chemotherapeutic agents and acting as a reservoir for sustained release, confirming previous pharmacologic observations that tissue concentrations exceed blood concentrations.[52] This was particularly illustrated with the new antibiotic agent azithromycin (Zithromax, Pfizer Laboratories, New York, N.Y.), although other drugs, such as clindamycin, roxithromycin, josamycin, clarithromycin, rokitamycin, and the macrolide erythromycin, have also been studied by means of PMNL-labeled radioisotopes.[53] Interestingly, the uptake times for erythromycin and azithromycin differ by about 24 hours, as the latter drug is more slowly absorbed. Moreover, initial passive delivery has been augmented with active transport through fibroblastic depot transfers of the drug by cell-associated phagocytosis.

In fact, animal models by Glaude et al have shown that macrophages loaded with azithromycin were (1) released slowly over a 24-hour period, (2) stimulated by rapid phagocytic release when induced with S. aureus, and (3) delivered as the only vehicle for drug transport.[54]

Parameters deleteriously altering accumulation, and hence bactericidal efficacy, included smoking, pH, temperature, metabolic activity, bacterial sequestration, and cellular functional activity. Therefore, migratory cells such as macrophages and fibroblasts may represent a biologic in vivo transportation vehicle for this, and other medications, with drug concentration, often approaching an intracellular-to-extracellular ratio of 100:1. This is distinctively different from the passive use of a biologic antibiotic-loaded autologous blood clot (hematoma), which is self-absorbed and acts as a lattice framework for future soft tissue infiltration and consolidation.

For example, in a recent clinical trial in the United Kingdom, Baldwin and colleagues demonstrated that patients undergoing fiberoptic bronchoscopy after receiving a 500-mg dose of azithromycin, had alveolar macrophages with peak levels of azithromycin on the order of 20 μg/ml 48 hours after administration. These peak concentrations were six times greater than those in bronchial mucosa and were well above the MIC for commonly encountered respiratory pathogens.[55] Postulated mechanisms of increased bactericidal action included effective opsonization and phagocytic engulfment of invading microorganisms, although motility remained neutral.

Intracellular infections with microorganisms that are susceptible to antibiotics in vitro, but refractory in vivo, represent a major therapeutic challenge for new antibiotics. The advent of new drug classifications, such as the azalides (Zithromax) and the 4-quinolones (Cipro, Miles Pharmaceuticals, West Haven, Conn.), that achieve high tissue and intracellular concentrations would seem to present opportunities for improving the treatment of such infections, in particular those caused by pathogenic intracellular organisms that resist intraphagocytic destruction.

Thus, according to McDonald and Pruul, the important factor in the treatment of intracellular tissue infections may be dealing with intracellular organisms through the concept of "tissue loading," rather than the traditional concept of treating extracellular pathogens with conventional antimicrobial agents.[56]

CONCLUSION

Several innovative antibiotic delivery systems have become available recently through innovative industrial and technologic processes. These modalities include external and implantable infusion pumps, antibiotic-impregnated PMMA and POP beads, and active phagocytic transport carriers. The practitioner is cautioned against the injudicious use of these modalities, however, since initial optimism regarding their use must be tempered by the current medicolegal climate.

REFERENCES

1. Dickinson B, Lipkin LA: Pharmacology and anesthetics for the foot specialist. In Marcinko DE, ed.: *Medical and surgical therapeutics of the foot and ankle,* Baltimore, 1992, Williams and Wilkins.
2. Kelly PJ, Wilkowske CJ, Washington, JA: Chronic osteomyelitis in the adult, *Curr Pract Orthop Surg* 6:120-130, 1975.
3. Hagen R: Osteomyelitis in a general surgical department, *Acta Orthop Scand* 40:673-674, 1969.
4. Neule HW, Stern PJ, Kreilein JG, Gregory RO, Webster KL: Complications of muscle-flap transposition for traumatic defects of the leg, *Plast Reconstr Surg* 4:512-517, 1983.
5. Ger R, Efron G: New operative approach in the treatment of chronic osteomyelitis of the tibial diaphysis: a preliminary report, *Clin Orthop* 70:165, 1970.
6. Bucholz HW, Engelbrecht H: Uber die Deportwirkung einiger Anibiotica bei Vermischung mit dem Kunstharz, *Palacos Chirurg* 41:511, 1970.
7. Walenkamp GH: Experiences in the treatment of osteomyelitis and infected endoprostheses with chains of gentamicin-PMMA beads. In van Rens F, Kayser M, eds: *Local antibiotic treatment in osteomyelitis and soft tissue infections,* Amsterdam, 1981, Excerpta Medica.
8. Weise K, Weller S: Indications and use of Septopal in chronic osteitis. In van Rens F, Kayser M, eds: *Local antibiotic treatment in osteomyelitis and soft tissue infections,* Amsterdam, 1981, Excerpta Medica.
9. Lindgren L: Basics in the treatment of orthopedic infections, with special reference to Septopal. In van Rens F, Kayser M, eds: *Local antibiotic treatment in osteomyelitis and soft tissue infections,* Amsterdam, 1981, Excerpta Medica.
10. Klemm K: Treatment of chronic bone infections with gentamicin-PMMA chains and beads, *Accid Surg* 1:20, 1976.
11. Dingeldein E: Bacteriological studies in patients treated with gentamicin-PMMA beads. In van Rens F, Kayser M, eds: *Local antibiotic treatment in osteomyelitis and soft tissue infections,* Amsterdam, 1981, Excerpta Medica.
12. Botticher R, Stretz HW: The treatment of infected tissues with the aid of local administration of gentamicin-PMMA chains: a new therapeutic concept. In van Rens F, Kayser M, eds: *Local antibiotic treatment in osteomyelitis and soft tissue infections,* Amsterdam, 1981, Excerpta Medica.
13. Vecsei V, Barquet A: Treatment of chronic osteomyelitis by necrectomy and gentamicin-PMMA beads, *Clin Orthop* 159:201-207, 1981.
14. Ritzerfeld W: Discussions on infection treatment. In Contzen H, ed: *Munich Symposium on Accident Surgery,* Erlangen, 1977, VLE Verlag.
15. Marks KE, Nelson CC, Lauterschleger EP: Antibiotic impregnated acrylic bone cement, *J Bone Joint Surg* 58A:358, 1976.
16. DeGroote W, Van Dooren J, Verdonk R, et al: The use of gentamicin-PMMA beads in the treatment of osteomyelitis. In van Rens F, Kayser M, eds: *Local antibiotic treatment in osteomyelitis and soft tissue infections,* Amsterdam, 1981, Excerpta Medica.
17. Serafin D, Sabatier RE, Morris RL, Georgiade NG: Reconstruction of the lower extremity with vascularized composite tissue: improved tissue survival and specific indications, *Plast Reconstr Surg* 66:230, 1980.
18. Goodell JA, Flick AB, Herbert JC, et al: Preparation and release characteristics of tobramycin impregnated polymethylmethacrylate beads, *Am J Hosp Pharm* 43:1454, 1986.
19. Wahlig H, Dingeldein E, Bergmann E, Reuss K: The release of gentamicin from polymethylmethacrylate beads: an experimental and pharmacologic study, *J Bone Joint Surg* 60B:270, 1978.
20. Levin PD: The effectiveness of various antibiotics in methylmethacrylate, *J Bone Joint Surg* 57B:234, 1975.
21. Heard GR, Oloff LM: Antibiotic impregnated bone cement: an "in vitro" comparative analysis, *J Foot Surg* 28:54, 1989.
22. Seligson D, Klemm K: Antibiotic bone cement combinations. In D'Ambrosia V, Maier E, eds: *Orthopedic infections,* Thorofare, NJ, 1989, Slack.
23. Trippel SB: Antibiotic impregnated cement in total joint arthroplasty, *J Bone Joint Surg* 68A:1297, 1986.
24. Marcinko DE: Gentamicin impregnated PMMA beads: an introduction and review, *J Foot Surg* 24:117, 1985.
25. Wassner UJ: Principles and results of the treatment of soft tissue infections with Septopal. In van Rens F, Kayser M, eds: *Local antibiotic treatment in osteomyelitis and soft tissue infections,* Amsterdam, 1981, Excerpta Medica.
26. Milatovic D: Intra-phagocytic activity of erythromycin, roxithromycin and azithromycin, *Eur J Clin Microbiol Infect Dis* 9:33-39, 1990.
27. Jacobs AM, Seifert AM, Kirisits TJ, Protzel HR: Antibiotic-loaded bone cement in the management of diabetic foot infections. In Frykberg RG ed: *The high risk foot in diabetes mellitus,* New York, 1991, Churchill Livingstone.
28. Nelson CL, Griffin FM, Harrison BH: "In vitro" elution characteristics of commercially and non-commercially prepared antibiotic PMMA beads, *Clin Orthop Rel Res* 284:303, 1992.
29. Koracevic B: A study on the problem of hematogenous osteomyelitis, *Dtsch Zentralbl Chirurg* 276:432, 1953.
30. Norden CW: Lessons learned from animal models of osteomyelitis, *Rev Infect Dis* 10:103, 1988.
31. Bouillet R, Bouillet B, Kadima N: The treatment of chronic osteomyelitis with antibiotic impregnated implants, *Acta Orthop Belg* 55:1, 1989.
32. Dacquet V, Varlet A, Tandogan R, et al: Plaster of Paris antibiotic pellets in the treatment of infections, *Clin Orthop Rel Res* 282:241, 1992.
33. Mackey D, Varlet A: Antibiotic loaded plaster of Paris pellets: an in-vitro study of a possible method of local antibiotic therapy in bone infection, *Clin Orthop* 167:135-141, 1995.
34. Oguachuba HN: Use of instillation suction technique in treatment of chronic osteomyelitis, *Acta Orthop Scand* 54:452, 1983.
35. Smith-Petersen MN: Local chemotherapy with primary closure of septic wounds by means of drainage and irrigation cannulae, *J Bone Joint Surg* 27:562, 1945.
36. Goldman MA, Johnson RK, Grossberry NM: A new approach to chronic osteomyelitis, *Am J Orthop Surg* 2:63, 1960.
37. Dilmaghani A, Close JR, Rhinelander FW: Method for closed irrigation and suction therapy in deep wound infections: Preliminary report, *J Bone Joint Surg* 51A:323, 1969.

38. Willenegger H: Klinik und therapie der Pyrogenen Knocheninfektionen, *Chirurg* 41:215, 1970.
39. Kawashima M, Tamura H, Tako K: Closed suction irrigation. In D'Ambrosia V, Maier E, eds: *Orthopedic infections,* Thorofare, NJ, 1989, Slack.
40. Pressman M: Continuous closed suction irrigation following postoperative infection of Silastic implant, *J Am Podiatry Assoc* 67:746, 1977.
41. Schwartz NH, Marcinko DE: Suction irrigation in podiatric surgery: construction and use of a dependable closed system, *J Am Podiatr Med Assoc* 74:216, 1984.
42. Downey MS: Osteomyelitis of the foot and ankle. In Abramson C, McCarthy DJ, Rupp M, eds: *Infectious diseases of the lower extremity,* Baltimore, 1991, Williams & Wilkins.
43. Dawyer RB, Eyring FJ: Intermittent closed suction-irrigation treatment of osteomyelitis, *Clin Orthop* 88:80, 1972.
44. Sorto LA: The infected implant, *Clin Podiatry* 1:199-209, 1984.
45. Compère EL, Metzger WI, Mitra RN: The treatment of pyogenic bone and joint infections by closed irrigation with a nontoxic detergent and one or more antibiotics, *J Bone Joint Surg* 49A:614, 1967.
46. McElvenny RT: The use of closed circulation and suction in the treatment of chronically infected, acutely infected, and potentially infected wounds, *Am J Orthop* 3:86-154, 1961.
47. Eliopoulos GM, Moellering RC: Principles of antibiotic therapy, *J Infect Dis* 60:213-222, 1980.
48. Hunt TK, Jawetz E: Inflammation, infection and antibiotics. In Dunphy JE, Way LE, eds: *Current surgical diagnosis and treatment,* Los Altos, Calif, 1979, Lange Medical Publications, pp 122-146.
49. Meyer TL, Kieger AB, Smith WS: Antibiotic management of staphylococcal osteomyelitis, with particular reference to antibiotic-resistance infections, *J Bone Joint Surg* 47A:285, 1965.
50. Nelson JP: Musculoskeletal infections, *Surg Clin North Am* 60:213-222, 1980.
51. Perry CR, Hulsey RE, Mann FA, Miller GA, Pearson RL: Treatment of acutely infected arthroplasties with incision, drainage, and local antibiotics delivered via an implantable pump, *Clin Orthop Rel Res* 281:217, 1992.
52. Glaude RP, Snider ME: Intra-cellular accumulation of azithromycin by cultured human fibroblasts, *Antimicrob Agents Chemother* 34:1056, 1990.
53. Van der Auwera P, Matsumoto T, Husson M: Intra-phagocytic penetration of antibiotics, *J Antimicrob Chemother* 22:185, 1988.
54. Glaude RP, Bright GM, Isaacson RE: In-vivo and in-vitro uptake of azithromycin (CP-62, 993) by phagocytic cells: possible mechanism of delivery and release at sites of infection, *Antimicrob Agents Chemother* 33:277, 1989.
55. Baldwin DR, Wise R, Andrew JM: Azithromycin concentrations at the site of pulmonary infection, *Eur Resp J* 3:886, 1990.
56. McDonald PJ, Pruul H: Phagocyte uptake and transport of azithromycin, *Eur J Microbiol Infect Dis* 10:1, 1991.

ADDITIONAL READINGS

Korkusuz F, Uchida A, Shinto Y, Araki N: Experimental implant–related osteomyelitis treated by antibiotic calcium hydroxyapatite ceramic composites, *J Bone Joint Surg* 75B:111, 1993.
Pearson ML: HICPAC Guidelines for prevention of intravascular device related infections, *Am J Infect Control* 24:262, 1996.
Perry CR, Rice S, Ritterbusch JK: Antibiotic administration using implantable drug pumps in the treatment of osteomyelitis: preliminary report, *Contemp Orthop* 10:45-52, 1985.
Tomczak RL, Lane J, Dowdy N: Use of ceftazidime PMMA beads in the treatment of *Pseudomonas* osteomyelitis, *J Foot Surg* 28:542-546, 1989.
Yassi A, McGill ML, Khokhor JB: Efficacy and cost-effectiveness of a needleless intravenous access system, *Am J Infect Control* 23:57, 1995.

Section Five

Special Concerns of the Infected Foot

16

Neuropathic Osteoarthropathy and Foot Infections

Michael J. DeMarco

In the thirty-ninth year of his reign, Asa was afflicted with a disease in his feet. Though his disease was severe, even in his illness he did not seek help from the Lord, but only from the physicians. Then, in the forty-first year of his reign, Asa died and rested with his fathers. 2 Chronicles 16:12-13

Neuropathic osteoarthropathy, also known as Charcot's joint, is a progressive and degenerative arthritic process that is found in conjunction with impaired pain perception or position sense. First described in patients with tabes dorsalis, neuropathic bone and joint disease is now known to be a destructive complication associated with many upper and peripheral lower motor neuron disorders. While often thought of today as a disease of the diabetic, Charcot's joint must be recognized as an associated pathology in spina bifida, meningomyelocele, and chronic alcoholism, as well as injuries of the spinal cord and peripheral nerves. The earliest description and understanding of the neuropathic joint were put forth by Jean-Martin Charcot, in 1868, in the treatise "On some arthropathies apparently related to a lesion of the brain or spinal cord."[1] Charcot, considered to be the "father" of neurology, presented four case studies of arthropathy associated with what he termed "l'ataxie locomotrice progressive" or tabes dorsalis.[1] It is remarkable to note that Charcot's original description of neuropathic joint disease has perhaps remained the best.[2]

Charcot developed the concept of "trophic" injury to nerves, suggesting that the joint changes were secondary to sclerosis of the posterior columns of the spinal cord.[1,3] This became known as the "French" theory of neuropathic joint disease. Strong opposition to this early theory came from Volkman and Virchow, who asserted that the origin of the neuropathic arthritis was mechanical in nature and secondary to repetitive subclinical trauma to insensitive joints.[3] This became known as the "German" theory. To this day, the battle has not been resolved, as it appears that both theories are valid and more interrelated than these early researchers were able to discern.

The first association of neuropathic arthropathy, in the foot and ankle, with diabetes mellitus was not reported until 1936. Jordan described a 56-year-old diabetic woman with a "rather typical, painless Charcot joint of the ankle."[4] The literature has since produced numerous reports of diabetic neuropathic osteoarthropathy.

Charcot's joint, as a clinical entity, is often approached with great apprehension by those who treat the foot and ankle. It is often viewed by physician and patient alike as a condition in which intervention is futile. The physician may be challenged on many levels by this destructive condition. Neuropathic osteoarthropathy must be diagnosed without delay or hesitation, and a thorough knowledge of the natural history of this pathology is paramount to the development of a treatment algorithm. The physician should be aware of both palliative and surgical treatment options. The clinical picture of a Charcot foot is often complicated by dermal ulceration and subsequent infections to both soft tissue and osseous structures (Figs. 16-1 and 16-2).

DISORDERS ASSOCIATED WITH NEUROGENIC ARTHROPATHY

Charcot joints have been associated with a wide variety of disorders affecting both the spinal cord and peripheral nerves. Although different disorders and injuries lead to specific patterns of destruction, it is not possible to distinguish one etiology from another on the basis of a single joint. The decline of syphilis, with its associated morbidity, has ushered in diabetes mellitus as the most predominant cause of the Charcot joint. The three most common conditions underlying Charcot arthropathy are diabetes mellitus, tabes dorsalis, and syringomyelia.[5] Other associated primary diseases include leprosy, multiple sclerosis, myelomeningocele, spinal cord injuries, and a variety of other conditions[5] (Table 16-1).

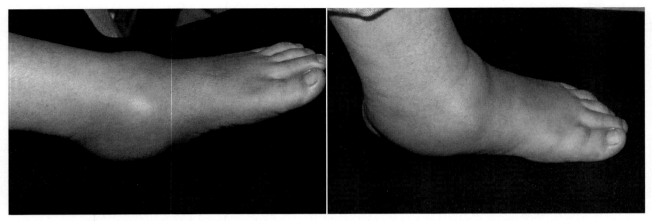

Fig. 16-1 An edematous, erythematous, and painless Charcot diabetic foot. Circulation and vascular perfusion were excellent. There was no history of trauma in this case.

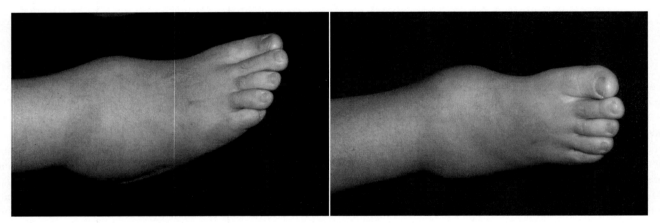

Fig. 16-2 The ankle, subtalar joint, and midtarsal joint subsequently proved to be dislocated. Differentiation of this foot from an infection may prove difficult, resulting in a battery of diagnostic tests. Often, the clinical presentation and history are of vital importance.

Tabes dorsalis

Tabes dorsalis is a form of syphilis in which the infecting spirochete, *Treponema pallidum,* invades the central nervous system, leading to degeneration of the posterior columns and root ganglia of the spinal cord. These lesions may result in lower extremity pain, ataxia, hyperesthesia, paresthesia, and loss of deep tendon reflexes.[2,3] Syphilis is most commonly screened by using the VDRL and RPR nontreponemal tests. When reactive, these tests should be followed by a specific treponemal test, such as the fluorescent treponemal antibody-absorption (FTA-ABS) test.

A neuropathic joint may be seen in as many as 10% of patients with tabes dorsalis. The presentation is often monarticular, involving the larger joints of the lower extremity, knee, and hip in 70% of cases and the lumbar spine in 20%.[6]

Syringomyelia

Syringomyelia is a neurologic disorder that involves abnormal fluid-filled cavities within the substance of the spinal cord. These lesions are congenital in about 50% of cases, while the rest are usually associated with tumors.[2,3] The relationship between syringomyelia and neuropathic joint disease was first described by Schultze and Kahler, in 1888.[7] It is estimated that as many as 25% of patients with syringomyelia will develop Charcot joints.[6] The upper extremity is usually affected, with the shoulder and elbow being the primary sites of involvement.[6,8]

Wastie reported that 29% of patients with leprosy, examined radiographically, had bone and joint changes characteristic of Charcot arthropathy.[9] Spinal dysraphism represents the most common cause of neuropathic joint disease in children. Such conditions may include open defects, such as myelomeningocele, as well as closed defects such as spina bifida.[10] The open defects can often be diagnosed in utero through amniocentesis and ultrasonography. Spina bifida most commonly manifests in the lower thoracic, lumbar, and sacral regions. These defects produce multisystem pathology, ranging from genitourinary disorders to orthopedic deformities and/or paralysis.[2,3]

TABLE 16-1 Conditions associated with Charcot's disease

Diabetes mellitus
Tabes dorsalis
Syringomyelia
Alcoholism
Leprosy
Spina bifida
Poliomyelitis
Multiple sclerosis
Pernicious anemia
Spinal cord trauma
Peripheral nerve lesions

Diabetic neuropathic joint disease

The incidence of diabetic neuropathic joint disease is still open to question. There are numerous reports in the literature, ranging from Bailey and Root's estimate of 0.08% to Cofield and associates' report of 29%.[11,12] This obvious disparity may be accounted for by differences in diagnostic criteria, as well as differences in study populations. The overall incidence is probably less than 5%. The incidence of diabetic Charcot joints may be increasing because diabetic patients are living longer and thus have a greater risk for developing these pathologic changes.

The onset of diabetic neuroarthropathy is most commonly reported to occur in the fifth and sixth decades of life. The average age at the time of diagnosis is 55 years, and there does not appear to be any sex preference.[13,14]

According to Sanders, the average duration of diabetes at the time of diagnosis of Charcot disease is 15 years.[15] In fact, it appears that the duration of diabetes is a more important risk factor than age. It is important to note that most of these patients are poorly controlled with respect to blood glucose levels.

Diabetic patients presenting with Charcot-related complaints usually have two characteristics. First, there may be a concurrent peripheral neuropathy. Most often this presents as a distal, bilaterally symmetric polyneuropathy that is primarily sensory. Physical examination will reveal diminished or absent pain sensation and decreased vibratory and proprioception sense, as well as a diminished Achilles reflex. It is possible, however, to have neuropathic joint pathology without an obvious neurologic deficit. Katz et al reported that as many as 20% of patients with neuropathic joint disease present without such deficits.[16]

The second characteristic, which is almost universal, is an abundant blood supply. These patients may present with bounding pulses. As will be discussed, it is this abundant blood supply that contributes to the vicious cycle of neuropathic joint disease. For example, Edelman et al reported on three cases of Charcot joints following revascularization procedures.[17] Based on their observations, they suggested that a neurally initiated vascular reflex leading to

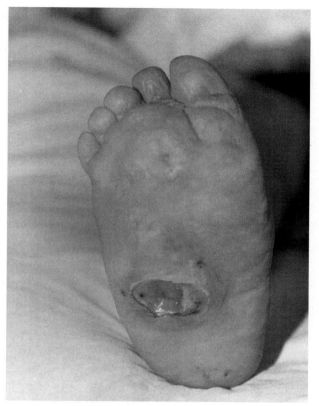

Fig. 16-3 Plantar ulceration in a patient with severe midfoot collapse. The potential for osteomyelitis in this foot is great. It also represents a diagnostic dilemma in many cases.

increased blood flow is the predominant mechanism in neuropathic joint disease, with mechanical trauma being only a secondary mechanism.[17]

Patients may present early in the disease process with swelling as the only manifestation of the underlying process. Other patients will already have suffered significant loss of the normal bony architecture of the foot by the time of initial evaluation. It is generally reported that these patients have little to no pain in spite of severe deformity. A typical presentation would be a patient with complete midfoot collapse (rocker-bottom foot) and plantar ulceration (Fig. 16-3). Patients with such open skin lesions should cause the clinician to have an increased suspicion of osteomyelitis. It is often difficult to differentiate between osteomyelitis and atrophic osteoarthropathy with osteolysis secondary to local hyperemia on the basis of plain radiographs alone.

RADIOGRAPHIC FINDINGS

Neuropathic joint disease has a variety of possible radiographic presentations, depending upon both the underlying condition and the point in the disease process to which the patient has progressed. The osseous changes of the Charcot joint have been classified in several ways. Perhaps the most useful system was described by Eichenholz.[18] He described three stages, beginning with "development" and progressing

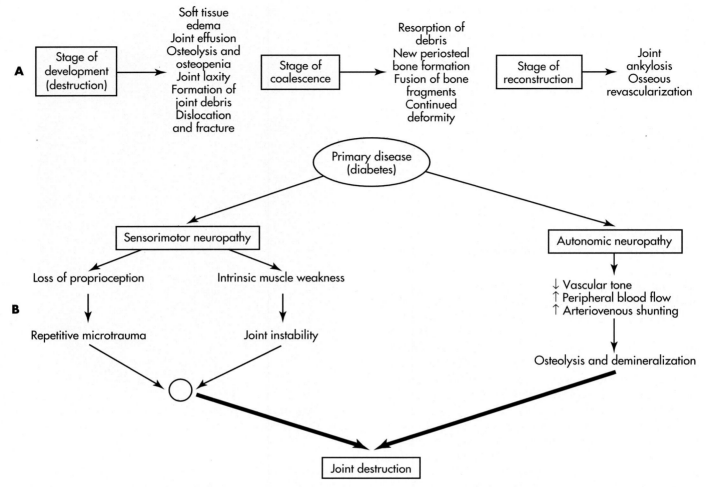

Fig. 16-4 A, Proposed stages of Charcot disease development. **B,** Factors leading to joint destruction in Charcot disease.

to "coalescence" and eventually reconstruction (Fig. 16-4). The first stage is essentially a destructive stage, while the last two stages may be thought of as healing stages. It has often been stated that upon gross evaluation, the changes seen in the Charcot joint closely parallel those of osteoarthritis, only to an exaggerated degree. From a pathophysiologic point of view, this is not entirely correct.

Early findings in the stage of development include soft tissue edema, joint effusion, and osteophytosis. As the condition progresses, intraarticular and extraarticular debris formation, subluxation, and osteochondral fragmentation may be observed.[5] These latter findings would not be consistent with osteoarthritis. Advanced changes in this first stage include complete loss of joint organization with fracture, dislocation, marked effusion, and severe angular deformities.[5] The stage of development involves a destructive cycle of ligamentous laxity leading to joint injury causing a hyperemic response. The hyperemia will cause resorption and softening of bone, which creates increased joint instability and injury.

The second stage of Charcot disease is a period of decreased destruction. During this time, there is resorption of debris with new periosteal bone formation and fusion of fragments. Osteosclerosis of bone ends is usually observed. Coalescence leads to the final stage of reconstruction as the body attempts to restore joint architecture.[5,18] Joint ankylosis and osseous revascularization occur in this final stage.[5]

Sanders has described five common anatomic patterns of bone and joint destruction in patients with neuropathic osteoarthropathy[15] (Table 16-2).

According to Sanders and Mrdjenovich, type I is a forefoot presentation, which may involve the phalanges, interphalangeal joints, metatarsals, and metatarsophalangeal joints. These changes are generally characterized as atrophic with osteoporosis, osteolysis, and subluxation. The dissolution of joints and absorption of diaphyseal bone give rise to deformities that have classically been described as the "sucked candy" appearance or the "pencil and cup" deformity. Some authors have contended that the forefoot presentation of osteolysis is an entity distinct from neuro-

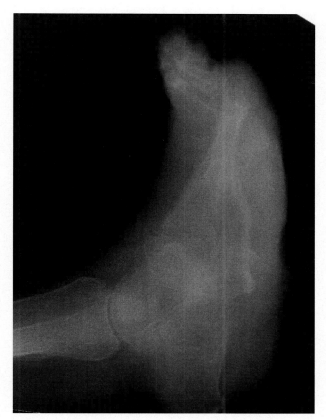

Fig. 16-5 Tarsal collapse in a Charcot foot.

TABLE 16-2	Anatomic patterns of Charcot's disease in the foot and ankle

I	Interphalangeal joints (IPJs) and phalanges
	Metatarsophalangeal joints (MPJs) and metatarsals
	Forefoot ulceration(s)
II	Tarsometatarsal joint (TMJ)
	Midfoot ulceration(s)
III	Talonavicular joint (TNJ)
	Naviculocuneiform joint (NCJ)
	Calcaneocuboid joint (CCJ)
IV	Ankle joint
V	Calcaneus

pathic osteoarthropathy. Most authors agree that the underlying pathophysiology is not different from that of the Charcot joint in the midfoot and ankle.

Charcot disease of the forefoot is complicated by the high association of plantar ulceration secondary to the sensory neuropathy and altered biomechanical patterns of weight bearing. Cofield et al reported ulceration in 91% of patients seen with forefoot osteolysis.[12] Isolated osseous changes with an associated ulceration dictate that the clinician consider osteomyelitis either as the source of destruction or as a complicating factor in a neuropathic joint. In many cases, resection of involved bone is indicated both for biopsy and as a therapeutic strategy for healing of the ulceration.

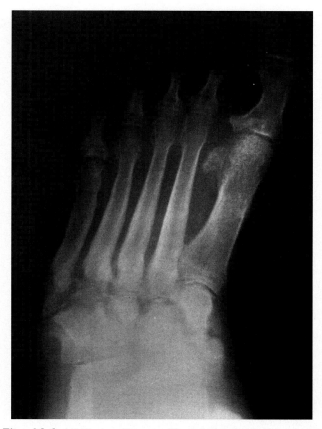

Fig. 16-6 Midfoot collapse with associated clinical plantar ulceration.

Type II is a neuropathic affliction of the tarsometatarsal joints (Lisfranc's joint). This type may present early on as osteoarthritis. Often there is fracture and dislocation of Lisfranc's joint, which may be spontaneous or the result of minor trauma (Fig. 16-5). Radiographically, a fracture or destruction of the base of the second metatarsal may be appreciated. Disruption of this important "keystone" articulation will allow the lesser metatarsals to dislocate laterally. These patients will frequently present with midfoot collapse and plantar ulcerations under the cuboid or cuneiform bones (Fig. 16-5).

Type III osteoarthropathy can involve the naviculocuneiform, talonavicular, and calcaneocuboid joints. Early radiographic signs of osteolysis at these joints should be taken very seriously, as continued weight bearing can bring about rapid disintegration and dislocation with midfoot collapse and a rocker-bottom deformity. Destruction may involve one or all of these joints (Figs. 16-6 to 16-8).

Type IV neuropathic osteoarthropathy is a pattern of ankle joint affliction. This presentation (Fig. 16-9) occurs much less frequently than the previously discussed patterns. Sanders reported ankle joint involvement in only 3% of diabetics in their study.[15] This pattern of Charcot has severe morbidity and disability associated with it. Type V neuroarthropathy involves the calcaneus and is the least frequently reported pattern of involvement.[15] This pattern may involve

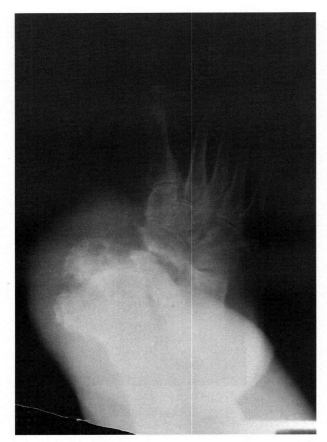

Fig. 16-7 Complete dislocation of the talonavicular joint. The potential for ulceration and infection, in this deformity, is obvious.

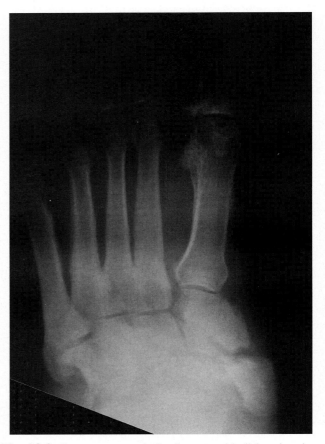

Fig. 16-8 Spontaneous navicular fracture with dislocation, in a diabetic patient.

fracture with complete avulsion of the posterior tubercle of the calcaneus.

PATHOPHYSIOLOGY

The pathophysiologic mechanisms of neuropathic osteoarthropathy are multiple and not entirely understood. If one is to have a full appreciation for the morbidity of Charcot disease, it is important to have an understanding of the underlying pathophysiology. Most of the evidence to date implicates a mixed neuropathy as the principal etiologic factor. This mixed neuropathy involves autonomic (sympathetic) dysfunction in conjunction with a sensorimotor peripheral neuropathy.

Increased peripheral blood flow and osseous hyperemias are consistent findings in the diabetic Charcot foot.[19] This is primarily accounted for by decreased sympathetic tone in vascular smooth muscle, which creates a situation of reflex vasodilation. This vascular reflex leads to an increased perfusion of bone, causing rarefaction and demineralization.[19,20] As bone minerals are depleted faster than they can be replaced, bone strength is decreased, making the bone more susceptible to abnormal stress loads. According to Nelms, shunting may allow a hundredfold increase in blood flow following sympathectomy.[21] Vessel wall stiffness due to calcification of the tunica media may also contribute to

blood flow abnormalities.[2] The presence of calcified vessels does not necessarily indicate decreased blood flow. Several cases of neuropathic osteoarthropathy, following revascularization of the lower extremity, have been reported.[17] Sensory neuropathy is a well-known finding in diabetic patients and is characterized by decreased vibratory, proprioceptive, and protective sensations.[19]

It is believed that the loss of proprioceptive feedback from the soft tissues surrounding joints results in poor postural control and decreased ability to off-load joints that are being subjected to pathologic stress levels.[19,20] Loss of protective sensations in conjunction with abnormal hemodynamics and bone metabolism is pivotal in the formation of a Charcot joint (Fig. 16-9).

The influence of peripheral motor neuropathy should not be underestimated. Clawtoe and hammertoe deformities develop as the intrinsic musculature weakens. These digital deformities create abnormal retrograde forces at joints that may already be compromised. These same forces can also produce plantar ulcerations. Weakness of the anterior leg muscles gives a mechanical advantage to the posterior muscles, leading to an ankle joint equinus with subsequent abnormal loading at the subtalar and midtarsal joints. Appreciation of muscular imbalance is essential to the success of any mechanical and surgical therapeutic strategies.

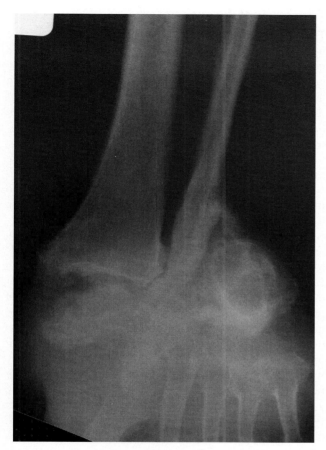

Fig. 16-9 Complete dislocation of the midtarsal, subtalar, and ankle joints.

HISTOLOGIC FINDINGS

The histologic findings in neuropathic osteoarthropathy have been compared to those seen in osteoarthritis, only exaggerated. Findings that differentiate the two entities are an active pannus formation and minute pieces of bone and cartilage imbedded in the synovium.[23] The latter finding is considered to be diagnostic of Charcot joint on biopsy. The microscopic picture is determined by the stage and severity of disease.

An interesting, but poorly understood, finding in the neuropathic joint is the coexistence of massive osseous disintegration and excessive production of periosteal new bone.[24] On gross inspection, intraarticular and extraarticular osteophytes may be seen in proximity to areas of osteolysis and erosion. O'Conner et al described pathologic findings in cartilage of dogs following transection of the anterior cruciate ligament after dorsal root ganglionectomy.[25] Findings included thinning of cartilage with decreased cellularity, while other areas demonstrated hypercellularity with thickened capsular tissue.

DIAGNOSTIC STUDIES

The diagnosis of diabetic neuropathic osteoarthropathy should be based on a complete history and physical as well as appropriate clinical testing. Noninvasive arterial studies are an essential part of the clinical evaluation. Since most Charcot patients have adequate peripheral circulation, it must be remembered that this may not be the case in patients who have had long-standing neuropathic changes. Documentation of segmental pressures, ankle and arm indices, and digital waveforms is important in the planning of surgical intervention. Circulatory status becomes of great importance for the patient with concomitant osteomyelitis, as this will affect the delivery of systemic antibiotics. Consultation with a vascular surgeon should also be considered. Plain radiographs are an important part of the overall evaluation, but may be too nonspecific for absolute diagnosis. It is not possible to distinguish between infective and noninfective processes with absolute certainty. Prompt differentiation between infective and noninfective processes is essential because of the different courses in therapy and prognosis. Since there may be a delay in radiographic changes of 2 weeks or more in both Charcot and osteomyelitis, nuclear imaging has become an essential diagnostic tool.

Currently, a suggestion for diagnosis is differential scintigraphy using technetium-99m phosphate and gallium-67-citrate in a sequential fashion. It must be remembered that the uptake of these radionuclides is nonspecific with respect to areas of infection, inflammation, and trauma. Interpretation of these studies must be made within the clinical context. The localization of technetium-99m phosphate complexes within bone is related to both reactive new bone formation (osteoblastic activity) and skeletal vascularity. The mechanism for bone concentration of the radionuclide is probably tracer binding to hydroxyapatite and organic matrix.[31] The mechanism of gallium-67 uptake involves binding of the complex to bacteria, neutrophils, and tissue protein.[31]

Technetium and gallium scans will be positive in patients with osteomyelitis; however, positive results may be seen in the presence of a Charcot joint as well. Positive uptake of technetium and gallium has been well documented in patients with neuropathic joints in the absence of ulceration.[26] The uptake of gallium in patients with Charcot may be variable. The uptake of both technetium and gallium will be focal in bone with acute osteomyelitis. The localization of gallium will be less focal and intense in chronic Charcot and chronic osteomyelitis.

The indium-111 scan has been proposed as a more specific indicator of infective processes, with a specificity of approximately 89%.[27] This technique appears to be the most specific diagnostic test next to bone biopsy. The gold standard, however, is still bone biopsy for culture and histologic evaluation. Although the literature has little to say about MRI evaluation of the Charcot foot, we have found it to be of little value in the evaluation of associated osteomyelitis. This is primarily the result of variation in technique and interpretation on the part of imaging centers. It is believed that this modality will increase in value with standardization of technique.

MANAGEMENT OF THE DIABETIC CHARCOT FOOT

The total management of the Charcot foot involves a multifaceted approach. A thorough understanding of the available biomechanical, surgical, and wound care modalities is a prerequisite to successful therapy. The most important aspect of managing the acute Charcot joint is strict cessation of weight bearing for approximately an 8- to 12-week period. Determination of when weight bearing is permissible should be based upon both clinical and radiographic signs of coalescence. Protected weight bearing may be initiated only with resolution of the clinical signs of edema, erythema, and calor. During periods of non–weight bearing, it is essential to closely follow the unaffected limb for signs of neuropathic joint disease. Some authors even suggest the use of a patellar tendon weight-bearing brace (PTB) or orthoses prophylactically.[28]

Long-term management with custom-molded accommodative orthoses is useful. These orthoses can be fabricated from a wide variety of materials and may be used in conjunction with an extra-depth shoe or custom-molded shoe. This type of management is often better tolerated and accepted by the patient than the use of a PTB. The use of custom-molded orthoses may be the most cost effective way to manage these patients.

Quantitative gait analysis is playing an increasing role in the long-term management of the Charcot foot. The need for an objective assessment tool for differential diagnosis, treatment planning, and treatment effectiveness is great. All too often, the first sign of abnormal plantar pressures in the diabetic foot is dermal ulceration. One such system is the F-Scan system, from Tekscan (Tekscan, Inc., Boston, Mass.). This instrument makes it possible to evaluate the reactive forces between foot and shoegear throughout the gait cycle. Bipedal plantar pressures are recorded from ultrathin (0.007 inch) insoles with 960 sensor locations distributed evenly across the entire plantar surface of the foot. Systems such as this are useful in evaluating patients prior to surgery or before the fabrication of molded shoes and accommodative orthoses. The clinician can immediately determine the effectiveness of devices that are designed to off-load various parts of the foot.

Local wound care should not be underestimated as an essential part of therapy. Ulcerations must be kept clean, with frequent debridement of necrotic and hyperkeratotic tissue. The main goals of wound care are to keep the ulcer free from infection and to provide an environment for wound healing through the formation of granulation tissue and epithelialization.

Patients with long-standing Charcot degeneration frequently have ulcerations associated with a deep fibrous plug of tissue. Such tissue limits the wound's ability to granulate and reepithelialize. Chronic wounds often necessitate deep debridement in the operating room. Vascular reconstructive surgical procedures are often needed, and partial foot or short leg amputation (SLA) may still be required in selected cases.

Charcot foot surgery

The decision to operate on patients with Charcot disease must take into consideration many factors. The patient's general medical condition should be evaluated, as these patients frequently have other complications associated with their neuropathy. A careful biomechanical examination of the patient is essential to a successful reconstruction. Specific patterns of muscle weakness must be assessed as well as the osseous deformities. The surgeon must also evaluate the patient's level of commitment to reconstruction, as these procedures can often involve significant convalescence. In some instances of severe deformity, an amputation may be considered as a viable therapeutic strategy because it will offer improved function for the patient.

Surgical approaches to Charcot reconstruction are many and range from digital stabilization to ankle arthrodesis.[29] Most often, multiple procedures are indicated and are often carried out in either a staged or a solitary manner. For example, if one were to address digital deformities without giving attention to a midfoot collapse, the patient would not be well served. In many patients, surgery to address bony prominences, with or without associated ulceration, may be all that is indicated. A rocker-bottom deformity with ulceration under the cuboid is common and usually responds well to plantar resection of the prominence with a debridement of the ulcer and aggressive local wound care. Forefoot procedures may involve digital stabilizations, possibly in conjunction with metatarsal head resections. These procedures may effectively eliminate retrograde forces causing plantar ulceration. Transmetatarsal amputation may be indicated in patients with severe deformity, and in some instances may be a more functional approach.[30-32] Midfoot arthrodesis at Lisfranc's joint is a common, but difficult, reconstructive procedure. The key to the success of this procedure is locating each metatarsal head on the same transverse plane. Ankle equinus is a fierce enemy of this procedure and must be addressed. Procedures performed in conjunction with the midfoot arthrodesis may be forefoot and/or rearfoot stabilizations.

In patients with collapse of the midtarsal or subtalar joints, a rearfoot stabilization may be indicated. These fusions are extensive and frequently necessitate bone grafting. Again, rearfoot fusions may be done in conjunction with other distal procedures, and any equinus must be addressed. Muscle and/or tendon procedures may be utilized in conjunction with stabilizations.

Gastrocnemius tendon recession or heel cord lengthening is often a key to successful reconstruction. Peroneus longus and tibialis posterior tendon transfers are often successful in patients with anterior muscle weakness and a drop-foot deformity. It must be remembered that Charcot reconstruction procedures are not without morbidity, and careful postoperative management is as important to success as the procedure itself.

Prevention and careful monitoring still constitute the best approach to management of the insensitive foot, regardless of etiology.

CONCLUSION

Charcot bone and joint degeneration is a process found in conjunction with impaired pain perception or position sense. It has many causes and is associated with upper and peripheral lower motor neuron disorders. Although it is important for the physician to diagnose and treat this enigmatic entity, it is vital to differentiate it from the infectious process. In this chapter, etiology, radiology, pathophysiology, histologic findings, diagnostic studies, and methods of management have been briefly reviewed. A rational approach to treatment of the infected Charcot foot has also been presented. It is hoped that this information will be valuable to all physicians who treat this condition.

REFERENCES

1. Charcot JM: Sur quelques arthropathies qui paraissent dependre d'une lesion du cerveau ou de la moelle epiniere, *Arch Physiol Norm et Pathol,* 1:161, 1868.
2. Charcot JM: On certain arthropathies apparently related to a lesion of the brain or spinal cord, Hoche GA, Sanders LJ, eds and trans, *J Am Podiatr Med Assoc.,* 82:403, 1992.
3. Delano PJ: The pathogenesis of Charcot's joints, *AJR* 56:189-200, 1946.
4. Jordan WR: Neuritic manifestations in diabetes mellitus, *Arch Intern Med* 57:307, 1936.
5. Frykberg RG, Kozak GP: Neuropathic arthropathy in the diabetic foot, *Am Fam Physician* 17:105, 1978.
6. Feldman F: Neuropathic osteoarthropathy. In Margulis AR, Gooding CA, eds: *Diagnostic radiology,* San Francisco, 1977, University of California Press, p 397.
7. Schultze F, Kahler O: Cited by Bruckner FE, Howell A: Neuropathic joints, *Semin Arthritis Rheum* 2:47-49, 1972.
8. Meyer GA, Stein J, Poppel MH: Rapid osseous changes in syringomyelia, *Radiology* 69:415-418, 1957.
9. Wastie ML: Radiological changes in serial x-rays of the foot and tarsus in leprosy, *Clin Radiol* 26:285, 1975.
10. Bruckner FE, Howell A: Neuropathic joints, *Semin Arthritis Rheum* 2:47, 1972.
11. Bailey CC, Root HF: Neuropathic foot lesions in diabetes mellitus, *N Engl J Med* 236:397, 1942.
12. Cofield RH, Morison MJ, Beabout JW: Diabetic neuroarthropathy in the foot: patient characteristics and patterns of radiographic change, *Foot Ankle* 4:15, 1983.
13. Clouse ME, Gramm HF, Legg M, Flood T: Diabetic osteoarthropathy: clinical and roentgenographic observations in 90 cases, *AJR* 121:22-34, 1974.
14. Sinha S, Munichoodappa CS, Kozak GP: Neuroarthropathy (Charcot joints) in diabetes mellitus, *Medicine* 57:191-210, 1972.
15. Sanders LJ: Diabetic neuropathic osteoarthropathy. In Frykberg RG, ed: *The high risk foot in diabetes mellitus,* New York, 1991, Churchill Livingstone.
16. Katz I, Rabinowitz JG, Dziadiw R: Early changes in Charcot's joints, *AJR* 86:965-974, 1961.
17. Edelman SV, Kosofsky EM, Paul RA, Kozak GP: Neuroosteoarthropathy (Charcot's joint) in diabetes mellitus following revascularization surgery, *Arch Intern Med* 147:1504-1508, 1987.
18. Eichenholtz SN: *Charcot joints,* Springfield, Ill, 1966, Charles C Thomas.
19. Frykberg RG, Kozak GP: The diabetic Charcot joint. In Kozak GP, Hoar CS, Rowbotham JL, eds: *Management of diabetic foot problems,* Philadelphia, 1984, WB Saunders, pp 103-112.
20. Frykberg RG: Neuropathic arthropathy: the diabetic Charcot foot, *Diabetes Educ* 9:17-20, 1985.
21. Nelms JD: Functional anatomy of skin related to temperature regulation, *Fed Proc* 22:933-936, 1963.
22. Edmans ME, Morrison N, Laws JW: Medial arterial calcification and diabetic neuropathy, *Br J Med* 284:928-930, 1982.
23. Floyd W, Lovell W, King RE: The neuropathic joint, *South Med J* 52:563-569, 1959.
24. King EJS: On some aspects of the pathology of hypertrophic Charcot's joints, *Br J Surg* 18:113-124, 1930.
25. O'Conner BL, Palmoski MT, Brandt KD: Neurogenic acceleration of degenerative joint lesions, *J Bone Joint Surg* 67A:562-572, 1985.
26. Sanders LJ, Murray-Leisure K: Infections of the diabetic foot. In Abramson C, McCarthy D, eds: *Infectious diseases of the lower extremity,* Baltimore, 1991, Williams & Wilkins.
27. Maurer AH, Millmond SH, Knight LCI: Infection in diabetic osteoarthropathy: use of indium-111 labeled leukocytes for diagnosis, *Radiology* 161:221, 1986.
28. Clohisy DR, Thompson RC: Fractures associated with neuropathic arthropathy in adults who have juvenile-onset diabetes, *J Bone Joint Surg* 70A:1192, 1988.
29. Banks AS, McGlamry ED: Charcot foot. *J Am Podiatr Med Assoc* 79:213, 1989.
30. Sanders LJ: Amputations in the diabetic foot. In Harkless LB, Dennis KJ, eds: *The diabetic foot,* Baltimore, 1987, Williams & Wilkins.
31. Lanatto L, Kaukonen JP, Laitinen R: Tc-99 HMPAO labeled leukocytes superior to bone scan in the detection of osteomyelitis in children, *Clin Nucl Med* 17:7-10, 1992.
32. Berkow R, ed: The Merck manual of diagnosis and therapy, Rahway, NJ, 1995, MSD Research Laboratories.

ADDITIONAL READINGS

American Diabetes Association: Position statement: foot care in patients with diabetes mellitus, *Diabetes Care* 18(S):26-27, 1995.

Armstrong DG, Lavery L, Houtman WH, Harkless LB: The impact of gender on amputation, *JFAS* 36:66-70, 1997.

Becker W, Palestro C, Winship J: Rapid imaging of infections with monoclonal antibody fragments (Leukoscan), *Clin Orthop Rel Res* 329 (8):263-272, 1996.

Giacalone VF, Armstrong DG, Ashry HR, Lavery DC, et al: A quantitative assessment of healing sandals and postoperative shoes in offloading the neuropathic diabetic foot, *JFAS* 36:28-31, 1997.

Haas LB: From research to practice, *J Am Podiatr Med Assoc* 86:518-520, 1996.

Hakki S, Harwood ST, Morrissey MA: Comparable study of monoclonal antibody scans in the diagnosis of orthopedics infections, *Clin Orthop Rel Res* 335(2):275-285, 1997

Harvey J, Cohen MM: Technetium-99 labeled leukocytes in diagnosing diabetic osteomyelitis in the foot, *JFAS* 36(3):209, 1997.

Kendall RW, Duncan CP, Smith JA: Persistence of bacteria on antibiotic laden acrylic deposits, *Clin Orthop Rel Res* 329(8):273-280, 1996.

Lau LS, Bin G, Suphaneewan J: Cost effectiveness of magnetic imaging in diagnosing *Pseudomonas aeruginosa* infection in a puncture wound, *JFAS* 36:36-453, 1997.

Lord M, Hosein BE: Pressure redistribution by molded inserts in diabetic footwear: a pilot study, *J Rehab Res Dev* 31:214-221, 1994.

Lutz S: Providers ponder impact of Medicare squeeze, *Mod Healthcare* 25:44-46, 1995.

Plummer ES, Albert SG: Foot care assessment in patients with diabetes: a screening algorithm for patient education and referral, *Diabetes Educ* 21:47-51, 1995.

Selby JV, Zhang D: Risk factors for lower extremity amputations in persons with diabetes, *Diabetes Care* 18:509-516, 1995.

Woolridge J, Moreno L: Evaluation of the costs to Medicare of covering therapeutic shoes for diabetic patients, *Diabetes Care* 17:542-47, 1994.

17

Psychiatric Considerations in Foot Infections

Kenneth J. Weiss
Elliot T. Udell

The duty of science is not to attack the objects of belief, but to stake out the limits of the knowable, and to center consciousness within them.   Virchow

Medical management of the infected foot requires insight into both the patient's mental state and his or her physical disorder. Patients with foot problems may also have psychological concerns ranging from excessive scar formation to disfigurement and death itself. Failure to appreciate and adequately address such perceptions of health, therapeutics goals, and expectations about what a specific treatment regimen will or will not accomplish may lead to a breakdown in the doctor-patient relationship and to poor medical management. The prudent physician should take into account the psychological factors that might produce either risk for infection or barriers to treatment.

This discussion will focus on clinical presentation and the psychology of the doctor-patient relationship in the treatment of complicated foot infections requiring prolonged care. Topics will be illustrated by case histories based on real situations with the potential for severe escalation producing tissue necrosis and/or osteomyelitis. Severe infections may require extensive surgical debridement and/or amputation of a portion or all of the lower extremity. Tremendous emotional involvement will ensue in the patient and family, and it is imperative that the physician be cognizant of this throughout the course of treatment.[1]

DENIAL, ANXIETY, DEPRESSION, AND RISK OF INFECTION

Human beings may adapt to "threat" by focusing on immediate survival issues and denying risk. This defense mechanism has been most publicized in the AIDS prevention movement. In this case, an "it can't happen to me" scenario is not an adapting attitude. Similarly, patients with ordinary foot infections may minimize the significance of their conditions, leading to noncompliance, missed follow-up care, and often disastrous consequences.[1,2] A typical psychological concern is denial. Denial itself can take several forms.

Normal denial

A certain measure of denial is an ingredient in optimism, a quality that bodes well for recovery. Denial is no longer adaptive, however, when it impedes treatment decisions.

Denial of extent of condition or its implications

This is a typical "shock" reaction to a new diagnosis or radical change in physical integrity. Such denial is transitory and is usually overcome by supportive counseling from clinicians and family.

Complete denial of illness or amputation

Complete denial may imply a departure from reality (psychosis) or an organic mental disorder, rendering the patient clinically incompetent and necessitating treatment with antipsychotic medication or appointment of a guardian. In the case of psychological denial in a patient requiring amputation, the clinical course is often complicated by depression once the denial subsides.

Anxiety and depression

In the common example of a patient with complications of diabetes mellitus, the clinician may see reactions of excessive concern (anxiety) and/or a sense of futility and hopelessness (depression). Anxiety presents as excessive and unrealistic worry, physical symptoms of autonomic overactivity, and often sleep and appetite disturbances. The typical thoughts of dread and doom among diabetic patients include dwelling on disfigurement and disability and fear of contracting AIDS from contaminated blood during surgery. Depression appears as a sense of self-defeat and loss of interest and pleasure. Whereas anxiety may interfere with the treatment of foot infections by paralyzing the patient's will, depression may be a prelude to passive suicide (giving up). In the foot-infected diabetic, the reality of a deteriorating organ may be unbearable. Many diabetics have spent years caring for themselves, only to find that they could not halt the progression of the disease. The presence of severe anxiety, and especially depression, should trigger referral to a psychiatrist.

PERCEPTIONS OF ILLNESS: THE DOCTOR AND THE PATIENT

The physician examining a patient with an ulceration, localized osteomyelitis, or gangrenous area may perceive the state of the patient's health very differently from the patient. The doctor, looking at the purulent toe of an insulin-dependent diabetic, may envision a treatment plan requiring many office visits, extensive vascular and radiologic evaluation, long-duration oral and/or intravenous antibiotic therapy, restriction of ambulation, and the possibility of surgical care. On the other hand, the patient may perceive a minor foot problem, being focused on work, shopping, children, or the next day's activities. There are key psychological factors that may contribute to perception of the illness. Awareness of these factors will enable the physician to better manage and lead the patient to acceptance rather than denial of a serious illness. The following two cases illustrate differences in attitude and outcome.

Case 1: Mr. Doe

Mr. Doe was an active 62-year-old man with diabetes mellitus, which had been controlled by oral hypoglycemic drugs and diet for 12 years. He was prophylactically treated by his foot specialist, every 8 weeks, with mycotic toenail and hyperkeratosis debridement. Initially, he self-administered treatment with over-the-counter "corn and callus" preparations, but his endocrinologist insisted that he see a professional regularly. One day, while the doctor was debriding a callus beneath Mr. Doe's third metatarsal head, a thick yellow exudate was noted. The foot specialist removed the remaining hyperkeratotic tissue and uncovered an infected ulceration. He cultured the exudate, ordered a complete radiologic workup, applied a dressing to the foot, and prescribed oral antibiotics. He also instructed the patient not to ambulate on the foot and offered Mr. Doe a pair of crutches. The doctor scheduled the patient for a follow-up visit in 3 days. Evaluation of the radiographs revealed soft tissue swelling. There were no signs of bone infection at the time.

The patient refused to use the crutches, as he had to shop for a sick wife at home and maintain a part-time job as a mail courier. Without hesitation, he thanked the doctor and walked out. He missed his next appointment and returned in 2 weeks. The infection appeared somewhat better. There was no exudate, but the ulcer was deeper. Once again the doctor

advised him to keep off of his feet, but Mr. Doe flatly refused. He also told the physician that he could come only every other week but would be meticulous in changing his dressing and taking his medicines.

Believing that some treatment was better than none, the doctor accommodated the patient. The ulcer remained unchanged for 8 weeks and then gradually deepened, invading the underlying osseous structures. The foot specialist called Mr. Doe's internist and admitted the patient into the hospital with a diagnosis of osteomyelitis and placed him on intravenous antibiotics. His condition required excision of a significant portion of the third metatarsal and surrounding necrotic tissue. Eventually he healed.

Case 2: Mrs. Stewart

Mrs. Stewart was a 65-year-old insulin-dependent diabetic. She presented to Dr. Gee with a small (less than 3 mm in diameter) ulceration distal to her right medial malleolus. The lesion was extremely painful and kept her up at night. Examination revealed a clean ulceration, and bacterial cultures did not reveal the presence of any pathogens. Trivalent bone scans were negative. The diagnosis of a superficial neurotrophic ulceration was confirmed. Treatment consisted of debridement with topical antibiotics, and careful attention to footwear that might constrict the area. Mrs. Stewart also limited ambulation according to Dr. Gee's advice. The patient saw Dr. Gee twice a week, and within 10 weeks the ulcer granulated completely and healed.

Discussion

Rhetorically, we may ask why Mrs. Stewart was so much more compliant than Mr. Doe. For one thing, she perceived her condition as more serious than he, as his use of denial to maintain his life-style ultimately worked against him. Another difference is that Mrs. Stewart was in constant pain. Even though her ulceration was not as severe as Mr. Doe's, she was kept up at night with pain and had daily discomfort. Her reaction was not one of denial, but of mild anxiety. She was willing to do anything to eliminate the pain and make her foot better. Mr. Doe, on the other hand, had advanced diabetic neuropathy. His foot was partly numb. He did not even feel the ulcer when it reached the bone. The absence of a normal alerting pain signal fostered his use of the denial mechanism. Because of his active life-style, he denied the severity of his condition and would have continued to deny it had he not been admitted to the hospital. Only then was a proper direct treatment plan formulated.

Types of doctor-patient relationships

There are methods that a physician can use to improve patient compliance. The first step is to understand the three types of doctor-patient relationships: active-passive, guidance-cooperation, and mutual participation. Each relationship has its place in the scheme of medical care, and choosing the right relationship for the proper situation will help ensure better patient management.

In the active-passive situation, the physician is active in giving orders and regulating the course of care, while the patient's role is one of passivity. The patient's understanding of the process is irrelevant. This type of situation works best when the patient may be totally impaired, such as following a cerebrovascular accident (stroke) or in Alzheimer's disease. It also is the doctor-patient relationship of choice in situations of acute illness. The doctor writes the orders, and a nurse or family member carries them out.

In the guidance-cooperation relationship, the patient might be a young agile person who has sustained a non-displaced fracture of the fifth metatarsal or suffered a mild to moderate lateral collateral ankle ligament tear. The treatment is given to the patient, who must follow it. The care is usually rendered on an outpatient basis, and the patient is able to comprehend and follow orders. The duration of therapy might be 6 to 8 weeks, and the patient can be seen infrequently to monitor progress or to apply or remove a cast.

Mutual participation works best if the patient is willing to be treated and capable of comprehending what is happening. The therapy will be of long duration, and the prognosis may be questionable. This would work best for a patient who has a diabetic ulcer or early osteomyelitis. In this scenario, the doctor and the patient are two thinking and reasoning adults who perceive the patient's true state of health and possible outcomes in the same way. They are functioning harmoniously and have open lines of communication. The patient realizes that the doctor is both knowledgeable and concerned for his or her welfare. If the patient is aware of this concern, there will be greater compliance, and even if the outcome is not optimal, the patient will not resent the doctor.

One way of demonstrating that the physician is both knowledgeable and caring is to be available to the patient. Another way is to appropriately obtain and interpret tests and explain the results to the patient. Tests such as bacterial cultures, radiographs, or vascular studies have their time and place. In addition to their actual clinical value, these tests demonstrate to the patient that the physician is "on top of things."[4]

Mr. Doe revisited

In Mr. Doe's case, the podiatrist opted to treat him in the guidance-cooperation mode. Instead of cooperation, the doctor encountered denial and noncompliance. Rather than let the patient have no treatment, the doctor settled for some treatment. This ultimately led to deterioration. The physician could have placed the patient in a hospital setting to temporarily adopt the active-passive doctor-patient relationship. After stabilizing the condition, and overcoming the patient's initial denial, Mr. Doe could have been discharged to the doctor's private care and a situation of guidance and acceptance or mutual participation could have been established. If it appeared in the hospital that the patient was still in a state of denial and would not follow outpatient orders,

the doctor could have consulted a liaison psychiatrist who specializes in managing the mental sequelae of chronic and acute medical conditions.

AMPUTATION AND DISFIGUREMENT

In clinical practice, the three most common conditions requiring amputation are gangrene, uncontrolled infection, and malignancy. A patient who may lose a portion of the foot or leg may react in one of several ways, depending on premorbid personality factors and current environment.

Low self-image

A young person who is threatened by an impending leg amputation will have great anxiety over potential disfigurement and how it may affect his or her appearance.[5] For example, he or she may wonder if an artificial leg will interfere with intimacy. Thoughts of how this change will affect his or her self-image may lead to noncompliance by way of denial. The physician, by virtue of having treated other amputees, might remember patients who adapted to artificial limbs. They might have been able to ski, go bowling, and attend to personal needs. In 1985, Lipowski suggested that the greater the subjective value of the body part or function affected by the disease or injury, the more intense and idiosyncratic will be the emotional reaction.[6] The practitioner is advised not to judge the patient's reaction to disfigurement or disability by his or her personal standards, since the symbolic meaning of the feet is subjective and individual.[2]

In treating patients, the objective should be mutual participation and explanation. For example, a study of postoperative amputees in Great Britain found that the level of compliance and cooperation improved if patients were given a great deal of information about their future prostheses and even allowed to participate in the decision-making process regarding the level of amputation and type of artificial limb.[7] Therefore, education may be an anxiety-reducing strategy to prevent depression.

Threat to homeostasis

Mr. Doe is a perfect example of a patient who perceives a threat to homeostasis, as his life revolved around taking care of his family and his job.[4] He led a very active life. Rather than confronting the facts of his medical condition and impending limb loss, he denied them. Patients relating from this mental framework may also be disposed to blaming others for their plight, including family and health care professionals.

Loss of control

The amputee or infection-scarred patient may feel helpless and hopeless, since modern medicine, with all of its wonders, could not cure the problem. He or she might feel isolated from friends and family or suddenly catapulted from a position of authority and control to being dependent on others for basic needs. Some patients respond to this situation by going into depression, acting childlike, or by expressing anger and hostility toward their medical providers. It is not uncommon for very caring and committed physicians to find themselves being sued or investigated by a patient's attorney even though they did not leave a leaf unturned in rendering proper patient care.[2]

Management of a patient who exhibits such thinking and behavior is twofold. If depression, regression, or isolation is exhibited, a mental health professional should be consulted. Psychotherapy, combined with short-term drug therapy, might be the answer. If anger is exhibited, every effort should be made to keep an open line of communication with the patient and the family. Hiding from an angry patient will only pour fuel on the fire.

Case 3: Mrs. Jones

Mrs. Jones was a 68-year-old diabetic. For the past 10 years she had been on renal dialysis and was treated for recurring ulcerations of the left heel for the last 2 years. Dressings and oral antibiotics managed the ulcers in all but one case. At that time, a 10-mm ulceration appeared medial to her left longitudinal arch. Although it was not deep, it was exquisitely painful. Dressings and antibiotics failed to bring her relief.

Because of Mrs. Jones's complaints of severe pain, the podiatrist referred her to a vascular surgeon. He evaluated her circulation and advised the podiatrist to continue with the same therapeutic regimen. After another week of oral cephalexin, the patient became anxious and fearful. She decided to seek the advice of a third surgeon. This physician decided to surgically excise the ulceration. Unfortunately, the surgical wound did not heal and additional surgery had to be performed. Eventually a below-the-knee amputation (BKA) was performed.

Because the patient had been in dialysis 3 times a week and now found herself unable to ambulate alone, she became angry and condemning. A month later, all physicians, including the vascular surgeon, the general surgeon, and the podiatrist, received letters from her attorney informing them that they were being sued.

Discussion

Initially, Mrs. Jones exhibited anxiety, fear, and frustration. She felt the podiatrist should have been more reassuring to her. Instead, the doctor focused on her foot, and when the condition did not improve, she sought second and third opinions. Moreover, had the third surgeon maintained the podiatrist's treatment plan, the patient might have sought the advice of a fourth doctor. When the surgery failed and rendered her condition worse, she became angry and depressed and ultimately vented her hostility at the entire medical community.

In this case, the patient's underlying personality structure was too strong to have cooperated with a single practitioner. Perhaps it was impossible to predict the outcome; perhaps not. However, if the podiatrist had been familiar with the psychiatric conditions that are associated with infection risk, a mental health professional could have been involved earlier in her treatment. In the next section, psychiatric conditions that might trigger a consultation are identified.

PSYCHIATRIC ANTECEDENTS OF FOOT INFECTIONS

Psychiatric patients may abuse their feet as a result of psychomotor agitation or frank self-destruction, inducing pathology that may range from abrasions to fractures. Although there is no specific correspondence between psychopathology and infection, there are several mental disorders in which abuse or neglect of the feet is a clinical consequence.[2] The following are examples that may serve as risk factors to alert the foot specialist.

Self-mutilation or the intentional disfigurement of a body part may be seen in a range of mental disorders, including depression (e.g., schizophrenia, command hallucinations), drug intoxication (e.g., PCP, angel dust), personality disorders (e.g., attention-seeking maneuver), factitious disorders (i.e., manufacturing or exaggerating an illness to assume the sick role), and mental retardation (severe and profound) with stereotypic foot banging. Anxiety or unrealistic worry may cause unintentional abuse of the feet as a result of increased sweating, pacing, and scratching, leading to "neurotic excoriations" and lichen chronicus simplex.[8] In the anxiety-prone patient, obsessive-compulsive disorder or ritualistic worrying may take the form of cleanliness rituals and the fear of contamination or AIDS. Mania, a severe state of overarousal, hyperactivity, and decreased need for sleep, may also lead to foot-stress pathology.

Infections can follow from psychopathology that includes pedal neglect due to apathy, loss or absence of intellect, and departure from reality (psychoses).[8] Deterioration from neglect may include hyperkeratosis formation, lacerations, abrasions, or bacterial infections. Therefore, mental illness can be seen as a host factor that, when influenced by environmental factors such as poor footwear or exposure, can produce pedal pathology.[9] Specific mental disorders include depression, schizophrenia, dementia, mental retardation, and drug or alcohol abuse.

CONCLUSION

The clinician must constantly be aware of the patient's mental status. This is especially true of patients presenting with foot infections. The clinician should appreciate the different doctor-patient relationships and must know the advantages and disadvantages of each. Finally, he or she must be aware of the range of possible patient reactions to various therapeutic outcomes.

The late Dr. Robert Rakow, an authority on managing the diabetic foot, once related to his residents that many patients called him an "angel" when their lesions responded to his treatment. The same patients demonized and even attempted to sue him when, due to no fault of his own, their conditions became worse. This was in spite of the hard work and care that went into treatment (personal communication, 1993). Although no clinician can be immunized against either a negative outcome or negative emotions, by recognizing the psychosocial factors presented in this chapter the clinician will be better equipped to handle a variety of difficult situations.

REFERENCES

1. Marcinko DE, Carlson R: Psychological consideration of the surgical patient, *J Am Podiatry Assoc* 74:441-444, 1984.
2. Weiss KJ: Psychiatric aspects of clinical practice. In Marcinko DE, ed: *Medical and surgical therapeutics of the foot and ankle,* Baltimore, 1992, Williams & Wilkins.
3. Szasz TS, Hollander A: A contribution to the philosophy of medicine: the basic models of the doctor-patient relationship, *Arch Intern Med* 97:585-590, 1956.
4. Udell E: Causes that trigger podiatric malpractice cases, *Curr Podiatr Med* March 1988, pp 22-26.
5. Lipkin M: Psychiatry and medicine. In Kaplan IH, Sadock BJ, eds: *Comprehensive Textbook of Psychiatry,* Baltimore, 1985, Williams & Wilkins.
6. Lipowski ZJ: *Psychosomatic medicine and liaison psychiatry,* New York, 1985, Plenum Medical Book Co.
7. Datta D: The psychology of limb loss, *Br Med J* 299:1287, 1989.
8. Doran AR, Roy A, Wolkowitz OM: Self-destructive dermatoses, *Psychiatr Clin North Am* 8:291-298, 1985.
9. Lemont H, Levy L: Osteomyelitis and the natural history of disease, *J Am Podiatry Assoc* 72:27, 1982.

ADDITIONAL READINGS

Donovan MI: Acute pain relief, *Clin Podiatr Med Surg* 11(1):147-161, 1993.

Wilkinson SV, Neary MT, Jones RO: The neuroanatomy of pain, *Clin Podiatr Med Surg* 11(1):1-15, 1993.

Woodburn SE: Postoperative pain management, *Clin Podiatr Med Surg* 11(1):55-65, 1993.

18

Medicolegal Implications of the Infected Patient

Isidore Steiner

An important phase of medicine is the ability to appraise the literature correctly.   Hippocrates

The infectious process is an unfortunate complication of disease or postoperative incident. Foot surgery and general surgery are equally likely to create this potentially debilitating problem. It is imperative that any physician treating the foot understand the legal ramifications of this problem and take every available medical, surgical, and legal measure to ensure that the art of medicine is practiced in the safest and most protective manner possible.

The purpose of this chapter is to review the general legal concepts of medical malpractice, and the more specific medicolegal precautions available to the practitioner in order to reduce the likelihood of malpractice claims when treating the infected foot. It will attempt to clarify the issues of importance and educate the clinician so that intelligent and appropriate medical and legal choices can be made without fear of detrimental repercussions. The chapter will also provide real case histories of foot and lower extremity infections. The elements of law for each particular case will be defined as they apply to the particular case. They will then be analyzed to enable the physician to apply appropriate legal principles to everyday practice.

GENERAL LEGAL CONCEPTS OF TORTS AND NEGLIGENCE

Intentional torts

The perpetrator of an intentional tort must cause either physical or mental harm to another person. The perpetrator does not necessarily have to possess desire to commit, or even commit, the intended tort. Intention to commit the tort is presumed and may be transferred.

Battery

Battery is the intentional infliction of damaging or insulting contact that causes pain and injury to the tissues or psyche. The injured person must establish damages, no matter how modest.

Assault

Assault is the intentional production of damaging or insulting contact, and the injured person need only believe that damage or offense has occurred. Usually, words alone are not sufficient, since words must be accompanied by some form of obvious act. Threats of potential future contact or injury are not sufficient. If the intended person is not cognizant of the threatened gesticulations, no assault has taken place.

Negligence

Negligence is not an intentional tort but rather the failure to appreciate or possess knowledge of the risks of personal behavior. There is a duty to act like a reasonable person under the same or similar circumstances, taking care to avoid unnecessary risks while maintaining a minimum standard of care. Additionally, there must be a close association between the act of the negligent person and the damage suffered by the injured party. Actual damages are required for a negligence claim, including such injury as lost wages, medical bills, disability, disfigurement, and pain and suffering. In the medical profession, the standard of care is now a national one, rather than the older community-based standard.

THE MALPRACTICE LAWSUIT

There are several parties to any lawsuit. The most obvious two are the injured patient (plaintiff) and the doctor (defendant). In addition, the judge calls the civil trial to order, acts as an unbiased referee, and directs the jury on issues of law. The lawyers are adversaries who direct the trial and frame facts to fit their purposes. Finally, the jurors act as fact finders who determine the outcome of a lawsuit, after considering the presented evidence. The jurors decide whether the plaintiff has proved the allegation of medical malpractice, not beyond a reasonable doubt, but by a

TABLE 18-1 Foot surgical complication rates

Infection, 14.45%
Amputation, 9.63%
Recurrence, 1.13%
Delayed healing, 0.28%
Osteotomy nonunion, 2.83%

From Podiatry Insurance Company of America: Annual Report, Brentwood, Tenn., 1996.

preponderance of the evidence. Whether the care was provided on a *pro bono,* or free, basis is irrelevant to the consideration of potential liability.

However, the most important party in a malpractice case is the practitioner's office or hospital records. The chart includes progress notes, test results, and consultation reports. Alteration of the records, through deletion, addition, or modification, is a critical offense, and proof of destruction or alteration strengthens the plaintiff's case and may prejudice the case against the defendant. Alteration can even shift the burden of proof to the defendant doctor. But, for judges and juries, the unaltered medical chart acts as the unbiased third party to the lawsuit.

The plaintiff would not be in litigation if it were not for the fact that he or she believes that a wrong has been performed. The plaintiff's attorney hires only experts who will testify as to the nature of the damages brought about by negligence. The defendant's expert believes the provider performed within the standard level of care in his or her profession and that circumstances beyond the defendant's control led to unfortunate results. The defendant's expert is hired to testify that the provided standard of care has been met and maintains an opinion in favor of the provider. A defense attorney who cannot procure such an expert is doing his client a grave injustice, as his opponent will make every effort to find the perfect plaintiff's medical expert. It is unfortunate when a plaintiff's attorney has found the perfect expert, but the defendant's counsel has decided to choose a so-called expert whose ego precludes rendering an opinion without criticism of the defendant.

The legal system, regarding malpractice, is an adversarial arena not unlike that of the gladiators of ancient Rome. Only the strongest survive. It is imperative to find the best defense attorney possible, who will procure the best possible defense expert.

LEGAL ISSUES AND CLAIMS

Frequently, a patient will seek medical care for a foot infection that needs immediate attention. Other times, referral to an appropriate physician, such as an infectious disease (ID) specialist or peripheral vascular surgeon, because of the severity and morbidity of the condition, is warranted. On occasion, an infection may develop postop-

eratively and require thoughtful and aggressive planning to sustain a medically and surgically acceptable result.

The points of law that plaintiffs and trial lawyers use when constructing a complaint are usually limited only by the imagination of the plaintiff's attorney. However, there are a number of points that generally appear in almost every complaint filed against a physician, in the United States, today. These include failure to diagnose, mistake in diagnosis, failure to obtain informed consent, lack of diligence, loss of chance, contributory negligence, improper surgical technique, and abandonment.

Failure to diagnose

The simple situation of "failure to diagnose" occurs when a physician fails to properly diagnose a certain condition. Since an infection is sometimes masked by other medical conditions, the practitioner may not anticipate the problem. The physician may also sometimes fail to appreciate the severity of the case because the problem manifests itself in an unusual manner. For example, the infection may precede or lead to vascular compromise. Because of physician negligence, the patient then suffers septic shock, amputation, or death. These three complications make for very substantial malpractice lawsuits. In the case of untimely death of a patient while under the care of a practitioner, it does not matter whether malpractice has occurred, since it is almost axiomatic that a lawsuit will follow.

Another typical example of "failure to diagnose" is the case of a diabetic patient, with an infected foot, who ultimately dies. After performing a cursory medical review, the provider's medical expert firmly testifies that the patient would have died no matter what the defendant would have done. Even with this testimony, the jury is not deterred from awarding the patient's family a very high settlement on the basis of their expert, who of course provided testimony on the negligent care the treating physician had rendered. Increasingly, juries are inclined to sympathize with families of individuals who die while under the care of a physician. Awards can range from several hundred thousand dollars to several million dollars. The merit of the case is usually irrelevant because the jury feels obligated to force the deep-pocket insurance companies to pay as society's retribution for suffering.

Failure to diagnose an infection can also lead to liability. Foot surgeons who consider themselves general diagnosticians are held to the same degree of skill as medical physicians who reside in the same geographic area. If a patient presents with an infection, it is the duty of the surgeon to perform a battery of tests to determine the scope and depth of the infectious process.

Failure to determine whether the infection is caused by a particular microbe or whether it has invaded the blood system may be cause for a malpractice suit. Improper treatment of an infection that results in amputation or death creates damages not only of negligence but also for causing the patient and the family severe pain and suffering.

Mistake in diagnosis

Related to the issue of failure to diagnose is "mistake in diagnosis." This occurs when a physician accepts a patient and undertakes the responsibility to correctly diagnose a condition or conditions. After a thorough examination, the diagnosis must be one that a reasonable practitioner, under similar circumstances, would have made. An incorrect diagnosis may lead to devastating results. If it is only an error in judgment, it may not be considered negligence. An improper diagnosis will cause the condition to deteriorate and needs to be reassessed within a reasonable period of time so that an alternative therapy may be instituted. Failure to make necessary changes in the treatment plan, or a failure to make a proper referral, may lead to allegations of negligence.

When a practitioner examines a patient and is unable to make a diagnosis or believes that treatment is beyond his or her scope of practice, it is his or her duty to immediately refer the patient to an appropriate specialist. For example, if a patient with multiple medical problems is seen with symptoms of a red, hot, swollen first ray segment, and it is difficult to ascertain whether the condition is caused by an offending ingrown toenail, a systemic disorder (e.g., acute gout), diabetes mellitus, or an infectious process such as osteomyelitis, the patient should be immediately referred to an appropriate specialist or admitted to the hospital for consultation with colleagues. It is the physician's duty to advise the patient to consult a specialist if the physician is unqualified to render an accurate diagnosis or give proper treatment. Should the practitioner know that the patient would receive superior care at the hands of another physician, whether of his or her own specialty or a different specialty, it is incumbent upon him or her to make the referral. A physician who fails to make this referral is held to the standard of what a reasonably careful and skillful physician, under like or similar circumstances, would have done with that particular patient in that particular situation. The practitioner's training must include the ability to assess at what point his or her treatment is ineffectual and that a need exists for a more qualified review of the case. This duty arises under two situations. First, if the physician does not own the necessary equipment to properly treat the patient, a referral must be made. Furthermore, if he or she does not have adequate knowledge or skill to treat that problem, the obligation is upon that physician to seek a specialist who possesses those qualifications. Similarly, when a physician realizes that his treatment is unsuccessful and the patient's condition is not improving, it is incumbent upon him or her to make a referral to a practitioner whose knowledge, training, or experience is superior.

Failure to obtain informed consent

Informed consent is an information exchange process between physician and patient, regarding the details of the anticipated procedure or proposed treatment regimen. Consent may be oral or written and should be documented in the medical record. Reasonable risks and alternative procedures must be disclosed, but remote risks need not be disclosed. Pertinent information must be supplied by the physician, but consent cannot be given by a minor or an incompetent adult. Explanations must be in language understood by the patient.

"Failure to obtain informed consent," in our contemporary society, usually does not win a malpractice lawsuit. However, a corollary of this issue, known as "failure to inform of risks," can very well lead to successful litigation. Nevertheless, each practitioner should construct comprehensive consent forms as well as a host of patient communication letters that should include, but are not limited, to the following:

  Failure to follow recommended treatment(s) form(s)
  Letter to subsequent treating physician
  Failure to keep appointment letter
  Withdrawal from patient care letter

This corollary suggests that whenever a physician is discussing surgery with a patient, a duty exists to inform the patient of the risks of that surgery, as well as the potential complications that may arise postoperatively. These risks include, but are not limited to, the infectious process, which occurs in a consistent percentage of patients on a regular basis. This is extremely important in dealing with cases of compromised circulation, since the patient may hesitate or defer surgical intervention if he or she is aware of the increased potential for infection resulting from the medical condition. Standardized consent forms are usually not acceptable for these kinds of patients. These patients require extensive explanations and more comprehensive and documented examination.

Lack of diligence

"Lack of diligence" is another possible area in the malpractice complaint. Lack of diligence includes situations in which failure to exercise proper diligence are involved in the treatment of a patient. For example, inadequate attention to a particular case, and/or making omissions in the course of treatment, can lead to this issue. In an infection situation, a practitioner has the duty to continue the necessary care until the infection is resolved. A delay in treatment or discharge before complete resolution of the condition has been considered negligence. Once a physician-patient relationship has been established, this duty begins, and does not end until the patient is discharged from the practice in a healthy condition or is referred to an appropriate specialist for continued care.

In the practice of medical and surgical foot care, infections are treated on a daily basis. However, postoperative infections require a special duty by the surgeon. The surgeon cannot withdraw from treatment until (1) the condition resolves and both parties consent to the discharge of the relationship, (2) the patient dismisses the surgeon, or (3) the surgeon provides adequate and reasonable notice by return receipt mail or by written referral to another specialist.

"Lack of diligence" also occurs when a physician fails to make a timely response to a patient complaint. An example of this type of negligence occurs when a postoperative patient calls the operating surgeon with certain symptoms and the physician suggests a lengthy delay until the next scheduled office visit. Since certain infections can result in severe morbidity if not treated immediately, it is imperative to treat every patient complaint, either by phone or personal contact, as though a potential infection could cause imminent death. Treatment in such situations should be no later than 24 hours and, most probably, within hours of contact. Typically, postoperative patients are encouraged to call the surgeon, either day or night, should they have potential problems or concerns. Obviously, these concerns may result in late night office or urgent hospital visits. Premature discharge of a patient from either the practice or the hospital can lead to allegations of medical negligence.

Loss of chance

The claim "loss of chance" occurs when a physician fails to properly diagnose or treat a condition and deprives the patient of a cure. For this element to exist in a lawsuit, there must be a preexisting condition. The patient's opportunity to recover from the condition must be reduced by improper care of the physician, or the chance for a successful recovery must be lost forever. When an infection leads to an amputation that could have been prevented, the ability to cure that condition is forever lost.

Contributory negligence

"Contributory negligence" is plaintiff conduct, or lack of conduct, that contributed to the harm suffered. Appropriate behavior is determined by what a reasonable person would have done in like or similar circumstances. There are two types of contributory negligence: classical and comparative. In the first case, any contributory patient negligence is an absolute obstacle to any recovery, while in the latter case, the patient's contribution is subtracted from the total monetary award.

Poor surgical technique

A surgeon has the duty to perform surgery at or above the level of a reasonably competent surgeon, of the same or similar specialty. "Poor surgical technique" can result in injury that is compensable, because the surgeon accepts the duty to perform competently when the patient is accepted as a surgical client.

Abandonment

"Abandonment" is the unilateral termination of a physician-patient relationship by the physician, when medical care is still deemed necessary, without reasonable notice to the patient, although claims of abandonment may occur when a patient unilaterally severs the professional relationship. Attorneys have been known to claim abandonment in a lawsuit when physicians act in a capricious manner and an

infection is not attended to within the time allowable for successful treatment.

FOOT INFECTION CASE REPORTS

This section will review five foot infection cases; each is followed by an explanation of how the specific situation might have been handled from a medicolegal perspective. They will be presented in case report format and are actual, real-life clinical situations.

Medicolegal case report 1

A 30-year-old man presented to an office-based practitioner, 24 days after a nail puncture through his left great toe. His chief complaint was swelling, redness, and unresolved pain in the affected area. Several days after the injury, the patient saw his primary care physician, who prescribed a 5-day course of oral antibiotics. When the symptoms did not resolve, the physician prescribed a regimen of parenteral antibiotics on an outpatient basis. When the condition still did not improve, the patient sought assistance from an internist who also provided foot care. Observations at the initial visit indicated a fulminating infectious process encompassing the extremely erythematous and warm first ray, as well as the medial plantar space. Palpation of the first metatarsal head, as well as hallucal movement, elicited severe pain. Radiographs revealed lytic changes of the first metatarsal head. Treatment consisted of hospital admission and another regimen of parenteral antibiotics. After 10 days of antibiotic treatment, minimal improvement was noted. At this stage, a foot surgeon evaluated the situation and performed excision and drainage of the first metatarsophalangeal joint with resection of the osteomyelitic metatarsal head, the next morning.[1]

Several months later, the patient served a lawsuit on the negligent physicians. The complaints of malpractice included (1) lack of informed consent, (2) failure to make a diagnosis, (3) failure to refer to a specialist, (4) poor surgical technique, (5) improper treatment, (6) abandonment, and (7) loss of chance.

In defending a malpractice lawsuit, the reply submitted by the doctor's defense attorney responds to each and every attack made by the plaintiff's counsel. A defense is an argument that attempts to absolve the physician of liability.

In this case, it may be suggested that the first physician did not recognize the severity of the situation and failed to adequately diagnose and treat the condition. Similarly, the second physician did not learn from the first physician's mistakes and errors. It is also possible that the delay could have been the difference between saving and losing the first metatarsal head and metatarsophalangeal joint. Both failed to adequately work up the patient and perform the necessary and available testing that a reasonable physician would have performed under like or similar circumstances. Numerous and serial radiographs should have been taken to determine the scope and extent of the infectious process. The assistance of a variety of medical specialists could have been elicited to help in the treatment process. Failure to diagnose the bone infection ultimately resulted in loss of the first metatarsophalangeal joint. Each treating physician established a physician-patient relationship, and each had a duty to make a correct diagnosis or refer the patient. Failure to make the diagnosis resulted in a breach of medical duty, which subsequently caused the patient to sustain an injury.

Medicolegal case report 2

A 74-year-old man with diabetes mellitus and alcoholic neuropathy presented with evidence of trauma to the left foot, showing erythema and cellulitis. Radiographs demonstrated increased soft tissue density and volume on the plantar-medial aspect of the foot, with air pockets suggesting potential abscesses and significant joint space changes. A culture taken from the abscess grew *Staphylococcus aureus.* The patient was treated with aspiration, followed by intravenous antibiotics for 30 days. He was then seen as an outpatient numerous times during the following 3 months.

By this time, the infection had spread to the bone, resulting in the necessity for a transmetatarsal amputation. The patient was suspected of being noncompliant because many office visits were missed and frequent telephone calls were received for lost prescriptions.[2] Several months after the amputation, the patient filed a malpractice lawsuit in Circuit Court. His complaints of alleged malpractice included (1) failure to diagnose, (2) failure to refer, (3) failure to inform of risks, (4) lack of diligence, (5) improper treatment, (6) abandonment, and (7) loss of chance.

In this case, the defense against the charge of abandonment was to cite the patient's failure to cooperate with the physician. It was argued that the ultimate result was not directly related to the physician's negligence but to the patient's noncompliance. However, it was the duty of the physician to contact the patient and have proof of those conditions in the medical record. The correspondence should have included the recommended mode of therapy, an explanation to the patient as to the severity of the condition, and the potential problems that could ensue with refusal to comply with instructions. This type of correspondence should be sent by certified U.S. mail with a return receipt request.

Another method of attacking this complaint is for the defense to counter that the patient is liable for contributory negligence. If the patient were found guilty of negligence that contributed to the resulting injury, it would then be left to the jury and judge to determine what percentage of that injury.

Medicolegal case report 3

A 42-year-old man presented to the office with a chief complaint of pain at the medial aspect of the right foot, centered over the tarsal navicular bone. He related that he noticed an area that appeared sunburned, on the inner foot, while playing tennis. When he ambulated, the area become swollen and painful. He recalled that on several occasions he had gone into the nearby woods to fetch his errant tennis balls. He had been seen by his family practitioner, who diagnosed an infection and placed him on oral antibiotics for 1 week. The symptoms initially subsided, only to return about 10 days later. The pain grew worse and spread to the ankle. Approximately 1 week after seeing the practitioner, he developed a strange skin lesion, which appeared flat and had a red outer border. Several concentric rings were noted within the lesion. In addition, the patient thought that perhaps he had developed the flu, as he experienced joint pain, a sore throat, and cough. The patient then sought care from a foot specialist, who did a thorough examination and found tenderness over the first, second, and third metatarsophalangeal joints, as well as the plantar fascia of the foot. Radiographs showed no osseous or soft tissue pathology. The patient was placed on an antiinflammatory agent, and appropriate laboratory studies were performed. The results of a complete blood count, SMA-12, HLA-B27 profile, RA latex, and antinuclear antibody titer level were all normal. The patient was told to return to the office in 30 days. At that time, the situation had not resolved, and the practitioner switched to another oral antiinflammatory agent and gave several steroidal joint injections. Six months later, the patient sought treatment from a rheumatologist because of increased edema in the foot, as well as generalized arthralgia. The rheumatologist performed a Lyme disease antibody test, which showed high levels of IgG and the microorganism *Borrelia burgdorferi,* which confirmed the diagnosis. Treatment was with tetracycline and medical management for potential cardiac and neurologic sequelae.[3]

Six months later, a lawsuit was served upon the family practitioner and the foot specialist. Included in the complaint were the following allegations: (1) failure to diagnose, (2) failure to refer, (3) failure to inform of risks, (4) lack of diligence, (5) *res ipsa loquitur,* and (6) loss of chance.

Both physicians had failed to diagnose the patient's condition within a reasonable time, which resulted in the chronic state of Lyme disease. They failed to refer to an infectious disease specialist or rheumatologist to determine the cause of the condition. Since the disease could lead to lifelong disability, both failed to understand the risks of their unsuccessful treatment, and were unable to inform the patient of his risks. A lack of diligence was also involved when they failed to give proper attention to the case and made significant omissions during their courses of treatment. Each accepted the case and developed a physician-patient relationship, but failed to properly diagnose the condition. The kind of injury sustained in this situation did not occur without the negligence of the two initial treating physicians. Their failure to properly diagnose and treat resulted in severe disability, which was not due to voluntary action or contribution on the part of the injured patient.

The doctrine of *res ipsa loquitur* ("the thing speaks for itself") allows an injured person to point to the injury and claim that its mere occurrence is enough to infer that the defendant (doctor) was culpable. Contributory negligence is not a part of this claim, since the origin of injury must be solely the defendant. For the claim to be successful, it must be demonstrated that the injury was such that it would not normally occur in the absence of the other party's negligence (i.e., below-the-knee amputation following an infection of a postoperative fifth digit arthroplasty procedure).

Finally, the patient and the prosecuting attorney believed that the doctors had failed to diagnose and treat the true condition within the required time frame and therefore had deprived the patient of a possible cure. In the loss of chance claim, there was a preexisting, treatable condition from which the patient could have recovered with proper care from the attending physician, and the loss chance for cure was forever. Since the cardiac and neurologic complications occurred, the damage was considered irreversible.

Medicolegal case report 4

The plaintiff, a 40-year-old man, fell approximately 4 feet from a log into some pine tree limbs piled on the ground. He fell on his right side and experienced foot, ankle, and back pain, but had no visible abrasions, contusions, or lacerations. The physician did not see any signs of injury on his body or any abnormalities to his lower extremities or back, so a muscle relaxant was prescribed and the patient sent home. The pain exacerbated, and he was sent to a public medical center because of financial constraints. Several hours later, a nurse reported normal body temperature and blood pressure. The medical resident examining the patient found severe muscle spasms in his right lower extremity, which he believed were posttraumatic reflex muscle spasms caused by either direct blunt trauma or straining of the musculature. The doctor did not take any x-rays because he was certain, absent cuts or abrasions, that no fracture was present. He consulted with another first-year resident, from a gynecologic training program, and they agreed that the patient should be given diazepam to reduce the muscle spasms. The patient went home but became so ill several weeks later that, his wife related, he was incoherent, could not walk, had a high fever, and had a visibly swollen and red leg and foot. He was taken to a local emergency room, where the resident in foot surgery examined him and immediately ordered blood studies and radiographs. X-rays showed gas in the tissues of the lower extremity, indicating a severe soft tissue infection. The patient was taken to surgery, where dead muscle tissue and rampant infection were noted throughout the foot and leg. Because of the severity of the infection, an orthopedic surgical consultation confirmed the necessity for hemipelvectomy. The leg was amputated 6 inches below the hip to save the patient's life. He was hospitalized for 6 more weeks and had at least four other surgeries to debride necrotic and damaged muscle in the contralateral extremity. The patient underwent several skin grafts, and purulent abscesses formed every few months at the right stump site

and the remaining left leg, requiring surgical drainage. The residual shortness of the left extremity and recurrent infections in the right stump precluded the use of a prosthesis, causing the patient to ambulate on crutches.[4]

A lawsuit was filed against the initial treating physician, the initial hospital, and the two residents employed by the hospital. The following elements were listed in the formal legal complaint: (1) failure to diagnose, (2) failure to refer, (3) lack of diligence, (4) loss of chance, (5) improper treatment, (6) mistaken diagnosis, (7) failure to exercise reasonable skill and judgment, and (8) loss of consortium.

It was quite clear that the first group of treating physicians, including the medical residents, were thoroughly negligent in the ability to diagnose and treat the patient's condition and in their failure to refer the patient to an appropriate specialist. They were guilty of a lack of diligence because they failed to give adequate attention to the case and made significant omissions in the course of their treatment. Once the patient was accepted and a physician-patient relationship was established, a duty existed between the parties, which was breached by the physicians. Their lack of diligence was the proximate cause of the injury. Their negligence led directly to the devastating result that ultimately occurred.

Medicolegal case report 5

The patient was a 35-year-old woman who fell at home and twisted her right ankle. She was unable to walk, and the amount of swelling in the foot caused her great concern.

She went to her family physician, who explained the commonness of ankle sprains and recommended an elastic bandage and generic antiinflammatory medication. After still being unable to walk a week later, she went to another physician, located several blocks from her husband's office. After a radiographic evaluation, this physician immediately scheduled an open reduction with internal fixation (ORIF) of the displaced ankle fracture. Following discharge from the hospital, the patient was instructed to return to the office in 3 weeks. One week later, she developed a burning sensation and a great amount of pain in her ankle. She noted a foul odor, which appeared to emanate from beneath the case. She returned to the surgeon a week early, and a wound discharge was noted, upon cast removal.

The site was probed, but no extension of the infection was noted. A new cast was applied, and the patient was instructed to return in several weeks. When her cast was removed at the next visit, the entire incision had broken down and purulence was everywhere. The operating physician told her not to be concerned, as this was a normal complication. Another cast was applied, even as the ankle grew progressively worse. She again returned to the office, and the surgeon removed the cast and indicated that the infection was healing, albeit slowly. The patient's husband suggested that she see another surgeon to evaluate the condition. Following an extensive examination and second opinion consultation, the new practitioner determined that she had developed osteomyelitis of the tibia and immediately admitted her to the hospital for further comprehensive evaluation and treatment.[5] Several months later, she filed suit against her family physician and the operating surgeon. The following elements were listed in the complaint: (1) failure to diagnose, (2) failure to inform of risks, (3) failure to refer, (4) failure to obtain informed consent, (5) lack of diligence (6) failure to advise of outcome of physical examination, (7) failure to treat, and (8) lack of consortium.

MEDICOLEGAL DEFENSIVE TECHNIQUES

The defensive posture taken by any physician regarding medicolegal self-protection begins on the first encounter with the patient. The patient must be assessed regarding his or her medical condition. An evaluation must also be made regarding circulatory status and whether it can sustain the rendered treatment. For example, in diabetic patients or those with peripheral vascular disease, special instruction books or written material might be reviewed with the patient. Vascular testing, if indicated, should be instituted both in the office setting and through outside referral to a vascular specialist. Affirmation by signature on the final page of the educational material indicates the patient's understanding of the situation. The patient's prior medical history should be carefully reviewed and any records of previous treating physicians acquired. After the treatment plan is instituted, careful monitoring of progress must be maintained to determine if any untoward results are occurring.

In cases of infection, the slightest change in condition may result in devastating circumstances. It is essential to perform necessary cultures, sensitivities, and blood and chemical studies. These should be repeated periodically when necessary, the required standard being the frequency another practitioner would use under like or similar circumstances. Follow-up telephone conferences with the patient, the family, and other supporting physicians are essential, especially in cases compounded by systemic medical compromise or those that may lead to morbidity. All conversations should be documented in the permanent medical record, and the patient may even be asked to sign the chart affirming that he or she was informed of the contents of the conversations. Written correspondence regarding the progress and condition of the situation should also become a regular habit of the practitioner. Should the infection take a sudden negative direction, the correspondence may be sent by registered mail with return receipt requested. For noncompliant patients, postcards may be sent to remind them of their appointments. The mailings should be documented within the body of the progress notes inside the office chart. Should the patient fail to return to the office for follow-up care, or disregard prescribed instructions, it is essential that a certified letter be sent immediately. Although the format of written correspondence is time consuming, it is the most protective method available to help defend against allegations of medical malpractice.

Although the risk of a claim of a lack of informed consent has recently been diminished by the prevalence of risk management seminars, it still may appear in formal complaints. All procedures performed in the office or hospital setting should be consented; including toenail and simple tendon procedures as well as more extensive forefoot and rearfoot surgical procedures. Within the body of the consent form, it is imperative that infection is listed as a possible complication that occurs with regularity in a small percentage of patients. The possible treatment of a major or minor postoperative infection should also be reviewed. If an infection does occur, the patient will not be so alarmed if he or she has been informed of the possibility. Obviously, such patients will be seen more frequently for follow-up care, and all rescheduled appointments, missed appointments, or areas of noncompliance should be thoroughly documented. Unfortunately, many otherwise well-maintained medical charts have significant flaws that can mean the difference between a no-cause action and an adverse judgment in the vicinity of several hundred thousand dollars. In today's litigious society, the adage "document, document, document" has never been more important.

At times, the practitioner will encounter a patient with conflicting symptoms that may make a specific diagnosis difficult or impossible. For the seasoned veteran practitioner, it is not difficult to refer the patient to another physician specialist. For the new practitioner who is building a practice, the financial incentives and potential community exposure may cause him or her to yield to the temptation of shotgun treatment for all possible diagnoses. Unfortunately, what may occur is not a successful resolution to the problem, but a nightmare of unyielding proportions. Therefore, the correct posture in this case is appropriate referral.

SUMMARY

Community-acquired, nosocomial, or postoperative foot infections pose a dilemma that ultimately challenges all providers of foot care, regardless of degree designation. Successful management requires careful legal documentation as well as appropriate medical care. Simple infections can be handled in the office by performing the necessary cultures and blood studies and giving the appropriate antibiotic prescriptions. Documentation verifies that reasonable care was rendered. More complicated infections may require specialized testing that may take place in the office or an outpatient or inpatient setting. Prior to performance of hospital debridement, resection, or amputation, it is important that a vascular or infectious disease specialist be consulted to document medical necessity. Failure to perform what is expected of the prudent practitioner is considered negligent, and, in certain jurisdictions, foot specialists have been held to a higher standard of care than the average medical practitioner.

CONCLUSION

The legal issues and claims possible from the diagnosis, treatment, and eventual outcome of the infected foot may be instigated at every potential twist and turn of the disease process. Proper understanding of the medical malpractice issues dealt with in this chapter, as well as knowledge of techniques that protect the practitioner, is necessary. The clinician must also recall that the attorney who examines a potential infectious disease malpractice lawsuit seeks to understand whether the practitioner rendered every possible diagnostic and treatment modality for his client. Depending on the quality of the law firm, even a small apparent indiscretion may lead to litigation and liability. Adopting some of the recommendations reviewed in this chapter will serve to reduce the risk of malpractice.

Every practitioner must be constantly vigilant, maintain an unremittingly defensive posture when treating any patient with a pedal infection, and use every possible modality to protect both the patient and practitioner from potential malpractice claims.

REFERENCES

1. Lavery L, Hasse K, Krych S: Hallux hammertoe secondary to *Pseudomonas* osteomyelitis, *J Am Podiatr Med Assoc* 81:608-612, 1991.
2. Lawson K, Schwarin J, Aubrey B: Septic bursitis of the foot: diagnosis, management and end-results, *J Foot Surg* 29:379-304, 1990.
3. Notari M, Mittler B: Lyme disease: a review and case report with pedal symptoms, *J Am Podiatr Med Assoc* 79:244-246, 1989.
4. *Allen v. State of Louisiana,* 535 So. 2d 903 (La App 2, Cir 1988).
5. *Jones v. Young,* 372, SW 2d 938 (No, App, 1987).

ADDITIONAL READINGS

Espino DV, Doty S: Age related changes in elderly individuals, *Clin Podiatr Med Surg* 10(1):7-23, 1993.

Helfand AE: Ethical considerations in podiatric care of the older patient, *Clin Podiatr Med Surg* 11(1):35-47, 1993.

Ries MD, Berrino JS, Nafziger AN: Distribution of orthopedic surgeons, lawyers and malpractice cases in New York, *Clin Orthop Rel Res* 337 (4):256-260, 1997.

Udell ET: Malingering behavior in private-medical practice, *Clin Podiatr Med Surg* 11(1):65-73, 1994.

Vincent C, Young M, Phillips A: Why do people sue doctors? *Lancet* 343: 1609-1613, 1994.

Internet Resources for Foot Infection Information

William P. Scherer

The evolution of the Internet can be traced back to 1962 when Paul Baran, an engineer at the Rand Corporation think tank, found a way for messages to move through a network of United States Department of Defense computers even if one communication line is destroyed during a war. In 1968, the Department of Defense commissioned the Advanced Research Projects Agency to build ARPAnet, a nationwide network of computers that would later become the backbone of the Internet. ARPAnet then became part of the National Science Foundation's NSFnet in 1986, as members of academic, government, and private research organizations joined the national infrastructure network.

When the National Science Foundation lifted its restriction against advertising and commercial use of the Internet in 1991, entrepreneurs formed companies to provide Internet access sites to the public. Because the Internet has a decentralized structure with no single managing body, the Internet Society was formed to make decisions about implementation of standards and software protocols for connecting different computers to the network.

Navigating the Internet was always a difficult task, even for a seasoned computer professional, until 1993, when the University of Illinois created a graphical user interface called the World Wide Web to provide easy access to the computer network. The World Wide Web is a unique linkage system for data contained in each of the different computer system networks on the Internet. The Web has links that are embedded in the documents known as hypertext in the form of underlined key words that allow access to other related documents or data with the click of a mouse button. Documents can be linked to photographs, sounds, video, or other Web sites around the world.

A graphical software application called a "World Wide Web browser" is needed to allow users to log onto and explore the world's largest computer network. The greatest advantage to this graphical interface is that it allows users to navigate the Internet without having to learn complicated computer languages. The Netscape Navigator for Windows or Macintosh computers is currently the most popular user-friendly Web browser; it is available at most computer stores and through some Internet access providers.

Three basic terms are used in exploring the Internet's World Wide Web. The communication language that permits the exchange of information across the Internet is called the HyperText Transmission Protocol (HTTP). The document itself is coded in HyperText Markup Language (HTML), which allows documents to be formatted for presentation using typefaces and graphics that are appropriate for the computer system on which they are displayed. A Uniform Resource Locator (URL) is the address and protocol that identifies a computer server on the Internet and a particular document on that computer system.

With all of the commercial interest, individuals all across the world can access the World Wide Web with their home or office computers by connecting their modems to an Internet provider. There are many sources of Internet access sites, including the largest public commercial online providers such as Prodigy, America Online, CompuServe, and Delphi, that provide user-friendly hourly connection rates. Regional Internet providers are smaller private companies that provide gateways to the Internet for heavy duty users in their geographic areas at extremely cost effective monthly rates, but require more computer expertise than the larger providers.

A Home Page is the introduction screen or welcome mat for a particular URL site on the World Wide Web that is set up by a corporation, school, hospital, or individual user. A Home Page usually provides a colorful logo to identify the site, introductory text to explain the purpose of the site, and hypertext links to documents, graphics, pictures, audio, or video on the site that the user can access or copy to his or her own computer. The interconnection of Home Pages and exchange of data between computers around the world constitute the pavement of the information superhighway.

There is no question that the Internet has become a powerful resource for physicians interested in accessing and retrieving information from companies, libraries, universities, online magazines, and government agencies. However, with millions of different World Wide Web sites located on more than a million Internet Web servers, finding needed material can be difficult. Fortunately, there are a variety of Internet directories and search tools that can assist in the quest for digital data.

The Internet is the largest and most complex computer network in the world, with over a billion pages of text, graphics, music, video, and programs scattered in a haphazard manner all over the globe with no centralized card catalog system. Additionally, the information is dynamic and constantly changing, making it impossible for anyone or any service to keep current on every topic. Although every effort has been made to ensure the accuracy of the information presented in this appendix, Internet resources may change without notice. The most common problem for both new and experienced Internet users is knowing that the information they are looking for is out there somewhere, but how do they find it.

Internet directory services and search engines are the two most popular ways computer users can search for information on the World Wide Web. An Internet directory is like an index of a book or a table of contents and is the easiest method to search and browse the Internet. World Wide Web sites, also known as Uniform Resource Locators (URL), are catalogued under general subjects like medicine, entertainment, and business. Each subject is further broken down into many stages of subcategories that narrow the focus of the subject. Most directories are interactive and allow users to enter a keyword or phrase to describe the topic they are interested in searching. To explore a particular Web site, a simple mouse click on the topic transports the user to that site.

The pioneer Internet directory and one of the most frequently accessed sites on the Internet is known as Yahoo!, http://www.yahoo.com. Founded in April 1994, by David Filo and Jerry Yang, Ph.D. candidates in electrical engineering at Stanford University, Yahoo! or "Yet Another Hierarchical Officious Oracle" quickly became the most comprehensive and widely used Web directory on the Internet. There are 14 main subjects that can be directly accessed from its home page, including Arts, Business, Computers, Education, Entertainment, Government, Health, News, Recreation, Reference, Regional, Science, Social Science, and Society.

Web directories are a great place to start searching the Internet, but search engines are the most powerful way to locate information on the World Wide Web. An Internet search engine is a general term that is used to cover a variety of online search and retrieval tools. Intelligent software agents called spiders and crawlers scour the Web on a frequent basis collecting information about existing Web sites located around the world. This information is then compiled into an accessible database that can be searched by anyone who logs into the search engine site.

The most common search engine option is known as a "keyword search." This allows the engine to hunt for any document or Web site that contains the exact word or phrase a user is searching for. A keyword match is known as a "hit"; the larger the number of hits, the more information that was found by the search engine. However, unlike Yahoo! where only the site name and address are displayed, a search engine can produce multiple hits from the same site and fragment the search.

Alta Vista, http://altavista.digital.com, is the result of a research project started in the summer of 1995 at Digital's Research Laboratories in Palo Alto, California. By combining a fast Web crawler with scalable indexing software, the team was able to build a large index of the Web in the fall of 1995. There are several billion searchable words and several million pages that can be accessed with the Alta Vista search engine. Alta Vista treats every page on the Web as a sequence of words. A word in this context means any string of alphabetics and digits delimited either by punctuation or by other nonalphabetic characters. This allows users to search the entire Internet for a single word or phrase.

Physicians' Online

In 1992, four health care experts, three of whom are board-certified physicians, formed Physicians' Online, http://www.po.com, a dedicated online service designed specifically for physicians. Through computer access, Physicians' Online allows physicians fast and easy use of credible and familiar clinical information. The core reference services, which include MEDLINE, AIDSLINE, and other diagnostic and therapeutic decision support tools, are provided free of charge to physicians through the sponsorship of pharmaceutical companies and managed care organizations.

Physicians' Online is a service developed by physicians and for physicians to address the information needs of doctors in the United States. Because Physicians' Online is a free service, it is gaining rapid acceptance in the general medical community and has become the largest physicians-only online service in the country.

The various services of Physicians' Online currently include MedEMail, Medical News, MEDLINE, AIDSLINE, CancerLit, QMR, Drug Interactions, Disease Center, Managed Care Center, and Medical Associations and Societies forums. During an online session, various sponsor messages are displayed at the bottom of the screen and can be further explored by using the mouse to click the sponsor button to get more detailed information.

Compiled and maintained by the National Library of Medicine, MEDLINE currently contains over seven million references dating back to 1966 from approximately 3,700 international medical journals. Natural language search technology makes MEDLINE on Physicians' Online fast and easy, requiring no special knowledge or commands. Simply enter your topic using plain English and the Easy Search technology will find your results within seconds. To keep the information as current as possible, the MEDLINE database is updated weekly.

AIDSLINE is also compiled and maintained by the National Library of Medicine and covers more than 80,000 abstracts from over 4,000 journals dating back to 1980. Content includes AIDS and related topics, as well as clinical and research information. Journal articles, conference proceedings, technical and government reports, meeting abstracts, and monographs are among the sources used to compile AIDSLINE.

Quick Medical Reference (QMR) is an in-depth information resource supporting the diagnosis of more than 600 complex diseases and 4,600 clinical findings in internal medicine. With QMR you can formulate differential diagnoses, determine the best lab tests to order, locate the most common findings in patients with a particular disease, and get a list of questions to ask which would either rule in or rule out a diagnosis. QMR also offers the capability to enter multiple diseases and/or findings so that you can explore the relationship among them.

The Drug Interactions section of Physicians' Online provides fast, easy access to the most up-to-date information for a single drug or multiple drugs. You can easily search all interactions for a single drug, or build a drug list and find their combined interactions. The information in Drug Interactions comes from FDA-approved prescribing information and is updated monthly.

National Institutes of Health

Composed of 24 separate Institutes, Centers, and Divisions, the National Institutes of Health (NIH), http://www.nih.gov, is one of eight health agencies of the Public Health Service, which in turn is part of the U.S. Department of Health and Human Services. The NIH's Web site is an extremely large site and contains timely information on news and events happening at the NIH's home office in Bethesda, Maryland, as well as health information for both physicians and the public, grants and contracts, and a variety of scientific resources.

HyperDOC, http://www.nlm.nih.gov, is a service of the National Library of Medicine (NLM) and can be accessed from the NIH home page. HyperDOC presents the resources of the world's largest biomedical library and allows fee-based access to every significant program that the library offers. One of the many databases in the NLM web site is MEDLARS, which includes over 40 online databases, such as MEDLINE, that contain about 18 million records. Other types of information in NLM databases include the complete text of practice guidelines for health professionals; information about toxic effects of chemicals; treatment for types of cancer; and lists of clinical trials for AIDS patients.

The Visible Human Project, http://www.nlm.nih.gov/ research/visible/visible_human.html, is an outgrowth of the NLM's 1986 long range plan. It is creating complete, anatomically detailed, three-dimensional representations of the male and female human bodies. The current phase of the project is collecting transverse CT, MRI, and cryosection images of representative male and female cadavers at 1-millimeter intervals. The long-term goal of the Visible Human Project is to produce a system of knowledge structures that will transparently link visual knowledge forms to symbolic knowledge formats such as the names of body parts. Images and animations of the project based on visible human data can be downloaded from the Web.

The Virtual Hospital

The University of Iowa College of Medicine, Department of Radiology, formed an interactive project with the Electric Differential Multimedia Laboratory called The Virtual Hospital (VH), http://vh.radiology.uiowa.edu. It is a continuously updated digital health sciences library that provides patient care support, distance learning to physicians, multimedia textbooks, teaching files, clinical guidelines, and assorted publications.

Multimedia textbooks (MMTB) are software programs that can be downloaded from the VH site; they pattern their user interface after a printed textbook. The MMTB incorporate multimedia functionality such as hypertext, free text searching, the ability to play video and audio clips, and the ability to display high resolution graphic images. This information is being planned to deliver continuing medical education to physicians' offices and homes.

Achoo Online Healthcare Services

One of the greatest hurdles for physicians who regularly use the Internet is the sheer volume of information available. Achoo, http://www.achoo.com, acts as a jump point and information resource for the medical community and all other Internet users interested in health care information. Achoo provides a link to Healthcare HeadlineNews, a comprehensive web-based health care news service. Hundreds of timely Healthcare headlines are categorized into over 150 news topics. Links to the full news stories are provided on each page.

The Achoo Internet Healthcare Directory's objective is to catalog, index, describe, and evaluate the mountain of health care information on the Internet and has over 6,300 links. There are three main categories of the directory: Human Life, Practice of Medicine, and Business of Health. Human Life categorizes the structures and functions of the human body; human health; the manifestation, recognition, and treatment of human disease; and the behavioral sciences. Practice of Medicine focuses on the issues relating to the professional practice of medicine. Business of Health provides up-to-date information on health care products and services for both health care professionals and consumers.

Center for Complex Infectious Diseases

The mission of CCID [http://www.ccid.org] is to determine the nature, origin, disease associations, modes of transmission, methods of diagnosis, and responses to therapy of complex infectious diseases, and to disseminate such information. CCID is currently specializing in the detection and characterization of viruses that have undergone a "stealth" adaptation to avoid elimination by the immune system. At present, the Web site provides information on stealth viruses cultured from patients with a spectrum of dysfunctional brain syndromes, including chronic fatigue, autism, severe encephalopathy, and bipolar psychiatric illness. The issue of live viral vaccines as a probable source of certain stealth viruses and a known source of SV40 virus is also addressed. The Web site also addresses new developments in SV40, parvovirus B19, and HHV-6 and will soon include sections on HIV, HCV, and prion mediated diseases. (From the Center for Complex Infectious Diseases Web site.)

The Infectious Diseases Society of America

The IDSA [http://www.idsociety.org] is an organization of physicians, scientists, and other health care professionals dedicated to promoting human health through excellence in research, education, prevention, and care of patients. The Society pursues and represents the concerns of its membership by its organizational structure, journals, meetings, and other activities. (From the Infectious Diseases Society of America Web site.)

The National Center for Infectious Diseases

The National Center for Infectious Diseases [http://www.cdc.gov/ncidod/ncid.htm] is committed to the prevention and control of traditional, new, and reemerging infectious diseases in the United States and around the world. (From the Centers for Disease Control/National Center for Infectious Diseases Web site.) Online information includes publications, brochures, fact sheets, selected prevention and control areas, resources, information networks and other information services, emerging infectious diseases, and a journal, published by NCID, on new, reemerging, and drug-resistant infections.

Emerging Infectious Diseases

Emerging Infectious Diseases [http://www.cdc.gov/ncidod/EID/eid.htm] is a quarterly, peer-reviewed WWW journal available from the Internet. Its mission statement is to promote the recognition of new and reemerging infectious diseases and to improve the understanding of factors involved in infectious disease emergence. *EID* has an international scope and is intended for physician professionals in infectious diseases and related sciences. It is composed of three sections: perspectives, synopses, and dispatches. (From Friede and O'Carroll, 1996.)

Association for Professionals in Infection Control and Epidemiology, Inc.

The Association for Professionals in Infection Control and Epidemiology, Inc. (APIC) [http://www.apic.org] is a multidisciplinary, voluntary international organization whose purpose is to influence, support, and improve the quality of health care through the practice and management of infection control and the application of epidemiology in all health settings. APIC is committed to improving patient care, preventing adverse outcomes, and minimizing occupational hazards associated with the delivery of health care. APIC's vision is to lead the field of infection prevention and control applied epidemiology in all health settings. (From the Association for Professionals in Infection Control and Epidemiology, Inc., Web site.) Its Web page contains the following nine sections: About APIC, Home, Infection Control and Your Life, What's New, Education, Professional Resources, Government Regulations, Publications, and Comments. (From Harr, 1996.)

Nosocomial and community-acquired infection surveillance databases

Many nosocomial and community-based infections can be tracked and monitored by various personal computer (PC) software programs. The national CDC database is available, but medical schools, hospitals, residency training programs and other infection control practitioners may obtain commercial database products, such as AICE (Infection Control & Prevention Analysts, Inc., Austin, Texas) and Q-Logic (Epi-Systematics, Inc., Fort Myers, Fla.). Other products to assist in infectious epidemiologic studies are Epi-Info, Inc., USD, Stone Mountain, Ga.), which is a system containing word processing database management, and epidemiological statistical databases, such as Epi-Map (USD), which is a program that produces maps from geographic boundary files. These databases also adjust for illness severity and represent a timesaving device for professional epidemiologists. (From Friedman, 1996.)

Miscellaneous electronic and internet infection information resource sites

The following telephonic, fax, or electronic resources are valuable information sites for those interested in treatment of the infected foot:

1. American Society for Microbiology: http://asmusa.org
2. Amputee Coalition of America, Jimmy Calloway, Ph.D.: phone, 888-AMP-KNOW; fax, 423-525-7917
3. APIC-NC Infection Control Newsletter: www.sandhills.org/org/bugline/
4. BJC Health Systems Infection Control Newsletter: http://osler.wustl.edu/~traynor/bjcicn.html
5. CDC Prevention Guidelines Database (PGDB; on diskette and CD-ROM): 404-332-4555
6. Foot and Ankle Research Consortium (FARC), Inc: board certification examination simulation study software for DPM's; phone 770-938-5974 and fax 770-939-7393
7. Infection Control Resources: www.hepnet.com/chica.html
8. Infectious Disease Newsletter: http://www.zilker.net/~medair/newslet.htm
9. Marcinko Business Associates (MBA), Inc.: practice management and financial planning; phone 770-448-0769 and http://www.footdoc.com/marcinko/davefram.html
10. National AIDS Clearinghouse: CDC NAC, PO Box 6003, Rockville, MD 20849-6003; phone 800-458-5231 or 800-243-7012 or fax 301-738-6616 or 800-243-7012 (deaf access); CDC information management resources office: Meade Morgan, Ph.D.,

Andrew Freede, M.D., Joseph A Reid, Ph.D., and Kenneth Williams

11. National Foundation for Infectious Diseases: http://www.medscape.com/Affiliates/NFID
12. National Institute for Occupational Safety and Health Information System (NIOSH): 800-356-4674
13. Society for Epidemiologic Research: http://phweb.sph.jhu.edu/pubs/jepi/ser.htm
14. University of Iowa Wound Care: http://www.nursing.uiowa.edu.chronicwound

Conclusion

The current Internet digital revolution allows almost instantaneous information to interested parties, virtually anywhere in the world. The most informative Web sites, organizations, and resources for the infection control practitioner have been listed in this section. This free flow of knowledge will prove useful to physicians, hospitals, and patients alike.

BIBLIOGRAPHY

Chapman KA, Moulton AD: The Georgia information network for public health official (INPHO): a demonstration of the CDC INPHO concept, *J Public Health Management Practice* 1:39-43, 1995.

Friede A, McDonald MC, Blum H: Public health information: how information age technology can strengthen public health, *Ann Rev Public Health* 16:239-252, 1995.

Friede A, O'Carroll PW: CDC and ATSDR electronic information resources for health officers, *Am J Infect Control* 24(6):440-454, 1996.

Friedman C: A brave new world of information and communication for infection control professionals, *Am J Infect Control* 24(6):417-420, 1996.

Harr J: Double-u, double-u, double-u dot apic, dot org: a review of the APIC World Wide Web site, *Am J Infect Control* 24(6):455-462, 1996.

Manangan LP: The infection control information system of Hospital Infections Program, Centers for Disease Control and Prevention, *Am J Infect Control* 24(6):463-467, 1996.

Pestonik SL, Classen DC, Evans RS: Implementing antibiotic practice guidelines through computer assisted decision support: clinical and financial outcomes, *Ann Intern Med* 124:884-890, 1996.

Scherer WP: Computerization of the medical office practice. In Marcinko DE: *Medical and surgical therapeutics of the foot and ankle,* Baltimore, 1992, Williams & Wilkins.

Scherer WP: Podiatry on the Information Superhighway, *Podiatry Management* 13:19-21, 1995. [Kane Communications, 7000 Darby Square, Suite 210, Upper Darby, PA 19082]

Scherer WP: On-line services: which one should you use? *Podiatry Management* 14:29-31, 1996.

Scherer WP: Computer software review, *Podiatry Management* 15:35-40, 1997.

Scherer WP: Internet search tools, *Podiatry Management* 15:55-58, 1997.

Skolnick AA: Experts explore emerging information technologies' effects on medicine, *JAMA* 275:669-670, 1996.

Sparks SM: Use of the internet for infection control and epidemiology, *Am J Infect Control* 24(6):435-439, 1996.

Index